Environmental Health Criteria 6

PRINCIPLES AND METHODS FOR EVALUATING THE TOXICITY OF CHEMICALS. PART 1

Published under the joint sponsorship of the United Nations Environment Programme and the World Health Organization

World Health Organization
Geneva 1978

ISBN 92 4 154066 4

PRINTED IN UNITED KINGDOM

CONTENTS

NOTE TO READERS OF THE CRITERIA DOCUMENTS

While every effort has been made to present information in the criteria documents as accurately as possible without unduly delaying their publication, mistakes might have occurred and are likely to occur in the future. In the interest of all users of the environmental health criteria documents, readers are kindly requested to communicate any errors found to the Division of Environmental Health, World Health Organization, Geneva, Switzerland, in order that they may be included in corrigenda which will appear in subsequent volumes.

In addition, experts in any particular field dealt with in the criteria documents are kindly requested to make available to the WHO Secretariat any important published information that may have inadvertently been omitted and which may change the evaluation of health risks from exposure to the environmental agent under examination, so that the information may be considered in the event of updating and re-evaluation of the conclusions contained in the criteria documents.

The use of chemicals in practically every aspect of life has grown very rapidly over the last few decades and international trade in bulk chemicals, specialty chemicals, and consumer products has increased proportionately, making imperative the need for continuous review and reappraisal of procedures for evaluating their safety. Concern about the possible health hazards that may arise from exposure to chemicals has increased throughout the world, especially in the industrialized countries. In many WHO Member States, this has resulted in new laws and regulations which, in turn, have created a need to assemble, analyse, and evaluate all available toxicological information with a view to assessing hazard. Toxicologists have responded by developing techniques for safety evaluation but these often differ from one country to another. The differences are sometimes slight, sometimes considerable; on occasion they have led to unfortunate misunderstandings, and often to needless duplication of work.

Ever since the World Health Organization started programmes on food safety and drug evaluation, the need for some degree of uniformity and for generally accepted principles and requirements for toxicological testing and evaluation has been recognized. This has resulted, in the last 20 years, in a number of technical reports and guidelines on such topics as the general principles and methods for the testing and evaluation of intentional and unintentional food additives (WHO, 1957, 1958, 1967a, 1974a) and drugs (WHO, 1966, 1968, 1975a), on the evaluation of teratogenicity (WHO, 1967b), mutagenicity, and carcinogenicity (WHO, 1961, 1969, 1971, 1974b, 1976a) and, more recently, on environmental and health monitoring and the early detection of health impairment in occupational health (WHO, 1973, 1975b), on chemical and biochemical methodology for assessing the hazards of pesticides to man (WHO, 1975c), and on the methods used in establishing permissible levels of occupational exposure to harmful agents (WHO, 1977). Several symposia have also been organized, to discuss, for example, the methods used in the USSR for establishing biologically safe levels of toxic substances (WHO, 1975d, 1975e), and screening tests in chemical carcinogenesis (IARC, 1976). All these publications remain a most useful source of information on selected aspects of toxicological evaluation.

The need for more uniformity in methods of environmental health risk evaluation was again raised at the 1973 World Health Assembly, in resolution WHA26.58 on human health and the environment which *inter alia* requested the Director-General to develop protocols for experimental and epidemiological studies, uniform terminology, and agreed definitions.

Harmonization of toxicological and epidemiological methods is also one of the objectives of the WHO Environmental Health Criteria Programme (WHO, 1976b), initiated in 1973 in collaboration with Member States and the United Nations Environment Programme (UNEP), while a very recent (1977) World Health Assembly resolution WHA30.47 requested the Director-General "to examine the possible options for international cooperation with a view to accelerating and making more effective the evaluation of health risks from exposure to chemicals, and promoting the use of experimental and epidemiological methods that will produce internationally comparable results".

Current concern about the health effects of chemicals is more intense in some countries than in others, with the consequent unevenness in political response reflected in variations in national safety regulations. This situation is likely to continue for some time. It is unrealistic and perhaps not really desirable at present, to seek international standardization in safety testing and evaluation as this might hinder the input of new ideas and the development of improved methods and might lead either to the application of needless tests or to failure to ask the essential questions. However, it is not too early for scientists and decision-makers to try to understand the similarities and differences in the safety evaluations made in different countries. The underlying objectives are the same everywhere, namely, to minimize harm and maximize safety and yet not impede the beneficial use of chemicals. Similarly, the basic scientific principles are globally accepted, so there is no reason why there should not be a gradual harmonization of methods and procedures for toxicological testing and evaluation.

With these views in mind and taking into account past work of WHO, an attempt was made to set forth, comprehensively and on an international basis, the principles and procedures for the safety evaluation of all types of chemicals. More than 50 distinguished experts from some 11 countries collaborated with the Organization and, in a series of meetings and individual consultations, planned, drafted, and revised this compilation of toxicological procedures, providing at the same time an excellent example of international cooperation. In addition, there was valuable support for the project from the WHO collaborating centres at: the Institute of Hygiene and Occupational Health, Sofia, Bulgaria; the National Institute of Public Health, Bilthoven, Netherlands; the Department of Environmental Hygiene, The Karolinska Institute, Stockholm, Sweden; the National Institute of Environmental Health Sciences, Research Triangle Park, North Carolina, USA; and the Sysin Institute of General and Communal Hygiene, Moscow, USSR.

The general approach in preparing this publication has been to present the underlying scientific principles, to evaluate the utility, strengths and weaknesses of various methods and procedures, to help the reader select the most suitable technique for a specific purpose (bearing in mind that circumstances will often dictate the most appropriate procedure) but not, as already mentioned, to prescribe standard tests. While aiming at agreement on purely scientific issues, it has not been sought on details of procedure, on the interpretation of results, or on methods for setting environmental health standards. Indeed, because there were often differences of opinion on these matters, the solution adopted has been to present the different viewpoints and interpretations. This explains a certain unevenness in the text, particularly in those chapters prepared jointly by many scientists from different countries.

Although an effort has been made to avoid inconsistency in terminology, uniformity has not been possible; indeed, this is something beyond the scope of the present monograph. However, WHO and UNEP recently initiated another project that aims at internationally agreed definitions for those terms most frequently used in toxicological evaluation. Until this project is completed, it is important to understand that some terms may have various meanings and implications in different countries or in different scientific circles and that it may be highly misleading to employ them outside the national pattern of use or outside the context of a specialized field, without precise definition. The reader is therefore warned to be wary of the uncritical transfer of technical terms from one set of circumstances to another.

Toxicology is a rapidly developing field, especially at this time; it is hoped, nevertheless, that this monograph provides a valid account of the present state of knowledge on the toxicity testing and evaluation of chemicals as practiced by some of the leading experts in the field. If it should also stimulate the exchange of knowledge and experience and so contribute to greater efficiency and reliability in toxicity testing and evaluation, it will have more than fulfilled its purpose.

The work has been divided into two separate publications. The first part contains the broad principles and more general aspects of toxicity testing, the planning and evaluation of acute, subacute, and chronic toxicity tests, chemobiokinetics and metabolism, morphological tests, inhalation studies, and tests for carcinogenicity and mutagenicity. Part 2 systematically covers some more specialized procedures for safety evaluation, i.e. functional studies of organs and systems, effects on reproduction, neurological and behavioural studies, effects on the skin and the eye, cumulation and adaptation, and finally discusses factors that could modify the outcome of toxicity testing and evaluation.

The main authors mutually reviewed the chapters of the treatise, which can therefore be considered to be a synthesis of various views and opinions, but this does not detract from the merit of their own contributions which are gratefully acknowledged. The WHO Secretariat at the Meeting of the Main Authors in Geneva (28 July to 1 August 1975)[a] and at the Scientific Group in Lyons (1 to 5 December 1975)[b] comprised: Dr M. El Batawi, Chief, Occupational Health[a]; Dr H. Bartsch, Unit of Chemical Carcinogenesis, IARC, Lyons[b]: Dr J. F. Copplestone, Vector Biology and Control[b]; Dr F. C. Lu, Chief, Food Additives[b]; Dr R. Montesano, Unit of Chemical Carcinogenesis, IARC, Lyons[a,b]; Dr H. Nakajima, Drug Evaluation and Monitoring[a]; Dr M. Vandekar, Vector Biology and Control[a]; and Dr G. Vettorazzi, Food Additives[a]. Dr V. B. Vouk, Chief, Control of Environmental Pollution and Hazards was the Secretary of the Geneva meeting, while Dr L. Tomatis, Chief, Unit of Chemical Carcinogenesis, IARC, Lyons, and Dr Vouk were the Joint Secretaries of the Scientific Group at Lyons. Representatives of other organizations who were present at the meetings include: Dr M. Marcus (US Environmental Protection Agency)[a]; Dr W. J. Hunter (Commission of the European Communities)[b]; Mr C. Prior (Organization for Economic Cooperation and Development)[b]; Dr V. Smirnyagin (International Council of Scientific Unions)[b]. Miss S. Braman, Technical Assistant, Control of Environmental Pollution and Hazards, serviced the two meetings and helped throughout with the preparation of the manuscript.

The final editing was carried out by a group headed by Professor N. Nelson who, indeed, presided over the whole project and to whom special thanks are due for, without his ideas, enthusiasm and, above all, profound knowledge of the subject, there would have been no treatise.

---

[a] Participated in the Meeting of Main Authors, Geneva, 28 July to 1 August 1975.
[b] Participated in the Scientific Group on Methods of Toxicity Evaluation of Chemicals, Lyons, 1–5 December 1975.

REFERENCES

IARC (1976) *Screening tests in chemical carcinogenesis—Proceedings of a Workshop organized by IARC and the CEC, Brussels 1975*. IARC Sci. Publ. No. 12.

WHO (1957) WHO Technical Report Series No. 129 (General principles governing the use of food additives: First report of the Joint FAO/WHO Expert Committee on Food Additives.) 22 pp.

WHO (1958) WHO Technical Report Series No. 144 (Procedures for the testing of intentional food additives to establish their safety for use: Second report of the Joint FAO/WHO Expert Committee on Food Additives.) 19 pp.

WHO (1961) WHO Technical Report Series No. 220 (Evaluation of the carcinogenic hazards of food additives: Fifth report of the Joint FAO/WHO Expert Committee on Food Additives.) 33 pp.

WHO (1966) WHO Technical Report Series No. 341 (Principles for pre-clinical testing of drug dafety: Report of a WHO Scientific Group.) 22 pp.

WHO (1967a) WHO Technical Report Series No. 348 (Procedures for investigating intentional and unintentional food additives: Report of a WHO Scientific Group.) 25 pp.

WHO (1967b) WHO Technical Report Series No. 364 (Principles for the testing of drugs for teratogenicity: Report of a WHO Scientific Group.) 18 pp.

WHO (1968) WHO Technical Report Series No. 403 (Principles for the clinical evaluation of drugs: Report of a WHO Scientific Group.) 32 pp.

WHO (1969) WHO Technical Report Series No. 426 (Principles for the testing and evaluation of drugs for carcinogenicity: Report of a WHO Scientific Group.) 26 pp.

WHO (1971) WHO Technical Report Series No. 482 (Evaluation and testing of drugs for mutagenicity: principles and problems—Report of a WHO Scientific Group.) 18 pp.

WHO (1973) WHO Technical Report Series No. 535 (Environmental and health monitoring in occupational health: Report of a WHO Expert Committee.) 48 pp.

WHO (1974a) WHO Technical Report Series No. 539 (Toxicological evaluation of certain food additives with a review of general principles and of specifications: Seventeenth report of the Joint FAO/WHO Expert Committee on Food Additives.) 40 pp.

WHO (1974b) WHO Technical Report Series No. 546 (Assessment of the carcinogenicity and mutagenicity of chemicals: Report of a WHO Scientific Group.) 19 pp.

WHO (1975a) WHO Technical Report Series No. 563 (Guidelines for evaluation of drugs for use in man: Report of a WHO Scientific Group.) 59 pp.

WHO (1975b) WHO Technical Report Series No. 571 (Early detection of health impairment in occupational exposure to health hazards: Report of a WHO Study Group.) 80 pp.

WHO (1975c) WHO Technical Report Series No. 560 (Chemical and biochemical methodology for the assessment of hazards of pesticides for man.) 26 pp.

WHO (1975d) *Methods used in the USSR for establishing biologically safe levels of toxic substances.* Geneva, WHO, 171 pp.

WHO (1975e) *Methods for studying biological effects of pollutants* (*A review of methods used in the USSR*). Copenhagen, WHO Regional Office for Europe, 80 pp. (EURO publication 3109(4).)

WHO (1976a) WHO Technical Report Series No. 586 (Health hazards from new environmental pollutants: Report of a WHO Study Group.) 96 pp.

WHO (1976b) *Background and purpose of the WHO Environmental Health Criteria Programme.* (Reprint from *Environmental Health Criteria 1 Mercury.*) Geneva, WHO, 9 pp.

WHO (1977) WHO Technical Report Series No. 601 (Methods used in establishing permissible levels in occupational exposure to harmful agents: Report of a WHO Expert Committee with the participation of ILO.) 68 pp.

PRINCIPLES AND METHODS FOR THE TOXICITY EVALUATION OF CHEMICALS

Editorial Group

15

PRINCIPLES AND METHODS FOR THE TOXICITY EVALUATION OF CHEMICALS

Contributors to Part 1

[b] Dr H. Bartsch, Unit of Chemical Carcinogenesis, International Agency for Research on Cancer, Lyons, France (Chapter 7)

Dr S. M. Charbonneau, Toxicology Research Division, Health Protection Branch, National Department of Health & Welfare, Ottawa, Canada (Chapter 3)

[a] Dr R. T. Drew, Medical Department, Brookhaven National Laboratory, Upton, NY, USA (Chapter 6)

[a] Dr H. L. Falk, National Institute of Environmental Health Sciences, Research Triangle Park, NC, USA (Chapter 2)

Dr V. J. Feron, Central Institute for Food Research, Zeist, Netherlands (Chapter 5)

[a] Dr P. Gehring, Toxicology Research Laboratory, Dow Chemical USA, Midland, MI, USA (Chapter 4)

[b] Dr H. C. Grice, Toxicology Research Division, Health Protection Branch, Department of National Health & Welfare, Ottawa, Canada

[a,b] Professor F. Kaloyanova, Institute of Hygiene & Occupational Health, Sofia, Bulgaria

[a] Dr G. N. Krasovskij, Laboratory of Water Toxicology, A. N. Sysin Institute of General & Communal Hygiene, Moscow, USSR (Chapter 1)

[a,b] Dr R. Kroes, Central Institute for Nutrition & Food Research, Zeist, Netherlands (Chapters 1 & 5)

Dr J. E. LeBeau, Toxicology Research Laboratory, Dow Chemical USA, Midland, MI, USA (Chapter 4)

[a,b] Dr S. Manyai, Biochemical Department, Institute of Occupational Health, Budapest, Hungary (Chapter 4)

[a,b] Dr R. Montesano, Unit of Chemical Carcinogenesis, International Agency for Research on Cancer, Lyons, France (Chapters 1 & 7)

[a] Dr I. C. Munro, Toxicology Research Division, Health Protection Branch, Department of National Health & Welfare, Ottawa, Canada (Chapters 1, 2 & 3)

[a] Professor S. D. Murphy, Division of Toxicology, Department of Pharmacology, The University of Texas Health Sciences Center, Houston, TX, USA (Chapters 1 & 2)

[a,b] Professor N. Nelson, Institute of Environmental Medicine, New York University, NY, USA (Chapters 1 & 7)

[b] Professor G. Nordberg, Institute of Hygiene & Social Medicine, Odense University, Odense, Denmark

[a,b] Professor D. V. Parke, Department of Biochemistry, University of Surrey, Guildford, England (Chapters 1 & 2)

[a,b] Dr E. A. Pfitzer, Department of Toxicology, Research Division, Hoffman-La Roche Inc., Nutley, NJ, USA (Chapters 1 & 2)

[a] Dr M. A. Pinigin, A. N. Sysin Institute of General & Communal Hygiene, Moscow, USSR (Chapter 1)

Dr J. C. Ramsey, Toxicology Research Laboratory, Dow Chemical USA, Midland, MI, USA (Chapter 4)

[b] Professor I. V. Sanockij, Department of Toxicology, Institute of Industrial Hygiene & Occupational Diseases, Moscow, USSR (Chapters 1 & 2)

Dr K. K. Sidorov, Department of Toxicology, Institute of Industrial Hygiene & Occupational Diseases, Moscow, USSR (Chapter 6)

[b] Dr L. Tomatis, Unit of Chemical Carcinogenesis, International Agency for Research on Cancer, Lyons, France (Chapter 7)

[b] Professeur R. Truhaut, Laboratoire de Toxicologie et d'Hygiène industrielles, Faculté des Sciences pharmaceutiques et biologiques, Université René Descartes, Paris, France

[a] Dr I. P. Ulanova, Department of Toxicology, Institute of Industrial Hygiene & Occupational Diseases, Moscow, USSR (Chapter 6)

[a,b] Dr V. B. Vouk, Control of Environmental Pollution and Hazards, Division of Environmental Health, WHO, Geneva, Switzerland (Chapter 1)

Dr Z. Zawidski, Toxicology Research Division, Health Protection Branch, Department of National Health & Welfare, Ottawa, Canada (Chapter 3)

[a] Participated in the Meeting of Main Authors, Geneva, 28 July to 1 August 1975.

[b] Participated in the Scientific Group on Methods of Toxicity Evaluation of Chemicals, Lyons, 1–5 December 1975.

17

1. SOME GENERAL ASPECTS OF TOXICITY EVALUATION

1.1 Introduction

Toxicology is concerned both with the nature and mechanisms of toxic lesions and the quantitative evaluation of the spectrum of biological changes produced by exposure to chemicals. Every chemical is toxic under certain conditions of exposure. An important corollary is that for every chemical there should be some exposure condition that is safe as regards man's health (Lazarev, 1938; Pravdin, 1934; Smyth, 1963; Weil, 1972a) with the possible exception of chemical carcinogens and mutagens (WHO, 1974a).

The quantitative evaluation of the biological changes caused by chemicals aims at the establishment of dose-effect and dose-response relationships that are of fundamental importance for health risk evaluation.

1.1.1 Defining toxicity, hazard, risk, and related terms

In a general sense, the toxicity of a substance could be defined as the capacity to cause injury to a living organism (NAS/NRC, 1970; Sanockij, 1970). A highly toxic substance will damage an organism if administered in very small amounts; a substance of low toxicity will not produce an effect unless the amount is very large. Thus, toxicity cannot be defined without reference to the quantity of a substance administered or absorbed (dose), the way in which this quantity is administered (e.g. inhalation, ingestion, injection) and distributed in time (e.g. single dose, repeated doses), the type and severity of injury, and the time needed to produce that injury.

There is no generally agreed definition of "hazard" associated with a chemical, but the term is used to indicate the likelihood that a chemical will cause an adverse health effect (injury) under the conditions in which it is produced or used (Goldwater, 1968; NAS/NRC, 1970; Pravdin, 1934).

Risk is a statistical concept and has been defined by the Preparatory Committee of the United Nations Conference on the Human Environment[a], as the expected frequency of undesirable effects arising from exposure to a pollutant. Estimates of risk may be expressed in absolute terms or in relative terms. The absolute risk is the excess risk due to exposure. The relative risk is the ratio between the risk in the exposed population and the risk in the unexposed population (BEIR, 1972; ICRP, 1966).

Safety is a term that has been used extensively but is difficult to define. One definition is that "safety" is the practical certainty that injury will not

---

[a] Preparatory Committee of the United Nations Conference on the Human Environment, Third Session, 13–24 September 1971 (A/Conf. 4818, pp. 45 & 46).

result from the substance when used in the quantity and in the manner proposed for its use (NAS/NRC, 1970). This definition is of little use unless "practical certainty" is defined in some way, for example, in terms of a numerically specified low risk. Another view is that "safety" should be judged in terms of socially "acceptable" risks. Such judgments are largely outside the scope of scientific evaluation but nevertheless require assessment both of the probabilities[a] of various adverse effects and of their severity in terms of human health or other concerns (NAS, 1975).

1.1.2 Laboratory testing

Human data on the toxicity of chemicals are obviously more relevant to safety evaluation than those obtained from the exposure of experimental animals (see section 1.4). However, controlled exposures of man to hazardous or potentially hazardous substances are limited by ethical considerations and information obtained by clinical or epidemiological methods must be relied on. Where such information is not available, as in the case of all new synthetic chemicals, data must be obtained from tests on experimental animals and other laboratory procedures. The degree of confidence with which human health risks can be estimated from laboratory data depends on the quality of the data, and the selection of appropriate laboratory testing procedures is the main subject of this monograph.

1.1.3 Toxicological field studies

In the laboratory, only a small number of animal species are available for testing. The testing of wild species, living in cages under field conditions, may be useful but sometimes presents a variety of problems. Successful trials require a large enough site (about 8 ha; 20 acres) with adequate and varied populations of birds, mammals, fish, insects, and other species, and the area studied must be considerably greater than that treated (Brown & Papworth, 1974). Data obtained from field trials of chemicals are of considerable value in supplementing data obtained with laboratory animal species and in validating the projection of experimental results to the ecosystem, including man. Studies of random events in natural ecosystems can also provide useful data.

Sensitive analytical techniques now make it relatively simple to conduct field studies in man by monitoring levels of a chemical or its metabolites in blood, urine, hair, or saliva; this biological monitoring together with environmental monitoring provides important information on the exposure

---

[a] i.e. the expected frequencies.

20

of man[a]. Regular periodic determination of the profile of certain plasma enzymes and other biochemical variables in the subject provides another valuable method for monitoring health effects particularly under occupational exposure conditions (WHO, 1973, 1975a, 1975b); changes in these profiles may provide early warning of damage by toxic chemicals (Cuthbert, 1974).

1.1.4 Ecotoxicology

A new subdivision of toxicology, "ecotoxicology", has emerged following observations that some persistent chemicals can exert toxic effects at several points in an ecosystem. The appearance of a chemical or the manifestation of a toxic effect may occur far away from its initial point of introduction into the environment. Methods for assessing the extent and significance of the movement of pollutants and their degradation products through the environment to target systems are discussed in a recent publication (NAS, 1975).

1.1.5 Priorities in the selection of chemicals for testing

In principle, all new chemicals require safety evaluation before manufacture and sale, but, because of the large number of chemicals that represent a possible hazard to human health and limited resources, it is necessary to give priority to those that are directly consumed by man, such as drugs and food additives, and those that are widely used such as pesticides or household consumer products. Industrial chemicals that can escape into the working or general environment or can contaminate other products are another category of concern.

Compounds of suspected high acute, chronic, or delayed toxicity (such as carcinogenicity) or of high persistence in the environment, or compounds which contain chemical groups known to be associated with these properties, deserve the highest priority. This also applies to compounds known to inhibit metabolic deactivation of chemicals as they may represent a more insidious form of toxicity.

Chemicals resistant to metabolism, especially metabolism by microflora, will have a high environmental persistence. Many halogenated compounds come into this category, and should, therefore, have some degree of priority. Compounds that accumulate in food chains or are stored in the body, e.g. methylmercury and DDT, will be a matter of concern. Such compounds are

---

[a] *Report of the Meeting of a Government Expert Group on Health Related Monitoring.* Unpublished WHO document CEP/77.6.

often highly lipid-soluble or strongly bound to tissue proteins, or may undergo enterohepatic recirculation with consequent slow excretion resulting in accumulation in the organism.

Physicochemical properties can be an important consideration in setting priorities for testing potential environmental pollutants. For example, biomagnification of stable, fat-soluble substances may lead to contamination of human food supplies as well as to adverse effects in wildlife at the higher levels of food chains, even though the intended use and sites of application of the substance would suggest that primary exposure of these species is unlikely (Edwards, 1970). Physicochemical properties such as vapour pressure, and particle size and density are important in predicting the atmospheric transport of chemicals (Fuchs, 1964; OECD, 1977). Adsorption of a chemical on soil particles may increase the likelihood that the material will become airborne or be transported by watercourses and subsequently deposited in areas remote from its site of application (Cohen & Pinkerton, 1966), or it may retard the movement of a chemical through ground water and thus reduce the likelihood of contamination of ground water supplies near the site of application (Edwards, 1970; Hamaker et al., 1966).

Even though certain predictions and comparisons of environmental distribution and biomagnification of chemicals in the environment may be made theoretically on the basis of the physicochemical properties of the substances in question, more definitive information of this nature can be obtained experimentally by the use of model ecosystems such as those described by Metcalf et al. (1971) and Lu & Metcalf (1975). These model ecosystems may be oversimplified, and they should not replace experimental field studies or programmes for monitoring environmental contaminants. However, their use in an early phase of the overall evaluation of the toxicity of environmental chemicals may: (a) help to determine order of priority of chemicals for study, (b) identify the components of the environment (food, water, air) most likely to be a source of human exposure and (c) suggest whether the chemicals are likely to accumulate in human tissues. Furthermore, the systematic application of such model systems to structure-distribution studies may help in determining with greater certainty those physicochemical properties of substances that are most useful in predicting the distribution and effects of chemicals in ecosystems (Lu & Metcalf, 1975).

Information on production, use, and disposal are of great importance in determining the sources and quantities of a chemical released into the environment, in assessing the possible extent of human exposure, and in identifying human populations that are likely to be exposed.

In conclusion, essential criteria for priority in the selection of chemicals for testing are: (*a*) indication or suspicion of hazard to human health and type and severity of potential health effects; (*b*) probable extent of production and use; (*c*) potential for persistence in the environment; (*d*) potential for accumulation in biota and in the environment, and (*e*) type and size of populations likely to be exposed. A chemical of first priority for testing would rate highly with respect to all or most of these criteria.

1.1.6 The extent of toxicity testing required

The extent of the toxicity testing required will depend on a variety of considerations, and generally valid procedures cannot be proposed. One scheme, proposed by Sanockij (1975a), for chemicals that are being developed, is shown in Table 1.1. As a first step, it may be useful to make an approximate estimation of toxicity based on the chemical structure and the physical and chemical properties of the substance, and on known correlations of these variables with biological activity (Andreyeshcheva, 1976; WHO, 1976a). These considerations may be of value for decisions on safety measures to be taken during initial laboratory work. Extrapolation and interpolation in homologous series may also be of value for decisions on safety measures to be taken during initial laboratory work (Ljublina & Miheev, 1974), but for some series of chemicals this is not applicable.

A preliminary evaluation of toxicity should start when chemicals are synthesized in the laboratory stage of the development of an industrial process. The full evaluation of the chemicals involved, both in respect to occupational and general population exposure, and assessment of possible air, water, and food contamination, should be initiated later, when it has been decided to proceed with full-scale production of the chemical. Toxicity data obtained during the development stages of a technological process could provide information concerning the health hazards not only of the raw materials and products, but also of the various other substances used or produced as intermediates in the technological process, and of gaseous and other wastes. Toxicological evaluation may also help in the selection of an alternative technological process, less hazardous to health.

Waste disposal by dispersion in air and water, the ease of environmental degradation of the chemical, and the toxicity of the degradation products, are other problems that need attention at an early stage in the toxicological evaluation of new chemicals. For example, resistance to degradation has to be taken into account when formulating health criteria regulating the application and disposal of pesticides (Medved & Spynu, 1970).

This phasing of toxicological studies may be useful in coordinating testing at national and international levels.

Table 1.1 The extent of toxicological evaluation required in relation to technological process development

Stages of technological development	Stages of toxicological evaluation	Toxicological studies
1. Theoretical concept and process flow diagram	Preliminary toxicological assessment	Analysis of literature data on toxicity and hazards of raw materials, reagents, catalysers, semiproducts and additives
		Assessment of toxicological parameters on the basis of metabolic analogies, persistence, the relationship between chemical structure, chemical and physical properties, and biological activity. Interpolation and extrapolation in homologous series
2. Laboratory development of the technological process	Acute toxicity	Acute and subacute experiments on animals. Toxicological evaluation of technological unit processes
3. Pilot plant stage	Subacute toxicity	Subacute toxicity experiments on animals. Studies of delayed effects. Medical examination of workers.
	Detailed toxicological evaluation	Chronic toxicity studies and, when indicated, effects on reproduction, carcinogenicity, mutagenicity. Formulation of medical and industrial hygiene requirements for full-scale production
4. Design of industrial scale process	Additional studies	Studies of the mechanism of action, early and differential diagnosis, experimental therapy
5. Production and use of chemicals	Field studies	Assessment of working and environmental conditions and of health status of workers and general population
		Epidemiological studies
		Clinical evaluation of experimental prophylactic, diagnostic and therapeutic methods
		Adjustment and correction of requirements for health and environmental protection

Environmental and health standards will need to be defined preferentially for those chemicals that show a significant degree of toxicity and represent a health hazard, and are likely to be used widely in industry, agriculture, or in consumer products.

Changes and developments in industrial processes, the development of new chemicals, and changes in the use of existing chemicals, may lead to new or increased hazards. This calls for a continuous re-evaluation of priorities.

1.2 Dose-Effect and Dose-Response Relationships

1.2.1 Dose

Most commonly, the term "dose" is used to specify the amount of chemical administered, usually expressed per unit body weight. If the dose is administered into the stomach, on the skin, or into the respiratory tract, transport across the membranes may be incomplete and the absorbed dose will not be identical with the dose administered. In environmental exposures, an estimate of the dose can be made from the measurement of environmental and food concentrations as a function of time, and involves the assessment of food intake, inhalation rate, and the appropriate deposition and retention factors.

The doses in the organs and tissues of interest may be estimated from:

(a) administered dose or intake;
(b) measurement of the concentrations in tissues and organ samples;
(c) measurement of concentrations in excreta or exhaled air.

The use of these three types of information for the purposes of tissue and organ dose estimation requires the postulation of models to describe the absorption, distribution, retention, biotransformation, and excretion of the original chemical or its metabolites, as a function of time (see Chapter 4).

When the site of toxic action is located at, or very near, the site of application, for example, the skin, then the tissue dose estimate may be very reliable. However, when the site of toxic action is remote, for example, a liver cell, then the estimates of toxicologically significant doses are much less reliable.

The presence of a chemical in the blood indicates absorption; however, the blood concentration of a chemical is in a dynamic state, reaching higher levels with increasing absorption but decreasing as the distribution, tissue storage, metabolic transformation, and excretion increase. The blood concentration of a chemical is useful as an indicator of the dose only when it is related in a defined manner to the concentration at the site or sites of action (organs and tissues) (Task Group on Metal Toxicity, 1976).

1.2.2 Effect and response

"Effect" and "response" are often used interchangeably to denote a biological change, either in an individual or in a population, associated with an exposure or dose. Some toxicologists have, however, found it useful to differentiate between an effect and a response by applying the term "effect" to a biological change, and the term "response" to the proportion of a population that demonstrates a defined effect (Pfitzer, 1976; Task Group on Metal Toxicity, 1976).

25

In this terminology, response means the incidence rate of an effect. For example, the LD_{50} value may be described as the dose expected to cause a 50% response in a population tested for the lethal effect of a chemical. This distinction will be made in the present monograph, although it should be recognized that this terminology is not generally accepted.

An effect can usually be measured on a graded scale of intensity or severity and its magnitude related directly to the dose. Certain effects, however, permit no gradation and can be expressed only as "occurring" or "not occurring". Such effects are usually called "quantal" (see for example, Finney, 1971). Typical examples of quantal effects are death or occurrence of a tumour[a].

The toxic action of chemicals usually affects the whole organism but the primary damage may be localized in a specific target organ or organs in which the toxic injury may manifest itself in terms of dysfunction or overt disease (NIEHS, 1977). According to Sanockij (1975a), the specificity of acute toxic action can be expressed in terms of a "zone of specific action" (Z_{sp}) which is the ratio between the threshold[b] dose of an acute effect at the level of the total organism and the threshold dose for an acute effect at a specific organ or system. If $Z_{sp} > 1$, the toxic action is specific; if $Z_{sp} < 1$, it is non-specific.

Acute effects are those that occur or develop rapidly after a single administration (Casarett, 1975) but acute effects may appear after repeated or prolonged exposure as well. Chronic effects may also result from a single exposure but more often they are a consequence of repeated or prolonged exposures. Chronic effects are characterized not only by their duration but also by certain pathological features. They may arise from the accumulation of a toxic substance or its metabolites in the body, or from a summation of acute effects. The latent period (or the "time-to-occurrence" of an observable effect) may sometimes be very long, particularly if the dose or exposure is low. Other aspects of the nature of toxic effects are discussed in section 2.6.

Not every effect is necessarily adverse or harmful. In some cases, a graded effect may be either within the so-called "normal" range of

---

[a] A similar classification of effects is used in radiological protection where a distinction is made between "nonstochastic" and "stochastic" effects (ICRP, 1977). Nonstochastic effects are those for which the severity of effect varies with the dose. Stochastic effects are those for which the probability of occurrence, rather than their severity, is regarded as a function of dose. Hereditary effects and carcinogenesis induced by radiation are considered to be stochastic.

[b] The threshold concept is discussed in section 1.3.2.

physiological variation, or an "adverse" effect, depending on its intensity. The distinction between a physiological change and a pathological effect (adverse effect) is sometimes very difficult to make and there is much disagreement on this subject which will be discussed in detail in section 1.3.1. The concept of biochemical lesion introduced by Peters and his collaborators (Gavrilescu & Peters, 1931; Peters, 1963, 1967), and based on the ideas of Claude Bernard (Bernard, 1898), is of fundamental importance in this respect. A biochemical lesion can be defined as the biochemical change or defect which directly precedes pathological change or dysfunction (Peters, 1967).

The Task Group on Metal Accumulation (1973) and the Task Group on Metal Toxicity (1976) have defined the critical concentration for a cell as the concentration (of a metal) at which undesirable (adverse) functional changes, reversible or irreversible, occur in the cell. Critical organ concentration has been defined as the mean concentration in the organ at the time any of its cells reaches critical concentration and critical organ as that particular organ which first attains the critical concentration of a metal under specified circumstances of exposure and for a given population. This definition of "critical organ" differs from the generally accepted use of the term, i.e. that the critical organ is the organ whose damage (by radiation) results in the greatest injury to the individual (or his descendants) (ICRP, 1965). However, some toxicologists question the usefulness of the concept of a critical organ or tissue because it diverts attention from the role that the various regulatory systems of the body may have in relation to a toxic injury.

1.2.3 Dose-effect and dose-response curves

Dose-effect curves demonstrate the relation between dose and the magnitude of a graded effect, either in an individual or in a population. Such curves may have a variety of forms. Within a given dose range they may be linear but more often they are not. Finney (1952a) has discussed various transformations that can be used to make dose-effect curves linear.

Dose-response curves demonstrate the relation between dose and the proportion of individuals responding with a quantal effect. In general, dose-response curves are S-shaped (increasing), and they have upper and lower asymptotes, usually but not always 100 and 0% (see for example Cornfield, 1954). One way of explaining the shape of dose-response curves is that each individual in a population has a unique "tolerance" and requires a certain dose before responding with an effect. There exists, in principle, a low dose to which none will respond and a high dose to which all will respond.

For each effect there will usually be a different dose-response curve. Loewe (1959) and Hatch (1968) have discussed the relationship between dose, effect, and response and its graphical representation in a three-dimensional model.

If the experiment or observation is well designed (Chapters 2 and 3), the dose-response relationship will be based on data from many individuals over a range of doses from minimum to maximum response. Mathematical and statistical procedures are then used to establish the curvilinear relationship that provides the best fit to all of the data, expressed as mean values with their standard deviations at different doses. Mathematical expressions for dose-effect and dose-response relationships and the merits of applying normal, log-normal, and other types of distributions are discussed in the Appendix.

It should be pointed out that the shape of the dose-response curve for the same substance and the same animal species may vary with changes in experimental conditions, such as changes in the way in which the dose is distributed in time (Weil, 1972a).

In evaluating human exposure to environmental chemicals, the dose will usually be estimated as a function of concentration and time. In some cases the concentration will be fairly constant and then the time-effect and time-response relationships will be similar to the dose-effect and dose-response relationships. However, in many cases the concentration will vary, as will the time of exposure to specific concentrations, and integrated relationships of dose-concentration-time must be considered as well as dose-effect and time-effect relationships (Druckrey, 1967; Golubev et al., 1973; Lazarev, 1963; Weil, 1972a).

Haber's rule ($ct = k$) states that the product of concentration (c) and time (t) results in a constant intensity of effect (k) for some gases. This formula was later changed to $ct^b = k$ (where b is constant) which fitted other biological data better (Lazarev & Brusilovskaja, 1934), although it also has its limitations. The extrapolation of concentration-time relationships has been used successfully to obtain predictions of response following long-term inhalation exposure to low concentrations (Pinigin, 1974).

Concentration-time relationships, such as the variation of the fraction of the dose with time as in combinations of short-term peak concentrations and prolonged low-level concentrations in air pollution, and variable cycles of exposure, may influence the toxic effect. Few systematic attempts to evaluate these factors have been made, although Sidorenko & Pinigin (1975, 1976) have described some principles for setting air quality standards from this viewpoint, and Pinigin (1974) has dealt with the problems of intermittent inhalation exposure. This problem has also been discussed by Ulanova et al. (1973, 1976).

28

1.2.4 Toxic effects due to a combination of chemicals

When an organism is exposed to two or more chemicals, their joint action may be:

(a) independent—when the chemicals produce different effects or have different modes of action;

(b) additive—when the magnitude of an effect or response produced by two or more chemicals is numerically equal to the sum of the effects or responses that the chemicals would produce individually;

(c) more than additive—often called potentiation or synergism;

(d) less than additive (antagonism, inhibition).

More specific terminology may be used when the mechanisms of joint action are known or when definite assumptions are made about them (Finney, 1971; Hewlett & Pluckett, 1961). The time intervals and sequences between exposures to different chemicals are extremely important, and the quality as well as the degree of joint action may depend on these variables (Kagan, 1973; Kustov et al., 1974; Williams, 1969). Furthermore, the joint action at lethal dose levels may be quite different from that at low dose levels, when the effects or responses are often only additive or independent (Smyth et al., 1969; Ulanova, 1969).

Most statistical models for joint action have been developed for situations in which two or more chemicals are administered simultaneously or within a short (few minutes) time interval. A model proposed by Finney (1952b, 1971) is often used for predicting the acute joint toxicity of chemicals. The model is strictly applicable to mixtures of chemicals that act at the same site, producing the same type of acute toxic effect and having parallel regression lines of probits against log doses (see Appendix). For a mixture of, for example, three chemicals, the equation for the median effective dose (ED_{50}) is

$$\frac{1}{ED_{50}(A,B,C)} = \frac{f_A}{ED_{50}(A)} + \frac{f_B}{ED_{50}(B)} + \frac{f_C}{ED_{50}(C)} \tag{1}$$

where f_A, f_B and f_C are the fractions of substances A, B, and C in the mixture. When all the values on the right hand side of equation (1) are known, a predicted ED_{50} (assuming additive joint action) can be calculated and compared with the actual ED_{50} of the mixture determined experimentally. A smaller than predicted ED_{50} demonstrates a more than additive response (synergism), a greater than predicted ED_{50} indicates a less than additive response (antagonism). Smyth et al. (1969) demonstrated that this equation can give satisfactory results under conditions that are less restrictive than stated above, for example in identifying the type of acute joint action among randomly selected industrial chemicals. Ball (1959) applied the equation to the estimation of maximum allowable concentrations for occupational exposure to mixtures of substances that exercise a "similar joint action", e.g. benzene and toluene. Another model for estimating the results of joint action has been developed using the isoeffective concentrations instead of ED_{50} in equation (1) (Pinigin, 1974).

The possibility of predicting the type of joint action is enhanced if there is information on the metabolism and disposition of the chemicals (Murphy, 1969; Williams, 1969). Basic principles concerning the kinetics of reactions of chemicals with primary sites (tissue receptor sites) and with secondary sites are important in considering the joint action of chemicals (Gaddum, 1957; Schild et al., 1961; Veldstra, 1956; Williams, 1969). The relevant factors seem to be the relative affinities at the sites of action (e.g. target enzymes, neuroeffector sites, and other vital target sites), and at the sites of loss or sinks (e.g. detoxifying enzymes, nonvital tissue binding sites, pathways of excretion, and storage sites), and the intrinsic activity at the sites of action[a]. Since there is a limited number of sites of action and sinks within any organism, there will be a limited dose range within which synergism or antagonism can be demonstrated. This, of course, is only one area where more information could help in predicting the effects of the joint action of chemicals. Other areas where knowledge is insufficient are the possible effects of low-level, prolonged exposures to mixtures of chemicals and the effects of multiple stresses including chemicals, physical factors such as heat and noise, and pre-existing disease (NIEHS, 1970).

Simultaneous exposures to the same chemical in different media (e.g. air, water, food) which is called "complex action" by some toxicologists (Korbakova et al., 1971; Kustov et al., 1974; Pinigin, 1974; Spynu et al., 1972) is another aspect of multiple stresses which has considerable practical importance.

1.3 Interpretation of Laboratory Data

It is essential that all experiments to evaluate toxicity should be designed to be scientifically meaningful, and should not be conducted merely to comply with statutory regulations. Thus, the evaluation of each new chemical will not be an identical task and procedures will differ, to some extent, from one compound to another. The protocol for an experiment will evolve gradually during the experiment, in accordance with earlier findings.

---

[a] Relative affinity—reciprocal of the dissociation constant for the chemical-receptor complex. Intrinsic activity—the capacity of the chemical to produce an effect when it combines with a reactive tissue site. For precise definitions see for example Ariëns et al. (1957).

It is useful to have laboratory data validated by a study of the mechanisms involved in the development of the toxic lesion. Furthermore, numerous endogenous and environmental variables can modify the toxicity of chemicals, as discussed in subsequent chapters. In some instances, the influence of these variables is known, and can be controlled, but often this is not the case and this may cause serious difficulties in the interpretation of laboratory toxicity data.

In the present context, we are mainly interested in the interpretation of laboratory data with a view to their application in the evaluation of the health risk to man. The discussion will therefore be limited to a few topics that are particularly relevant in this respect.

1.3.1 Distinction between adverse and nonadverse effects

An adverse, or "abnormal" effect has often been defined in terms of a measurement that is outside the "normal" range. The "normal" range, in turn, is usually defined on the basis of measured values observed in a group of presumably healthy individuals, and expressed in statistical terms of a range representing 95% confidence limits of the mean or, for individuals, in terms of 95% "tolerance" limits[a] established with a derived degree of confidence (95% or 99%). An individual with a measured value outside this range may be either "abnormal" in fact, or one of that small group of "normal" individuals who have extreme values. According to Sanockij (1970), the distinction between "normal" and "abnormal" values based on statistical considerations may be used as a criterion for adverse effects, if the exposed population consists of adult, generally healthy individuals, subject to periodical medical examination, such as workers. Departures from "normal" values associated with a given exposure will then be considered as adverse effects, if the observed changes are:

(a) statistically significant ($P < 0.05$) in comparison with a control group, and outside the limits ($m \pm 2s$) of generally accepted "normal" values;

(b) statistically significant ($P < 0.05$) in comparison with a control group, but within the range of generally accepted normal values, provided such changes persist for a considerable time after the cessation of exposure; and

---

[a] Tolerance limits are defined as $m \pm ks$ where m is the sample mean, s is the sample standard deviation and k is a coefficient that depends both on the size of the sample (N) and the required degree of confidence. If the "normal" mean has been determined on the basis of a very large sample, the 95% limits will be equal to $\mu \pm 1.96\sigma$ where μ and σ are the "true" or population values of the mean and the standard deviation, respectively (see for example Owen, 1955).

(c) statistically significant ($P < 0.05$) in comparison with a control group, but within the "normal" range, provided statistically significant departures from the generally accepted "normal" values become manifest under functional or biochemical stress.

This statistical definition of adverse effects is less suitable for the general population which includes some groups that may be specially sensitive to environmental factors, particularly the very young, the very old, those affected with disease, and those exposed to other toxic materials or stresses. In this case, it is practically impossible to define "normal" values, and any observable biological change may be considered as an adverse effect under some circumstances. For this reason, attempts have been made to set criteria for adverse effects based on biological considerations and not only on statistically significant differences with respect to an unexposed population (control group). Although there is no general agreement on such criteria and the ultimate decision on what is an adverse effect will have to depend, in each case, on experience and expert judgment, it may nevertheless be useful to give examples of such criteria, which illustrate at the same time how different such criteria may be.

A Committee for the Working Conference on Principles of Protocols for Evaluating Chemicals in the Environment (NAS, 1975) defined nonadverse effects as the absence of changes in morphology, growth, development, and life span. Furthermore, nonadverse effects do not result in impairment of functional capacity or impairment of the capacity to compensate for additional stress. They are reversible following cessation of exposure without detectable impairment of the ability of the organism to maintain homeostasis, and do not enhance susceptibility to the deleterious effects of other environmental influences.

On the other hand, adverse effects may be deduced as changes that:

"1. occur with intermittent or continued exposure and that result in impairment of functional capacity (as determined by anatomical, physiological, and biochemical or behavioural parameters) or in a decrement of the ability to compensate additional stress;

2. are irreversible during exposure or following cessation of exposure if such changes cause detectable decrements in the ability of the organism to maintain homeostasis; and

3. enhance the susceptibility of the organism to the deleterious effects of other environmental influences."

Soviet toxicologists emphasize that criteria for differentiating between adverse and nonadverse effects should not be based on overt pathology (e.g. inflammation, necrosis, hyperplasia), and have proposed, *inter alia*, a number of criteria based on metabolic and biochemical changes. Such changes are considered to be adverse if:

(a) the metabolism of a substance becomes less efficient or the elimination of a substance (expressed in terms of biological half-time, $T_{\frac{1}{2}}$) slows down with increasing doses of the substance (Sanockij, 1956);

(b) enzymes that have a key significance in metabolism are inhibited (Kustov & Tiunov, 1970);

(c) the inhibition of a certain enzyme results in an increase in the concentration of the corresponding natural substrate in the body and/or in a decreased capacity to metabolize the specific substrates in a loading test (Kustov & Tiunov, 1970);

(d) the relative activities of different enzyme systems are changed (e.g. the ratio of the activities of asparagine and alanine transaminases (Kustov & Tiunov, 1970)).

Pokrovskij (1973) also attaches great importance to the changes in the pattern of isoenzymes in the blood, and to the changes in the subcellular membranes (e.g. lysosomal membranes) resulting from the action of toxic substances.

Differentiation between "nonadverse" and "adverse" effects requires considerable knowledge of the importance of reversible changes and subtle departures from "normal" physiology and morphology in terms of the organism's overall economy of life, ability to adapt to other stresses, and their possible effects on life span. Newer and improved methods of research have increasingly provided more sensitive tests for subtle biological deviations such as induction of enzymes of the smooth endoplasmic reticulum of the liver, or reversible hypertrophy of the liver. These types of changes are produced by relatively low doses of many chemicals and they are considered by some authors to be adaptive and generally useful to health, and by others to be indicative of injury (Hermann, 1974; Kustov & Tiunov, 1970; Parke, 1975). One of the most challenging areas for basic research in toxicology today is the acquisition of data that can be used to estimate whether, or under what conditions, subtle changes in enzyme activities, nerve action potentials, altered behavioural reaction etc. indicate impairment of physiological function or predict impending development of more serious irreversible injury, should exposure to the chemical continue.

In addition to all these considerations, the possibility must be kept in mind that an effect may not be seen because the number of animals studied was inadequate, the observation time was too short, or for other reasons.

1.3.2 Threshold: practical and theoretical considerations

The concept of "threshold" is complex and the term has to be carefully defined, so that statements concerning this concept in relation to the protection of human health are not confused by semantic differences. A distinction should be made between the threshold for individuals and thresholds for limited groups of individuals or general populations.

The dependence of effect or response on the dose of a chemical has already been discussed (section 1.2). As a rule, the intensity of the effect or response decreases with reduction in dose, and a biological reaction often reaches zero before the dose becomes equal to zero. Below a certain limiting exposure level, or dose, i.e. below the threshold, a chemical substance may not elicit a toxic effect. The threshold for an adverse effect of a chemical is defined by some toxicologists as the minimum exposure level or dose that gives rise to biological changes beyond the limits of homeostatic adaptation. True homeostatic adaptation should be carefully distinguished from pathological processes (Sanockij, 1975a).

The existence of a threshold for all adverse effects is, however, still a matter for discussion. Sanockij (1975b) has provided data which show that small quantities of environmental chemicals may not reach their receptor because the rate of elimination or metabolic degradation is relatively more effective with smaller doses. It has also been suggested that where effective repair processes are present, even if a substance interacts with the receptor, it need not necessarily produce an adverse effect.

For some toxic effects, such as neoplastic disease or mutations of genetic material, it has been assumed by some authors that a single molecule of a chemical is sufficient to initiate a process that may progressively lead to an observed, harmful effect. For this reason, it may not be possible to demonstrate that a threshold dose for a carcinogen or a mutagen exists (Saffiotti, 1973).

Other scientists view carcinogenic or mutagenic chemicals as toxic entities that may have special properties with regard to the nature and characteristics of their adverse effects, but are subject to the same physicochemical and biological interactions that are considered to result in a threshold dose for other chemicals (Dinman, 1972; Sanockij, 1970; Stokinger, 1972; Weil, 1972a).

The question of the existence of a threshold for carcinogens and mutagens was recently discussed by a WHO Scientific Group (WHO, 1974a), which concluded that "the existence of a threshold may be envisaged. Nevertheless, the difficulties of determining a threshold for a population are great. Therefore, mathematically derived conclusions that it is impossible to demonstrate no-effect levels experimentally cannot be ignored". A "no-effect" level for a group of animals may occur because the dose is really below the theoretical no-effect level (i.e. below the threshold) or because the number of animals is too small. For example, in an experiment with 20 animals, it is possible that none of the animals will show an effect whereas in an experiment with 100 animals some response might be seen. However, an upper limit for the probable response can be estimated statistically. For instance, if in an experiment with 100 animals, no response has been observed, it can be shown that there is a 95% probability that, under the conditions of the experiment, the upper limit of response is 3%, and that there is a 99% probability that the response will not exceed 4.5%. Even in an experiment with 1000 animals showing no response, the upper 95% confidence limit of response is 3 animals showing an effect per 1000 treated animals (Food & Drug Administration, 1970).

Another reason for not having seen a response in an experiment may be that the time of observation was too short. This may be the case, for example, when the quantal effect considered is a cancer, with a long latent period between exposure and appearance of tumours.

For these reasons the "no-effect level" has no real meaning and a better term is "no-observed-effect level" (NAS, 1975).

1.3.3 Extrapolation of animal data to man

In many cases, studies with laboratory animals make it possible to predict the toxic effects of chemicals in man. However, it is important to realize that experimental animal models have their limitations, and that the accuracy and reliability of a quantitative prediction of toxicity in man depend on a number of conditions, such as choice of animal species, design of the experiments, and methods of extrapolation of animal data to man.

Hoel et al. (1975) considered the criteria for the adequacy of an experiment to be used for the extrapolation of animal data to man. They include: test animal species and strain (the animal should be susceptible to induction of the effects under consideration); the number of animals; the route of administration (which should include the routes of human exposure); and the physical state and chemical form of the agent. The side effects of the chemical and its organ specificity should also be taken into account in the design of the experiment. In interpreting the results, attention should be paid to adequate survival of the animals, to possible intercurrent disease, the quality and extent of pathological data, the quality and extent of relevant data collection during the experiment, and the availability of data at the time of interpretation.

1.3.3.1 *Species differences and related factors*

The most difficult problem in the extrapolation of animal data to man is the conversion from one species to another. For most substances, the pathogenesis of poisoning is the same in man and other mammals, and for this reason the signs of intoxication are also analogous. Thus, quantitative rather than qualitative differences in toxic response are most common. Man may be more sensitive than certain laboratory animals but there are also many cases where some animal species are more sensitive than man. For example, the mouse is most sensitive to atropine, the cat is less sensitive, while the dog and the rabbit tolerate atropine in doses 100 times higher than the lethal dose for man. However, the dog is more sensitive to hydrocyanic acid than man (Elizarova, 1962).

Species differences in sensitivity can often be explained by differences in metabolism, in particular by quantitative and qualitative differences in the ability of an enzyme to detoxify chemicals, and also by differences in the rates of absorption, transport, distribution, and elimination of chemicals (Curry, 1970; Ecobichon & Cormeau, 1973; Flynn et al., 1972; Hucker, 1970; Portman et al., 1970; Sato & Moroi, 1971). Rall (1970) discussed various factors to be considered in the selection of animal models for pharmacotherapeutic studies in relation to the steps that intervene between administration of the drug (or chemical) and the arrival of the compound at the ultimate sites of action. After oral administration, absorption in standard laboratory animals is generally considered to be very similar to man, although there are quantitative differences for some compounds. For example, species differences in the absorption and action of some compounds are related to differences in the bacterial flora of the gastrointestinal tract (Williams, 1972). Rall further concluded that the distribution and storage of drugs are reasonably consistent in mammalian species, including man, although plasma binding tends to be more extensive in man than in small mammalian species. Urinary excretion in different animal species depends to some extent, on their different diets, since diet influences urinary pH and thus the extent of ionization of compounds. Biliary excretion is quite variable from species to species and apparently is more extensive in mice and rabbits than in rats or man. Species differences in response to chemicals appear to be mainly related to rates of biotransformation which are generally more rapid in small laboratory animals than in man.

One of the most potent bladder carcinogens, 2-naphthalenamine (2-naphthylamine), produces bladder cancer in the dog, hamster, and man, but not in the rat, rabbit, or guineapig. Species differences in the carcinogenicity of 2-fluorenylacetamide (2-acetaminofluorene) have been attributed to the different extents of metabolism to the proximate carcinogen, the N-hydroxy derivative (Miller et al., 1964). Similarly, strain differences in metabolism may also affect toxicity (Mazze et al., 1973).

If metabolic information is available, differences in absorption, distribution, biotransformation, and elimination of toxic substances in man and animals should be taken into account when selecting experimental animals.

Species differences in toxicity may also be due to differences in cellular transport. Aflatoxin, which is more toxic to rats than to mice, both as an acute poison and as a carcinogen, is transported more slowly into the liver cells and is metabolized more rapidly in the mouse than in the rat (Portman et al., 1970).

In determining the required duration of an animal experiment, it is often useful to compare the life span of the animal with that of man. Using the "body weight rule", the average life span for 70 species of mammals showed a linear correlation with body weight, but the average life span of man was found to be an exception (Krasovskij, 1975). The regression equation obtained from a study of many mammals showed that the average life span for a mammalian representative, having the same body weight as man (70 kg) was equal to 15 years. Thus, if this assumption is accepted the average life span of a rat (about 2.5 years) corresponds to only 15–17 years of a man's life. This inconsistency in the life spans of man and experimental animals should be taken into account in the design and interpretation of animal experiments for the evaluation of toxicity to man.

There are other problems in the evaluation of toxicity to man from experiments on animals, such as where an effect is difficult to measure or where similar conditions are difficult to obtain in animal models, for example, intelligence and the more esoteric behavioural changes. Furthermore, in animal experiments, the effects of social factors, so important to man, cannot be evaluated.

For these reasons, when extrapolating from animals to man it is prudent to apply a species conversion factor which should be determined on the basis of biological considerations and the available information on the test species (Hoel et al., 1975). There is no definite rule for the species conversion factor. If the extrapolation of data is based on the most sensitive species tested, some toxicologists use a factor of 1 (Šabad et al., 1973), but others recommend a factor as large as 10 (Weil, 1972a).

The unit of dose to be used has also to be considered in the extrapolation of data to man and it has recently been recommended that the dose per unit surface area approximately equivalent to the weight raised to the power 2/3 should be used. If the dose is given in terms of dietary concentration, there seems to be no need to make the surface area adjustment (Hoel et al., 1975; Mantel & Schneiderman, 1975).

A separate problem, to which there appears to be no satisfactory answer at present, is the conversion from an inbred animal strain to a genetically highly heterogeneous human population (Hoel et al., 1975).

1.3.3.2 *Safety factors*

In almost all instances, laboratory data on the toxicity of chemicals are drawn from experiments in which the adverse effect occurs at a considerably higher incidence rate than would be acceptable in man. For this reason alone, and apart from the biological differences between laboratory species and man, an extrapolation from a known dose-response range to an unknown range is necessary. Indeed, essentially the same problem arises when a human accident or epidemiological data are used as the starting point.

Traditionally, a safety factor has been introduced to provide for uncertainties in extrapolation from animals to man, and from a small group of individuals to a large population. Such safety factors have ranged from 1 to as much as 5000. Because of the current uncertainty regarding the mathematical and biological reliability of methods for extrapolating from high doses to low doses, primary dependence on somewhat arbitrary safety factors continues. However, means of extrapolating from high to low doses are being intensively studied at the present time, especially with respect to carcinogenicity.

Most regulatory authorities rely on the use of safety factors but there are no precise guidelines for deciding the appropriate size of such a factor. Sanockij (1962) and Sanockij & Sidorov (1975) have discussed the rationale for different safety factors. In general, the size of the safety factor will depend on (a) the nature of the toxic effects, (b) the size and type of population to be protected, and (c) the quality of toxicological information available. A factor of 2 to 5 or less may be considered as sufficient if the effect against which individuals or a population are to be protected is not regarded as very severe, if only a small number of workers are likely to be exposed, and if the toxicological information is derived from human data. On the other hand, a safety factor as large as 1000 or more may be required if the possible effect is very serious, if the general population is to be protected, and if the toxicological data are derived from limited experiments on laboratory animals. In some cases, the safety factor may be a value that has been used with reasonable success and is, therefore, perpetuated.

For most food additives that are not considered to be carcinogenic, it has been the accepted practice to divide the no-adverse-effect dose (i.e., the maximum ineffective dose) in animals by 100, to arrive at an acceptable daily intake (ADI) for man (Vettorazzi, 1977; WHO, 1958). For pesticides and certain environmental chemicals, safety factors ranging from less than 100 to several thousand have been used (Vettorazzi, 1975). For some occupational exposures, and for certain air pollutants (WHO, 1977) much smaller safety factor have been proposed in the range of 2–5. Safety factors have also been proposed for carcinogenic chemicals ranging from 100 (Druckrey, 1967; Janyševa,1972) to about 5000 (Weil, 1972a) but they have not been generally accepted.

1.3.3.3 *Low-dose extrapolation*

Low-dose extrapolation is based on mathematical models that are used to predict the response at a given low dose or to predict that dose which gives a predetermined low response. Such models may relate the incidence of a quantal effect to dose, or they may consider the distribution of the "time to occurrence" of a condition and its relation to dose. In both cases, the results of extrapolation are strongly dependent on the choice of the model. For example, the Advisory Committee on Food Additives (FDA, 1970) noted that dose-response data may fit several models equally well in the 2% to 5% range, but the doses extrapolated to very low responses would differ very strikingly: the ratio of ED_1 to $ED_{0.000001}$ would be either 100, 100 000, or 1 000 000 for the probit, logistic, or one-hit curves, respectively.

Several extrapolation procedures have been proposed which will give an upper limit to the dose corresponding to a low response. In other words, the result of extrapolation will not be the best estimate of the unknown dose required to give the desired response but a dose that is most likely to be below the dose required to give this response. Two procedures based on this approach have received particular attention: one is based on the one-hit model, the other on the probit model.

The one-hit model assumes that an effect can be induced after a single susceptible target has been reached by a single biologically effective unit of dose (see for example Cornfield, 1954). At low doses, this model is numerically equivalent to the linear dose-response model which is compatible with animal data for some carcinogens (Druckrey, 1967) and with some human data such as the incidence of lung cancer in relation to the number of cigarettes smoked per day (Doll, 1967). In their simplest form (i.e. when the true response at zero dose is assumed to be zero), the currently used extrapolation procedures based on this model (Gross et al., 1970; Hoel et al., 1975; Schneiderman, 1971) operate as follows: (1) the upper 99% confidence limit (UCL) is estimated for the observed response at a dose d; (2) a desired limit is set for a low response (R) e.g. 1 in 1 000 000; and (3) the dose (d_e) that would produce a response which is, with a 99% probability, lower than R is calculated from the equation $d_e = d \cdot R/(\text{UCL})$. Such procedures are more conservative than the procedures based on any other currently used dose-response model (probit, logit, or extreme-value models). In addition, the one-hit model seems to have a reasonable biological basis for carcinogenesis at low doses (Hoel et al., 1975).

Mantel & Bryan (1961) proposed the use of probits (see Annex to this Chapter) and a log-normal distribution to describe the variability of the sensitivities (tolerances) of individuals in a population. The probit model gives a dose-response curve that is concave at low-dose levels, and is less conservative than the linear model based on the one-hit hypothesis. The Mantel–Bryan procedure (see for example Schneiderman & Mantel, 1973) involves (1) the choice of a desired limit of response (R) (e.g. 1 in 1 000 000); (2) the estimation of the upper 99% confidence limit (UCL) for the observed response at dose d, and (3) imposing a probit-log dose straight line through UCL, with a slope (β) equal to 1 (i.e. one probit per 10-fold dose-range). The choice of the slope (β) is critical in this procedure. $\beta = 1$ has been proposed because a slope greater than 1 is usually (but not always) observed in carcinogenesis experiments. The Mantel & Bryan procedure has been modified to take into account response levels in control groups (Mantel et al., 1975).

A second category of models is based on the observation that the median "time to occurrence" (latent period) of an effect such as cancer may increase as the dose decreases but not proportionally. A thousand-fold change in the dose usually causes an approximately ten-fold change in the median time to tumour appearance and, with decreasing dose levels, a dose may be reached which would predict tumour occurrence beyond the life expectancy of the exposed individuals. This would still be consistent with the hypothesis that molecular changes in the cells, occurring in proportion to the concentration of carcinogens, are the initiating event (for a recent review see Jones & Grendon, 1975). One model (Altschuler, 1973; Blum, 1959; Druckrey, 1967) considers a log-normal distribution of the time-to-occurrence with median time depending on dose but with standard deviation independent of the dose. The dose d is related to the median time (t) by $d = c/t^n$, where n is assumed to be greater than one, and c is a constant. Peto et al. (1972) compared this model with another model in which the time to occurrence is considered to have a Weibull distribution (Day, 1967; Peto & Lee, 1973). They found that the Weibull distribution agreed with experimental data better than the log-normal, but this no doubt depends on the type of cancer involved. The low-dose extrapolation using these models would also be strongly dependent on the choice of the model (Chand & Hoel, 1974). Dose-"time-to-occurrence"-response relationships in cancer risk assessment have also been considered by Janyševa & Antomonov (1976).

The application of all these procedures presents practical difficulties (Hoel et al., 1975). Low-dose extrapolation is thus a very difficult problem that cannot be solved by statistical methods alone. Great caution should be exercised in using the existing methods and their inherent limitations should always be kept in mind. Good experimental data, combined with human data if available, and an understanding of the mechanisms of toxic action are essential if the task of low-dose extrapolation is to be accomplished satisfactorily.

1.3.3.4 *Other methods of extrapolation*

A method for extrapolation from one species to another based on an established relationship between the indices of toxicity and body weight for different animal species has also been suggested (Krasovskij, 1976a). In mammals, the weights of internal organs, and many physiological variables (pulse and respiration rates, consumption of oxygen, food, and water, liver microsomal enzyme activity) show a log-log linear relationship with body size of the animals (allometric ratios). This regularity appears to be valid for more than 100 different variables including the period of gestation, litter size, erythrocyte life span, and latent period of tumour development but there are also other variables to which it does not apply. This "body weight rule" (Krasovskij, 1975) may be expressed as follows: the logarithms of biological variables of mammals show a linear regression to the logarithms of the body weight.

Krasovskij (1976b) showed that values for the lethal dose for dogs of several chemicals obtained from regression analysis of toxicity in four other species of small mammals compared well with predictions made from direct extrapolation from albino rats or from the most sensitive animal species, or from the relationship of body surface area, and also with predictions obtained by the method of Ulanova (1969) and Van Noordwijk (1964). For the calculation of extrapolation coefficients from regression equations, see Krasovskij (1976b).

1.4 Human Data

1.4.1 Ethical considerations

In research involving human subjects, a number of elements, such as the assessment of risk, potential benefit, and quality of consent, have to be evaluated to ascertain whether ethical considerations are satisfied. The essential provisions for protecting human subjects in experimentation and research have been expounded by many international and national organizations. Key factors include the right to informed consent and freedom from coercion. The international instruments in dealing with this matter are the Declaration of Helsinki (as revised in Tokyo in 1975) and Article 7 of the International Covenant on Civil and Political Rights, adopted by the United Nations General Assembly, December 1966. Article 7 provides that "no-one shall be subjected without his free consent to medical or scientific experimentation" (Cranston, 1973; WHO, 1976b). Some countries possess specific codes of ethics relating to human experimentation, and special problems of experimentation that involve the

41

use of fetuses, children, the mentally ill, and prisoners require special consideration.

It is essential that human experimentation should only be undertaken when there is adequate evidence from animal and other studies that both the chemical and the circumstances of administration are safe. Every experiment with human volunteers should be subject to prior review and approval by a local ethical committee in order to ensure that the intended study complies with the ethical principles embodied in the Declaration of Helsinki and with other requirements of national and local bodies.

Ideal conditions of truly informed consent may not always be achieved in practice, consequently the burden of responsibility rests mainly with the investigator and, to a lesser extent, with the peer review body. Because of these difficulties, the guidelines and procedures for the protection of human subjects should be constantly reviewed and updated (WHO, 1976b).

In any case, collection of data from human subjects must be accomplished with due respect for human rights and dignity. The use of ethics committees with broad representation to review and approve all such experimentation is recommended to protect the rights of human subjects and to ensure responsible investigation.

1.4.2   Need for human investigations

Although there is general repugnance at the idea of using human subjects to assess the safety of environmental chemicals, the question is not whether or not human subjects should be used in toxicity experiments but rather whether such chemicals, deemed from animal toxicity studies to be relatively safe, should be released first to controlled, carefully monitored groups of human subjects, instead of being released indiscriminately to large populations with no monitoring and with little or no opportunity to observe adverse effects (Paget, 1970).

The prediction and prevention of possible toxic hazards that may arise from the introduction of chemicals into the environment can be made more valid if data from studies of the chemical in human subjects are available. Three particular aspects of human toxicology have need of such information, namely: (a) the selection, through comparative consideration of metabolism, of the most appropriate animal species for studies to predict the human response; (b) investigation of a specific, reversible effect of the compound in the most sensitive animal species, to determine whether there is a correlation with a similar effect in man; and (c) study of effects specific to man.

Certain types of information about the effects of chemicals can only be obtained by direct observations on man. Often, carefully controlled experiments can provide significant information at doses well below those anticipated to be "safe"; measurement of subtle changes of reaction time, behavioural functions, and sensory responses may be examples. In other cases, useful information may be obtained by careful studies on human cells or tissue maintained by culture techniques.

Human toxicological data include both the data obtained from epidemiological surveys of populations exposed to a toxic chemical under normal conditions of use, in cases of acute accidental poisoning and in occupational exposure, and the data from experiments in volunteers. Although an experiment is defined as observations under controlled conditions of exposure, there is, at times, only a grey area that distinguishes an experiment with human subjects from observations on human subjects under natural conditions. For example, some segments of human populations are at higher risk and should be particularly closely monitored, e.g., those exposed to chemicals at work or those receiving continuous treatment with medicines. The periodic clinical evaluation of workers is normally the responsibility of the employer and careful records of these examinations coupled with measurement of exposure conditions often exist. If accidental excessive exposure of an individual or a population should occur, it is both ethical and pertinent to learn as much as possible, recognizing always the right of the patient. Because of the wide individual variation in the toxicity of chemicals to man, the final evaluation should be based on information obtained from as widely varied a human population as is compatible with the various ethical principles involved.

1.5 The Use of Toxicological Data in Establishing Environmental Health Standards

1.5.1 Environmental health standards

The aim of environmental health standards is to protect individuals, human populations, and their progeny from the adverse effects of hazardous environmental factors, including chemicals. A sound principle of health protection is to keep all exposures as low as reasonably achievable, subject to the condition that the appropriate exposure limits, defined by the standard, are not exceeded.

Environmental health standards for chemicals may be formulated either in terms of concentrations in environmental components (e.g., air, water, food, consumer products) or in terms of amounts of substances that may be taken into the body. These concentrations and amounts should be sufficiently low that the threshold dose (if it exists and can be determined) will not be reached, or that the population of concern will not be subject to "unacceptable" risk, even following life-time or working life-time exposure. In some cases, as for irritant air pollutants, the distribution of exposure concentrations in time should also be considered. Standards may also prescribe the quantity of a substance to be used at any time and the manner of its use.

Social, cultural, and economic considerations should be taken into account in setting standards, but never to the detriment of health protection which should be of primary concern.

It is obvious that a standard setting process will necessarily involve many considerations besides toxicology. This process is often very different in different countries and different types of society. In general, however, it involves appraisal of toxicological data, particularly of dose-response relationships, including the effects on non-human targets (plants, animals, materials); social and economic analysis, policy analysis and review of experience elsewhere, leading eventually to an administrative or policy decision concerning the standard. Other relevant questions include the technological feasibility of achieving a standard, the cost and benefit of implementing it, means of enforcement, other public health priorities etc. Many of these topics are outside the scope of the present monograph.

1.5.2 Assessment of health risk and evaluation of benefits

Assessment of health risk from a given exposure to an environmental factor is an essential step in any procedure for setting environmental health standards. Assessment of health risk involves more than routine application of "safety factors", or low dose extrapolation which provides estimates of response that are, strictly speaking, applicable only to the conditions of the experiment. The application of a "species conversion" factor has been discussed and the difficulties pointed out (section 1.3.3.2). Questions such as the incidence of effects in various age groups and the degree of life shortening in affected individuals are all relevant to standard setting. For this reason the study of "time-to-occurrence" models in the extrapolation of data should be encouraged (Albert & Altschuler, 1976; Hoel et al., 1975). In addition, the seriousness of adverse effects will have to be evaluated from the public health and social viewpoint. Attention should also be paid to the heterogeneity of human populations, and, at present, it is not clear how the existence of susceptible groups, and the influence of nutrition and pre-existing disease in human populations should be taken into account. The existing methods of extrapolation from animal data to man deal with exposures to single substances whereas the actual human environment contains a large number of hazardous chemicals and other factors that can interact and considerably modify the effects, for example, in cancer induction (Bingham & Falk, 1959; Montesano et al., 1974). From this viewpoint, the importance of epidemiology and systematic surveillance of high risk groups cannot be overemphasized.

The acceptability of a given risk should also be considered in standard setting. This, as well as the judgment on safety (which involves decision on the acceptability of risk) exceeds the expertise of toxicologists. This is a domain where society at large has a role to play. Political decisions are also required on various social, economic, and ecological concerns. The same applies to the evaluation of benefits. As pointed out by a WHO Expert Committee (WHO, 1974a) "the expertise needed for the evaluation of risk is different from that needed for benefit evaluation. On the risk side, concern is focused on adverse health effects on man, damage to the environment, and misuse of natural resources. On the benefit side, the emphasis is on value to the consumer and the country". The interaction of all these factors is often described by the term "risk and benefit analysis" (see for example Falk, 1975), which is only partly within the area of toxicological expertise. The final judgment as to whether the benefit does or does not justify a risk is for society to make.

1.5.3 An example of toxicological information used in standard setting

Although standard setting procedures will differ from country to country, and the requirements for toxicological information will vary to a considerable extent, it may be useful, nevertheless, to describe, as an example, the procedure used in the USSR for setting standards for chemical pollutants in surface waters (Sysin, 1941; WHO, 1975a).

Information is first obtained on the likely concentrations of the chemical in industrial waste waters and the physical and chemical properties of the chemical. The stability of the substance under environmental conditions is then evaluated by standard analytical methods and the influence of the chemical on the self-purification processes of natural waters is studied.

The toxicological investigations required include LD_{50} studies for mice, rats, guineapigs and rabbits (Krasovskij, 1965) and subacute experiments lasting 1–2 months, to provide data on functional disturbances of organs and systems and on any cumulative properties of the chemical (Krasovskij, 1970). These tests are followed by chronic toxicity experiments lasting 6–8 months. Study of specific effects of chemical water pollutants (e.g., mutagenicity, teratogenicity, and effects on reproductive function) is also a necessary component of toxicological investigations.

The subthreshold (maximum ineffective) concentration determined by chronic experiments is then compared with the threshold concentrations established for the other two indices of water quality (i.e. effects on the self-purification of water and its organoleptic properties), and the smallest concentration is assumed to be the "hygienic" standard.

The total number of hygienic standards for hazardous substances in water, developed in the USSR, has reached 500; of these, about 60% have been established according to organoleptic criteria and 30% according to the toxicological hazard index. These standards have been incorporated in the water legislation of the country and serve as the basis for practical control measures in protecting water bodies from chemical pollution.

1.6 Limitations of Safety Evaluation

Experimental toxicology is a highly complex, multidisciplinary science. The extrapolation of animal data to man requires well-informed contributions from several scientific disciplines. Absolute proof of safety for man of a chemical substance cannot be obtained from the results of toxicological tests (Coon, 1973). However, toxicological tests do provide guidance on the relative toxicity of a compound and help in identifying likely modes of action in man.

Acute toxicity studies in animals are of value in predicting potential toxic effects of a chemical in human beings exposed to near fatal doses. From the results of such studies, the nature of acute responses in man may be anticipated with a view to initiating life-supporting measures or first-aid or therapeutic procedures.

Short-term and subacute studies are particularly valuable in determining the more subtle toxic effects of a chemical, whether or not it has potential for cumulative toxicity and whether or not the toxic effects are reversible upon cessation of exposure. These tests are of value in estimating the potential hazard to man following exposure of intermediate duration, usually 2–7 years.

Of greatest concern to toxicologists, regulatory officials, and the general public are the possible chronic toxic effects of chemicals. Chronic toxicity tests assist in establishing the degree of risk to man that may be expected from low-level long-term exposure to a chemical substance. Chemicals that tend to persist or concentrate in the biosphere and as a result have the potential to affect large segments of the population are of particular concern.

In extrapolating animal data to man, several factors must be taken into consideration. These include the "no-effect level" derived from animal experiments, the nature of the dose-response curve and the nature of the toxic effects produced (Friedman, 1969). The known or anticipated level of exposure in man and the potential number of exposed individuals must also be considered (NAS, 1975). It is worth pointing out that the so-called "no-effect level" is a statistically derived value usually estimated within a 95% confidence interval and that a 5% probability exists that the value is in error. It has been noted, for example, that if a toxic effect occurs in only 1% of the test animals, the effect will be entirely missed 37% of the time if only 100 animals are used in each test (Friedman, 1969). In addition, if the same effect occurs spontaneously in control animals, the chances of detecting that response in treated animals becomes even more remote.

Predictions of toxicity from laboratory animal studies are dependent on the relevance of these studies to man, to wild-life, and to environmental ecosystems. They are also dependent on the genetics, nutrition, general health, and environmental circumstances of the individuals exposed.

There may be a hereditary disposition in man to an increased susceptibility to toxic chemicals, such as an increased tendency to malignant tumours (Kellerman et al., 1973). Similarly, persons under stress or treatment with immunosuppressive drugs may also be at greater risk to chemical toxicity and chemical carcinogenesis. These individuals will constitute abnormal populations for which the degree of risk may not be predictable from animal studies or from human studies carried out on healthy subjects, but these abnormal populations may be of sufficient magnitude to merit special consideration. Furthermore, genetic variations in laboratory animals are paralleled by variations in the toxic response to chemicals, and this puts additional limitations on predictions of possible human toxicity from such animal data.

Similarly, the nutritional status of individuals may also result in wide variation in susceptibility to toxic chemicals because malnutrition may lead to reduction of natural protection afforded by detoxication mechanisms.

Safety evaluation of chemicals is too frequently empirical and there is often a tendency to mistake quantity of data for quality. Regulatory agencies and toxicologists must be flexible and keep abreast of new experimental techniques and methods and of fundamental developments in the understanding of the mechanisms of toxicity. The application of new methods could be more relevant and informative than the routine use of old traditional ones, but these new methods should not necessarily be expected to replace traditional procedures, nor should they be applied routinely until adequately evaluated for significance and reliability.

Whether new or old procedures are employed, it is very important that the specific conditions under which the experiments are conducted should be accessible to other scientists, so that the results from different laboratories may be compared. Where it is not possible to set forth such details in publications of toxicological investigations, a central listing of detailed experimental procedures and conditions would be desirable.

MATHEMATICAL EXPRESSIONS OF DOSE-EFFECT AND DOSE-RESPONSE RELATIONSHIPS

Dose-effect and dose-response relationships may be plotted and an empirical "best fit" of a curvilinear correlation may be expressed as a mathematical equation. Alternatively, a visual inspection of the graph may suggest a mathematical equation, such as linear, exponential, or power function, and then the best-fit of the data points to the equation may be calculated. A single set of data could fit several mathematical equations equally well when the range of data is limited. Therefore, care must be taken not to assume that biological events follow a specific mathematical model unless the data have been collected over a wide range of values.

Whenever possible, it is useful to develop a hypothesis for a mechanism of toxic action on biological grounds, to derive the general mathematical expression for the mechanism, and then to fit the data to the equation to obtain the values for the constants in the equation that will be specific for the conditions of the experiment. For example, one mechanism of action may indicate that the law of mass action (or chemical equilibrium) applies to the dose-effect relationship. If one assumes 1) that one molecule of the chemical binds reversibly with one receptor site; 2) that effect (E) is directly proportional to the fraction of the total receptors bound by the chemical; and 3) that the amount of bound chemical is very small compared to the total concentration or dose (D), then the application of the law of mass action leads to a relationship: $E = K_1 D/(K_2 + K_1 D)$ where K_1 and K_2 are constants specific to the experiment. Clark (1933) noted that this mathematical equation, which gives an equilibrium curve asymptotically approaching the maximum effect, has a very similar shape, over certain dose ranges, to a logarithmic curve, such as $E = K_1 \log(K_2 D + 1)$, or a power function curve, such as $E = K_1 D^{K_2}$.

The sigmoid or S-shaped curve is a commonly observed curvilinear expression for some dose-effect and most dose-response relationships. The biological basis for this relationship may be partially understood by the nature of the frequency distribution of individual susceptibilities or resistances in a population. Most of the individuals in a population will respond close to a central dose level, and a few will respond only at very low or at very high dose levels. This leads to a frequency distribution for the individual responders as a function of dose. A frequency distribution, however, does not describe a biological mechanism for susceptibility or resistance, but the random occurrence of individuals with different susceptibilities.

Fig. 1.1 shows a normal frequency distribution; the curve is symmetrical around a central point. Its cumulative frequency distribution provides the often observed sigmoid curve. A dose-response relationship will be observed as a cumulative frequency distribution because an individual who responds at a low dose will, of course, also respond at higher doses. Thus the frequency of responders at a given high dose includes all those that respond at that and all lower doses.

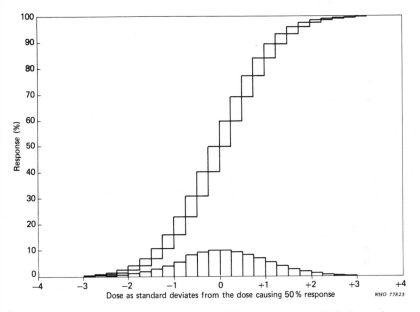

Fig. 1.1 A hypothetical dose-response relationship as a frequency distribution and as a cumulative frequency distribution.

Fig. 1.2 presents a distribution which is skewed towards the high-dose levels. This distribution is often described as log-normal because a logarithmic transformation of dose values results in a normal frequency distribution (Fig. 1.3). In nature, many frequency distributions are log normal in shape. This shape is also observed in distributions where the central point is near zero; since the dose level cannot be less than zero, there is only a narrow range in which the more susceptible responders will cluster. The logarithmic scale expands the zero point towards negative infinity, thus producing a more symmetrical distribution around the central point. In

49

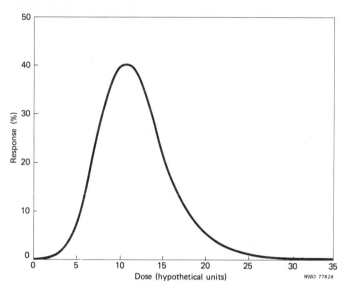

Fig. 1.2   Skewed frequency distribution for hypothetical data.

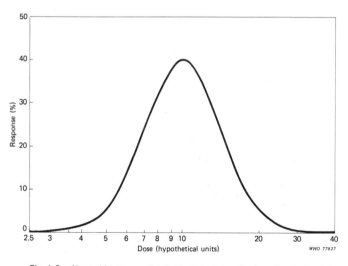

Fig. 1.3   Normal frequency distribution when dose is plotted on log scale.

addition to normal and log-normal distributions, there are various other types of skewed distributions.

The mathematical equation for the S-shaped curve is difficult to handle and it is therefore often transformed into a straight line for the presentation and evaluation of data. It is a mathematical characteristic of the normal distribution that the points of inflection of the curve on either side of the peak (or mean value) are at values equal to plus and minus one standard deviation (S.D.) from the mean (*m*). The integration of the normal distribution function shows that the area under the curve from *m* − 1 S.D. to *m* + 1 S.D. includes 68.3% of all members of the population. Thus 15.9% of the population will be responders at doses equal to or less than the mean minus 1 S.D., and 84.1% will be responders at doses equal to or less than the mean plus 1 S.D. It may also be calculated that approximately 95.4% of the population will respond within a dose range given by the mean ± 2 S.D., and approximately 99.9% will respond between the mean ± 3 S.D.

Since *m* − 3 S.D., *m* − 2 S.D., *m* − 1 S.D., *m*, *m* + 1 S.D., *m* + 2 S.D., and *m* + 3 S.D. indicate equal dose intervals, the corresponding percentage of responders, i.e. 0.1, 2.3, 15.9, 50, 84.1, 97.7, and 99.9 respectively, will give a straight line when these percentages are plotted at equidistant intervals. Fig. 1.4 illustrates this transformation; both the percent scale and the commonly used "probit" scale are presented. Finney (1971) has presented the history of the development and the utility of probit transformation[a]. Many toxicologists use log-probability graph paper to

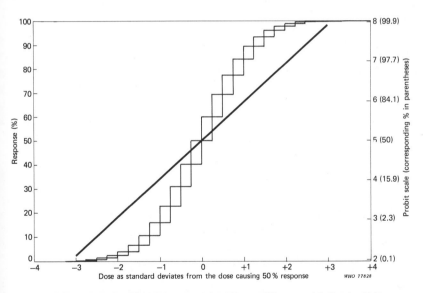

Fig. 1.4   Transformation of the normal sigmoid curve (%) to a straight line (probit).

---

[a] "Probit" = probability unit. Probit is the "standard deviate" or the "normal equivalent deviate" (NED) increased by 5. The NED is defined as the abscissa corresponding to a probability *P* in a normal distribution with mean 0 and standard deviation 1.

express dose-response relationships as a linear function for log-normal distributions of an effect.

Fig. 1.5 shows two dose-response curves on the log-probability graph paper. The ED_{50} (50% effective dose) value for chemical A is 10 dose units, while that for chemical B is 0.01 dose units. ED_{50} data are sometimes presented in the literature as a single dose value, without providing confidence limits or the slope of the dose response curve. It is clear in Fig. 1.5 that for chemicals A and B, not only are the ED_{50} values three orders of magnitude apart but the test systems respond in a very different manner.

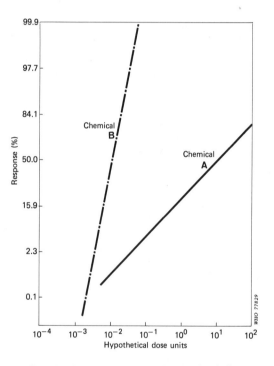

Fig. 1.5   Dose-response curves for two chemicals.

As an example of the necessity for taking into account the slopes, the practice of some toxicologists to study the effects of repeated doses at $\frac{1}{10}$ of the single dose ED_{50} can be considered. For chemical A an effect would already be seen in 16% of the population (ED_{16}) after the first of the repeated doses, while for chemical B it is quite probable that an effect will never be seen even after many repeated doses (Fig. 1.5). This is predictable, if the slopes of the dose-response curves are known.

Flat slopes, as for chemical A, are often indicative of such factors as poor absorption, rapid excretion or detoxication, or of toxic effects that become manifest some time after administration. Steep slopes, as for chemical B, most frequently indicate rapid absorption and rapid onset of toxic effects, as for example with hydrogen cyanide or irritant gases. While slope is not an absolutely reliable indicator of physiological or toxicological mechanisms, it is useful to the experienced toxicologist, and should always be reported along with its confidence limits.

Fig. 1.6 illustrates the importance of parallelism of dose-response curves for making any general statements about relative effects. Chemicals C and D have identical ED_{50} values. However, any statement about the relative equality of effect would only be true at that particular dose. In fact, at higher doses, chemical C would be more effective than D, and at lower doses, chemical D would be more effective. Chemicals E and F, on the other hand, show relative equi-effects in the ratio of 1 to 10 dose units over the entire dose range. This parallelism of dose-response curves is essential for

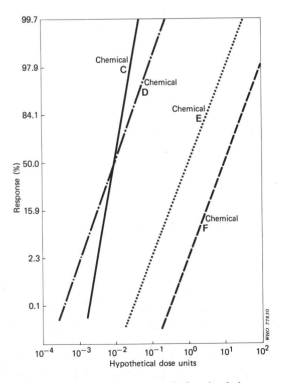

Fig. 1.6   Dose-response curves for four chemicals.

the validity of general statements about relative toxicities. Special note should be made, however, that the curves for chemicals E and F apply only to one specific effect and one set of experimental conditions. Observations of response for a different toxic effect, or administration by a different route or to a different species may not produce parallel dose-response curves for the same chemicals.

REFERENCES

ALBERT, R. E. & ALTSCHULER, B. (1973) Considerations relating to the formulation of limits for unavoidable population exposures to environmental carcinogens. In: Ballon, J. E., ed. *Radionuclide carcinogenesis*, Springfield, Va, NIIS, pp. 233–253 (AEC Symposium Series CONF-72050).

ALBERT, R. E. & ALTSCHULER, B. (1976) Assessment of risks in terms of life shortening, *Environ. Health Perspect.*, **13:** 91–94.

ANDREYESHCHEVA, N. G (1976) Predicting biological effect as a function of the chemical structure and the primary physical and chemical properties of organic compounds. *Environ. Health Perspect.*, **13:** 27–30.

ARIËNS, E. J., VAN ROSSUM, J. M., & SIMONIS, A. M. (1957) Affinity, intrinsic activity and drug interactions. *Pharmacol. Rev.*, **9:** 218–236.

BALL, W. L. (1959) The investigation of present-time definitions and conceptions of maximum allowable concentrations in different countries. *Pr. Lék.*, **11** (3): 127–128.

BEIR (1972) *The effects of population exposure to low levels of ionizing radiations—Report of the Advisory Committee on the Biological Effects of Ionizing Radiation.* Washington, DC, National Academy of Sciences—National Research Council, 217 pp. (Govt. Printing Office Publication 0-489-797).

BERNARD, C. (1898) [*Introduction to the study of experimental medicine.*] Paris, Librairie Delagrave (in French).

BINGHAM, E. & FALK, H. L. (1959) Environmental carcinogens—the modifying effect of co-carcinogens on the threshold response. *Arch. environ. Health,* **19:** 779–783.

BLUM, H. F. (1959) *Carcinogenesis by ultraviolet light.* Princeton, NJ, Princeton University Press.

BROWN, B. M. & PAPWORTH, D. S. (1974) Environmental chemical hazards to wildlife. In: Boyland, E. & Goulding, R., ed. *Modern trends in toxicology,* London, Butterworths, Vol. 2, ch. 3, pp. 70–85.

CASARETT, L. J. (1975) Toxicologic evaluation. In: Casarett, L. J. & Doull, J., ed. *Toxicology, the basic science of poisons.* New York, Macmillan Publishing Co. Inc.

CHAND, N. & HOEL, D. G. (1974) A comparison of models for determining safe levels of environmental agents. In: Proschan & Sefling, ed. *Reliability and biometry,* Philadelphia, SIAM, pp. 382–401.

CLARK, A. J. (1933) *Mode of action of drugs on cells.* Baltimore, Williams & Wilkins.

COHEN, J. M. & PINKERTON, C. (1966) Widespread translation of pesticides by air transport and rain-out. In: Gould, R. F., ed. *Organic pesticides in the environment,* American Chemical Society, pp. 163–176 (Advances in Chemistry Series, vol. 60).

COON, J. (1973) Toxicology of naturally-occurring chemicals: a perspective. In: *Toxicants occurring naturally in foods* (2nd ed.). Washington, DC, National Academy of Sciences.

CORNFIELD, J. (1954) Measurement and comparison of toxicities: the quantal response. In: Kempthorne, O., Bancroft, T. A., Gowen, J. W., & Lush, J. L., ed. *Statistics and mathematics in biology,* Ames, The Iowa State College Press, pp. 327–344.

CRANSTON, M. (1973) *What are human rights?* New York, Taplinger Pub. Co. Inc., p. 111.

CURRY, S. H. (1970) Theoretical changes in drug distribution resulting from changes in binding to plasma proteins and to tissues. *Pharm. Pharmacol.*, **22:** 753–758.

CUTHBERT, J. W. (1974) Industrial toxicology. In: Boyland, E. & Goulding, R., ed. *Modern trends in toxicology.* London, Butterworths, pp. 86–115.

DAY, T. D. (1967) Carcinogenic action of cigarette smoke condensate on mouse skin. *Br. J. Cancer,* **21:** 56–81.

DINMAN, B. D. (1972) "Non-concept" of "no-threshold" chemicals in the environment. *Environ. Sci.*, **175** (4021): 495–497.

DOLL, R. (1967) *Prevention of cancer: pointers from epidemiology.* London, Nuffield Provincial Hospital Trust.

DRUCKREY, H. (1967) Qualitative aspects of chemical carcinogenesis. In: Truhaut, R., ed. *Potential carcinogenic hazards from drugs, evaluation of risks,* New York, Springer-Verlag, pp. 60–78. (UICC Monograph Series, Vol. 7.)

ECOBICHON, D. J. & CORMEAU, A. M. (1973) Pseudocholinesterases of mammalian plasma: physiochemical properties and organophosphate inhibition in 11 species. *Toxicol. appl. Pharmacol.,* **24:** 92–100.

EDWARDS, C. A. (1970) *Persistent pesticides in the environment.* Cleveland, Ohio, CRC Press.

ELIZAROVA, O. N. (1962) In: *Opredelenie porogovyh doz promyšlennyh jadov pri peroral'nom vvedeni,* Moscow, Medicina, pp. 107–108 (in Russian).

EPSTEIN, S. S. (1973) The Delaney amendment. *J. prev. Med.,* **2:** 140–149.

FALK, H. L. (1975) Consideration of risks versus benefits. *Environ. Health Perspect.,* **11:** 1–5.

FOOD & DRUG ADMINISTRATION (1970) Food and Drug Administration Advisory Committee on Protocols for Safety Evaluation: Panel on Carcinogenesis Report on Cancer Testing in the Safety Evaluation of Food Additives and Pesticides. *Toxicol. appl. Pharmacol.,* **20:** 419–438.

FINNEY, D. G. (1952a) *Statistical method in biological assay,* London, Charles Griffin Ltd, 661 pp.

FINNEY, D. G. (1952b) *Probit analysis* (2nd ed.). London, Cambridge University Press.

FINNEY, D. G. (1971) *Probit analysis* (3rd ed.). London, Cambridge University Press.

FLYNN, D. I., LYNCH, M., & ZANNONI, V. G. (1972) Species differences and drug metabolism. *Biochem. Pharmacol.,* **21:** 2577–2590.

FRIEDMAN, L. (1969) The role of the laboratory animal study of intermediate duration for the evaluation of safety. In: Symposium on the evaluation of the safety of food additives and chemical residues. *Toxicol. appl. Pharmacol.,* **16:** 498–506.

FUCHS, N. A. (1964) *The mechanics of aerosols,* Oxford, Pergamon Press, pp. 270–287.

GADDUM, J. H. (1957) Theories of drug antagonism. *Pharmacol. Rev.,* **9:** 211–217.

GAVRILESCU, N. & PETERS, R. A. (1931) Biochemical lesions in vitamin B deficiency. *Biochem. J.,* **25:** 1397–1409.

GOLDWATER, L. J. (1968) Toxicology. In: Sax, N. I., ed. *Dangerous properties of industrial materials,* New York, Amsterdam, London, Reinhold Book Corporation, pp. 1–23.

GOLUBEV, A. F., LJUBLINA, A. E., TOLOKOIČEY, N. A., & FILOV, V. A. (1973) In: *Količestvennaja toksikologija.* Leningrad, Medicina, p. 217 (in Russian).

GROSS, M. A., FITZHUGH, O. G., & MANTEL, N. (1970) Evaluation of safety of food additives: an illustration involving the influence of methyl salicylate on rat reproduction. *Biometrics,* **26:** 181–194.

HAMAKER, J. W., GORING, C. A. L., & YOUNGSON, C. R. (1966) Sorption and leaching of 4-amino-3,5,6-trichloropicolinic acid in soils. In: Gould, R. F., ed. *Organic pesticides in the environment,* American Chemical Society, pp. 23–37 (Advances in Chemistry Series, Vol. 60).

HATCH, T. F. (1968) Significant dimensions of the dose-response relationship. *Arch. environ. Health,* **16:** 571–578.

HATCH, T. F. & GROSS, P. (1964) *Pulmonary deposition of inhaled aerosols.* New York, Academic Press.

HERMAN, R. S. (1974) Induction of liver growth by xenobiotic compounds and other stimuli. *CRC crit. Rev. Toxicol.,* **3** (1): 97–158.

HEWLETT, P. S. & PLACKETT, R. L. (1961) Models for quantal responses to mixtures of two drugs. In: Jonge, H. de, ed. *Symposium on quantitative methods in pharmacology.* Amsterdam, North Holland Publishing Co., pp. 328–336.

HOEL, D. G., GAYLOR, D. W., KIRSCHSTEIN, R. L., SAFFIOTTI, U., & SCHNEIDERMAN, M. S. (1975) Estimation of risks of irreversible delayed toxicity. *J. Toxicol. environ. Health,* **1** (1): 133–151.

HUCKER, H. B. (1970) Species differences in drug metabolism. *Ann. Rev. Pharmacol.,* **10:** 99–118.

ICRP (1965) *Principles of environmental monitoring related to the handling of radioactive materials. Report of Committee IV of the International Commission on Radiological Protection.* London, Pergamon Press.

ICRP (1966) *The evaluation of risk from radiation, a report prepared for Committee I of the International Commission on Radiological Protection.* Oxford, London, Edinburgh, New York, Toronto, Paris, Braunschweig, Pergamon Press (ICRP Publication 8).

ICRP (1977) *Recommendations of the International Commission on Radiological Protection* (ICRP Publication 26 (in press)).

JANYŠEVA, H. JA (1972) [On the establishment of MPCs of benz(a)pyrene in the ambient air of built-up areas.] *Gig. i Sanit.,* No. 7, pp. 87–91 (in Russian).

JANYŠEVA, H. JA & ANTOMONOV, JU G. (1976) Predicting risk of tumour occurrence in terms of life-shortening. *Environ. Health Perspect.,* **13:** 95–100.

JONES, H. B. & GRENDON, A. (1975) Environmental factors in the origin of cancer and estimation of possible hazards to man. *Food cosmet. Toxicol.,* **13:** 251–267.

KAGAN, Y. S. (1973) [Methods of quantitative estimation of combined and complex action on the organism of physical and chemical factors in the environment.] *Gig. i Sanit.,* No. 2, pp. 89–92 (in Russian).

KELLERMANN, G., SHAW, C. R., & LUYTEN-KELLERMANN, M. (1973) Aryl hydrocarbon hydroxylase inducibility and bronchogenic carcinoma. *New Engl. J. Med.,* **289:** 934–937.

KORBAKOVA, A. K., ŠUMSKAJA, N. I., ZAEVA, G. N., & NIKITENKO, T. K. (1971) In: *Naučnye osnovy sovremmenyh metodov gigieničeskogo normirovanija himičeskih veščest'v v okružajuščej srede.* Moscow, Institut gigieny truda i profzabolevanija AMN SSSR, pp. 35–39.

KRASOVSKIJ, G. N. (1965) [Methodology for conducting an acute experiment and for evaluating the results, and its basis.] In: *Sanitarnaja ohrana vodoemov ot zagrjaznenija promyšlennymi stočnymi vodami.* No. 7, 247–268 (in Russian).

KRASOVSKIJ, G. N. (1970) [On methods for studying the cumulative properties of toxic compounds.] *Gig. i Sanit.,* No. 3, pp. 83–88 (in Russian).

KRASOVSKIJ, G. N. (1975) Species and sex differences in sensitivity to toxic substances. In: *Methods used in the USSR for establishing biologically safe levels of toxic,* Geneva, WHO, pp. 109–125.

KRASOVSKIJ, G. N. (1976a) [General standardization of biological parameters for mammals according to body weight, and some practical aspects of investigations.] In: *Trudy MMI im Sečenova T.80—Novoe v metodah issledovannija, diagnostiki, lečenii i profilaktiki važneišíh zabolevanii.* Pp. 64–88 (in Russian).

KRASOVSKIJ, G. N. (1976b) Extrapolation of experimental data from animals to man. *Environ. Health Perspect.,* **13:** 51–58.

KUSTOV, V. V. & TIUNOV, L. A. (1970) [Enzyme system activity as a means of estimating thresholds of the effects of toxins.] In: *Metody opredelenija toksičinosti i opasnosti himičeskih veščestv.* Moscow, Medicina, pp. 231–234 (in Russian).

KUSTOV, V. V., ŽDANOV, A. M., & JUNOVSKIJ, G. D. (1974) [On the evaluation of the combined effect of factors by the method of partial regression.] *Gig. Tr. Prof. Zabol.,* **16:** 33–36 (in Russian).

LAZAREV, N. V. (1938). *Obščie osnovypromyšlennoj toksikologii.* Moscow & Leningrad, Medgiz.

LAZAREV, N. V. (1963) *Rukovodstvo po gigiena truda,* Moscow, Medgiz.

LAZAREV, N. V. & BRUSILOVSKAJA, A. I. (1934) *Fiziol. Ž. SSSR,* **XVII,** pp. 611–619 (in Russian).

LJUBLINA, E. I. & MIHEEV, M. I. (1974) [Scientific bases for establishing tentative safe levels of substances affecting man.] In: *Žurnal Vsesjuznogo Občestva im. D. I. Mendeleeva,* **XIX** (2): 142–145 (in Russian).

LOEWE, S. (1959) Relationships between stimulus and response. *Science,* **130:** 692–695.

LU, P. Y. & METCALF, R. (1975) Environmental fate and biodegradability of benzene derivatives as studied in a model aquatic ecosystem. *Environ. Health Perspect.,* **10:** 269–284.

MANTEL, N. & BRYAN, W. R. (1961) Safety testing of carcinogenic agents. *J. Natl Cancer Inst.*, 27: 455–470.

MANTEL, N. & SCHNEIDERMAN, M. (1975) Estimating "safe" levels, a hazardous undertaking. *Cancer Res.*, 35: 1379–1386.

MANTEL, N., BOHIDAR, N., BROWN, C., CIMINERA, J., & TUKEY, J. (1975) An improved "Mantel-Bryan" procedure for "safety" testing of carcinogens. *Cancer Res.*, 35: 865–872.

MAZZE, R. I., COUSINS, M. J., & KOSEK, J. C. (1973) Strain differences in metabolism and susceptibility to the nephrotoxic effects of methoxyflurane in rats. *J. Pharmacol. exp. Therapy*, 184: 481–488.

MEDVED, L. I. & SPYNU, E. I. (1970) [Principles and methods of hygienic standardization of pesticides. In: *Principles and methods of establishing maximum permissible concentrations of harmful substances in the air of production premises.*] Moscow, Medicina (in Russian).

METCALF, R. L., KAPOOR, I. P., LU, P. Y., SCHUTH, C. K., & SHERMAN, P. (1973) A model ecosystem for the evaluation of pesticide biodegradability and ecological magnification. *Environ. Sci. Technol.*, 5: 709–744.

MILLER, E. C., MILLER, J. A., & ENOMOTOR, M. (1964) The comparative carcinogenetics of 2-acetylaminofluorene and its N-hydroxy metabolite in mice, hamsters and guinea pigs. *Cancer Res.*, 24: 2018–2032.

MONTESANO, R., MOHR, U., & MAGEE, P. N. (1974) Additive effect in the induction of kidney tumours in rats treated with dimethylnitrosamine and ethylmethanesulfonate. *Br. J. Cancer*, 29: 50–58.

MURPHY, S. D. (1969) Some relationships between effects of insecticides and other stress conditions. *Ann. NY Acad. Sci.*, 160: 366–377.

NAS/NRC (1970) *Evaluating the safety of food chemicals.* Food Protection Committee, Food and Nutrition Branch, Division of Biology and Agriculture, National Research Council, Washington DC, National Academy of Sciences. 55 pp.

NAS (1975) *Principles for evaluating chemicals in the environment—A report of the Committee for the Working Conference on Principles of Protocols for Evaluating Chemicals in the Environment.* Washington, DC, National Academy of Sciences.

NIEHS (1970) *Man's health and the environment, some research needs—Report of the Task Force on Research Planning in Environmental Health Science US Department of Health, Education and Welfare, Public Health Service, National Institutes of Health, National Institute of Environmental Health Sciences.* Washington, DC, US Govt Printing Office.

NIEHS (1977) *Human health and the environment, some research needs—Report of the Second Task Force for Research Planning in Environmental Health US Department of Health, Education and Welfare, Public Health Service, National Institutes of Health, National Institute of Environmental Health Sciences.* Washington, DC, US Govt Printing Office (DHEW Publication No. NIH77-1277).

OECD (1977) *The OECD programme on long range transport of air pollutants. Measurements and findings.* Paris, Organisation for Economic Co-operation and Development, 268 pp.

OWEN, D. B. (1955) *Handbook of statistical tables,* London, Paris, Pergamon Press, pp. 127–137.

PAGET, G. E. (1970) The design and interpretation of toxicity tests. In: Paget, G. E., ed. *Methods in toxicology,* Philadelphia, F. A. Davies, pp. 1–10.

PARKE, D. V. (1975) Induction of the drug-metabolizing enzymes. In: Parke, D. V., ed. *Enzyme induction,* London, Plenum Press, pp. 207–272.

PETERS, R. A. (1963) *Biochemical lesions and lethal synthesis.* Oxford, London, New York, Paris, Pergamon Press.

PETERS, R. A. (1967) The biochemical lesion in thiamine deficiency. In: Wolstenholme, G. E. W. & O'Connor, M., ed. *Thiamine deficiency, biochemical lesions and their significance,* London, J. & A. Churchill Ltd, pp. 1–8.

PETO, R. & LEE, P. N. (1973) Weibull distribution for continuous carcinogenesis experiments. *Biometrics*, 29: 457–470.

PETO, R., LEE, P. N., & PAIGE, W. S. (1972) Statistical analysis of the bioassay of continuous carcinogens. *Br. J. Cancer*, 26: 258–261.

PFITZER, E. A. (1976) General concepts and definitions for dose-response and dose-effect relationships of toxic metals. In: Nordberg, G., ed. *Effects and dose-response relationships of toxic metals*. Amsterdam, Oxford, New York, Elsevier Scientific Publishing Company.

PINIGIN, M. A. (1974) [Current problems of community toxicology in relation to chemical air pollution.] In: *Itogi nauki i tehniki. Serija farmakologija. Himioterapevtičeskie sredstva. Toksikologija. Problemy toksikologii.* Vol. 6, Moscow (in Russian).

POKROVSKIJ, A. A. (1973) [Biochemical approaches to the evaluation of toxic factors in the environment. In: *Documentation of the Conference on Methodological Approaches to the Study and Evaluation of Toxic Factors in the Environment.*] Moscow (in Russian).

PORTMAN, R. S., PLOWMAN, K. M., & CAMPBELL, T. C. (1970) On mechanisms affecting species susceptibility to aflatoxin. *Biochim. Biophys. Acta*, 208: 487–495.

PRAVDIN, N. S. (1934) *Rukovodstovo promyšlennoi toksikologii.* Moscow, Biologija i Medicina.

RALL, D. F. (1970) Animal models for pharmacological studies. In: *Proceedings of the Symposium on Animal Models for Biomedical Research III,* Washington, DC, National Academy of Sciences, pp. 125–146 (ISBN 0-309-01854-4).

ŠABAD, L. M., SANOCKIJ, I. V., ZAEVA, G. N., BUREVIČ, T. C., KACNELSON, B. A., JANYŠEVA, H. JA, & SUGAEVA, B. V. (1973) [On the possibility of establishing MPCs for benz(a)pyrene in the air of industrial premises.] *Gig. i Sanit.*, No. 4, pp. 78–81 (in Russian).

SAFFIOTTI, U. (1973) Comments on the scientific basis for the "Delaney Clause". *J. Prev. Med.*, 2: 125–132.

SANOCKIJ, I. V. (1962) [The calculation of a safety factor for experimentally based maximum permissible concentrations of industrial poisons. In: *Industrial toxicology and clinical aspects of occupational diseases of chemical etiology.*] Moscow, Medgiz (in Russian).

SANOCKIJ, I. V. (1970) In: Sanockij, I. V., ed. *Metody opredelenija toksičnosti i opasnosti himičeskih veščestv.* Moscow, Medicina, pp. 11–12 (in Russian).

SANOCKIJ, I. V. (1975a) Investigation of new substances: permissible limits and threshold of harmful action. In: *Methods used in the USSR for establishing biologically safe levels of toxic substances,* Geneva, WHO, pp. 9–18.

SANOCKIJ, I. V. (1975b) [*The threshold concept for the reactions of living systems to environmental influences and its consequences. Soviet-American Symposium, Tbilisi.*] Gidrometeoizdat, pp. 112–120 (in Russian).

SANOCKIJ, I. V. & SIDOROV, K. K. (1975) [The current status of the problem of safety factors in establishing the maximum permissible concentrations of substances in the components of the general environment.] *Gig. i Sanit.*, No. 7, pp. 93–96 (in Russian).

SATO, T. & MOROI, K. (1971) Species and age differences in the activity of isocarboxazid hydrolysing enzyme. *Arch. int. Pharmacodyn. Ther.*, 192: 128–134.

SCHILD, H. O., ARIENS, E. J., SIMONIS, A. M., DIKSTEIN, S., DE JONGH, S. E., HEWLETT, P. S., & PLACKETT, R. L. (1961) Section on mixtures of drugs. In: De Jonge, H. ed. *Quantitative methods in pharmacology, Proceedings of a Symposium held in Leyden on May 10–13, 1960,* Amsterdam, North Holland Publishing Company, pp. 282–334.

SCHNEIDERMAN, M. A. (1971) A method for determining the dose compatible with some "acceptable" level of risk. In: *Chemicals and the future of man—Hearings before the Sub-Committee on Executive Reorganization and Government Research of the Committee on Government Operations, US Senate, Ninety-Second Congress, First Session, 6 and 7 April 1971.* Washington, DC, US Govt Printing Office.

SCHNEIDERMAN, M. A. & MANTEL, N. (1973) The Delaney Clause and a scheme for rewarding good experimentation. *Prev. Med.*, 2: 165–170.

SIDORENKO, G. I. & PINIGIN, M. A. (1975) Establishment of safe levels of chemicals in communal hygiene: methodological approaches. In: *Methods used in the USSR for establishing biologically safe levels of toxic substances,* Geneva, WHO, pp. 126–138.

SIDORENKO, G. I. & PINIGIN, M. A. (1976) Concentration-time relationship for various regimens of inhalation of organic compounds. *Environ. Health Perspect.,* **13:** 17–21.

SMYTH, H. F., JR (1963) Industrial hygiene in retrospect and prospect—toxicological aspects. *Am. Ind. Hyg. Assoc. J.,* **24:** 222–226.

SMYTH, H. F. JR, WEIL, C. S., WEST, J. S., & CARPENTER, C. P. (1969) An exploration of joint toxic action: twenty-seven industrial chemicals intubated in rats in all possible pairs. *Toxicol. appl. Pharmacol.,* **14:** 340–347.

SPYNU, E. I., VROČINSKIJ, K. K., ZOR'EVA, T. D., & MAL'KO, N. N. (1972) [Complex hygienic standardization of new organophosphorus pesticides in environmental components.] *Gig. i. Sanit.,* No. 11, pp. 96–99 (in Russian).

STOKINGER, H. E. (1972) Concepts of thresholds in standards setting. *Arch. environ. Health,* **25** (3): 153–157.

SYSIN, A. M., ed. (1941) [*Maximum allowable concentrations of toxic substances in water bodies.*] Moscow and Leningrad, Stroizdat (in Russian).

TASK GROUP ON METAL ACCUMULATION (1973) Accumulation of toxic metals with special reference to their absorption, excretion and biological half-time. *Environ. Physiol. Biochem.,* **3:** 65–107.

TASK GROUP ON METAL TOXICITY (1976) Consensus report for an international meeting organized by the Sub-committee on the Toxicology of Metals of the Permanent Commission and International Association on Occupational Health, Tokyo, 18–23 November 1974. In: Nordberg, G., ed. *Effects and dose-responses relationships of toxic metals,* Amsterdam, Oxford, New York, Elsevier Scientific Publishing Company, pp. 7–111.

ULANOVA, I. P. (1969) [Problems of hygienic standardization of mixtures of gases and vapours of chemical substances. In: *The toxicology of new industrial chemicals.*] Moscow, Medicina, pp. 33–39 (in Russian).

ULANOVA, I. P., AVILOVA, G. G., BAZAROVA, L. A., MAL'CEVA, N. M., MIGUKINA, N. V., HALEPO, A. I., & EITINGTON, A. I. (1973) [Experimental data on adaptation to poisons under different conditions of their action. Pharmacology, chemotherapeutic substances, toxicology.] *Itogi nauk i teh.,* No. 5, pp. 64–75 (in Russian).

ULANOVA, I. P., AVILOVA, G. G., MAL'CEVA, N. M., & HALEPO, A. I. (1976) [Comparisons of reactions of the organism to continuous and intermittent action of some chlorinated hydrocarbons.] *Gig. Tr. Profzabol.,* No. 7, pp. 22–25 (in Russian).

VAN NOORDWIJK, J. (1964) Communication between the experimental animal and the pharmacologist. *Stat. Neerl.,* **18** (4): 403–416.

VELDSTRA, H. (1956) Synergism and potentiation. *Pharmacol. Rev.,* **8:** 339–387.

VETTORAZZI, G. (1975) Toxicological decisions and recommendations resulting from the safety assessment of pesticide residues in food. *Crit. Rev. Toxicol.,* **4** (2): 125–183.

VETTORAZZI, G. (1977) Safety factors and their application in toxicological evaluation. In: Hunter, W. J. & Smeets, J. G. P. M., ed. *The evaluation of toxicological data for the protection of public health.* Oxford, Pergamon Press (for the Commission of the European Communities) pp. 207–223.

WEIL, C. S. (1972a) Statistics versus safety factors and scientific judgment in the evaluation of safety for man. *Toxicol. appl. Pharmacol.,* **21:** 454–463.

WEIL, C. S. (1972b) Guidelines for experiments to predict the degree of safety of a material for man. *Toxicol. appl. Pharmacol.,* **21:** 194–199.

WHO (1958) WHO Technical Report Series, No. 144 (Procedures for the testing of intentional food additives to establish their safety for use—Second Report of the Joint FAO/WHO Expert Committee on Food Additives.) 19 pp.

WHO (1973) WHO Technical Report Series, No. 535 (Environmental and health monitoring in occupational health—Report of a WHO Expert Committee.) 48 pp.

WHO (1974a) WHO Technical Report Series, No. 546 (Assessment of carcinogenicity and mutagenicity of chemicals—Report of a WHO Scientific Group.) 19 pp.

WHO (1974b) WHO Technical Report Series, No. 554 (Health aspects of environmental pollution: planning and implementation of national programmes—Report of a WHO Expert Committee.) 57 pp.

WHO (1975a) WHO Technical Report Series, No. 571 (Early detection of health impairment in occupational exposure to health hazards—Report of a WHO Study Group.) 80 pp.

WHO (1975b) WHO Technical Report Series, No. 560 (Chemical and biochemical methodology for the assessment of hazards of pesticides for man—Report of a WHO Scientific Group.) 26 pp.

WHO (1975c) *Methods for studying biological effects of pollutants (a review of methods used in the USSR). Report of a Working Group, Moscow, November 1974.* Copenhagen, WHO Regional Office for Europe.

WHO (1976a) WHO Technical Report Series No. 586 (Health hazards of new environmental pollutants—Report of a WHO Study Group.) 96 pp.

WHO (1976b) *Health aspects of human rights with special reference to developments in biology and medicine.* Geneva, World Health Organization, pp. 25–27.

WHO (1977) *Environmental Health Criteria 4: Oxides of nitrogen.* Geneva, WHO, 79 pp.

WILLIAMS, R. T. (1969) The fate of foreign compounds in man and animals. *Pure appl. Chem.,* **18:** 129–141.

WILLIAMS, R. T. (1972) Toxicological implications of biotransformation by intestinal microflora. *Toxicol. appl. Pharmacol.,* **23:** 769–781.

2. FACTORS INFLUENCING THE DESIGN OF TOXICITY STUDIES

2.1 Introduction

The choice and sequence of toxicity tests will depend on the questions or hypotheses that are developed. The nature and sequence of tests used to satisfy requirements of regulatory agencies may differ markedly from those used in an investigation of the basic mechanisms of toxic action. Differences in approach will also depend on whether the investigation is initiated to evaluate the toxicity of a chemical prior to its introduction into use, i.e. prospective toxicology, or to confirm in laboratory animals an epidemiological association that suggests chemical-induced disease in man, i.e. retrospective toxicology. Under ideal conditions, prospective toxicology will eliminate the need for retrospective toxicity evaluation.

National or international regulatory or advisory bodies have developed fairly specific guidelines or test protocols which are expected to be applied to the toxicity evaluation of certain groups of chemicals, introduced deliberately into our environment, e.g. food additives and pesticides (Council of Europe, 1973; FDA, 1959; WHO, 1967). The development of guidelines for the systematic evaluation of the toxicity of chemicals to which man is exposed, through his occupation or through incidental contamination of the ambient environment, is less common. Where specific guidelines have been formulated, they usually require: test information on acute toxicity in several species of experimental animals; some knowledge of the biochemical disposition of the compounds; various short-term toxicity tests; tests of the effects of the chemical on reproductive function; chronic toxicity tests in one or more species; special tests on organ function, clinical biochemistry and haematology, and other specific tests as determined by the particular type and intended uses of the chemical under consideration. Some commercial firms have developed their own guidelines for toxicity tests and their sequence in the premarket toxicological evaluation of products. Often the sequence of tests will have certain checkpoints at which decisions will be made as to whether continued development of the product (and more extensive toxicity testing) is warranted.

In this chapter, various topics will be discussed from the standpoint of the usefulness of certain types of information and the influence that various factors may have in designing protocols for the interpretation of data obtained in toxicity evaluation programmes.

2.2 Chemical and Physical Properties

2.2.1 General considerations

The late Horace Gerarde stated in an address that "toxicity is the capacity of a substance to cause injury. It is an inherent, unalterable molecular property which is dependent upon chemical structure. There is nothing we can do about the toxicity of a chemical except to know it"[a].

The nature or quality of the toxic action inherent in a chemical will depend to a large extent upon the functional group or groups present in the molecule. Knowledge of the reactions that these functional groups may undergo with reactive groups in critical endogenous biochemical constituents provides a means of predicting the nature of the toxic effects that may be expected. Smyth (1959) used the permanence of threshold limit values over a period of years as a criterion for evaluating various types of information used in setting safety limits for industrial chemicals. For a limited number of compounds, occupational threshold limit values (TLVs) had been established on the basis of analogy with better known substances and the permanence of these TLVs appeared to equal that of TLVs based upon data from experimental toxicity studies and from human experience. However, evaluation of toxicity by analogy with chemically-related substances contains considerable potential for error, and requires a great deal of toxicological information on very closely related chemical substances. Very minor changes in structure may be accompanied by profound changes in toxicity. The relationships between physicochemical characteristics and toxicity, including the biological activities of homologous series, have been reviewed by Ljublina & Filov (1975).

2.2.2 Physicochemical properties and the design of toxicity studies

Zbinden (1973) included fourteen chemical and physical variables in a check list of types of information useful in the toxicity evaluation of new drugs. Although some of these variables may be determined in the course of a toxicological evaluation, all of them apply equally as well to environmental chemicals as to therapeutic chemicals.

Knowledge of the chemical structure is essential for the preliminary prediction of the nature and site of toxic action, assuming, of course, that some prior knowledge of the toxicity of chemically-related compounds is available. It is also essential for developing extraction and assay procedures

---

[a] Presented at the Flavor Manufacturers' Association of the United States. Fall Symposium, 16 November 1972, Washington, DC.

for the determination of tissue concentrations and allows for logical estimates of the nature of metabolites that may be found. Indeed, without such knowledge, logical design of an experiment is impossible.

The stability of the chemical at various pH values and the photochemical properties are variables that must be considered as soon as a substance arrives for testing in the toxicology laboratory, as they may determine the manner in which the chemical should be stored prior to administration to test animals or indicate the stability of residues in tissue extracts. Many organic chemicals undergo photochemical reactions that lead to either more or less toxic products (Crosby, 1972) and organic esters are often readily hydrolysed under conditions encountered during their laboratory investigation (Eto, 1974). It may be necessary to exercise special precautions to avoid chemical reactions during the preparation and storage of test solutions or diets and during the analysis of tissues and metabolic reaction mixtures. Furthermore, if a chemical is likely to become activated by photochemical reactions, special tests for phototoxicity may be required.

The organic solvent/water partition coefficient and pK are physical properties of particular importance in the determination of the absorption and distribution of a compound in living organisms as well as in the development of appropriate extraction and assay procedures for the chemical. Hansch & Dunn (1972) reviewed numerous studies which suggest that characterization of the lipophilic nature of compounds may allow systematic predictions of their relative biological activities. Dillingham et al. (1973) applied these principles when they compared the toxicity of substituted alcohols in a tissue culture with their acute toxicity in mice and concluded that tissue culture test systems may be useful in determining predictive correlations between *in vivo* toxicity and the physicochemical properties of compounds.

The extent of ionization of an organic compound will influence its passage through lipoidal membranes (La Du et al., 1971). In general, the unionized lipid-soluble form of an organic compound will most readily pass through biological membranes. Although most of the physicochemical principles of absorption and distribution have been developed through systematic studies on medicinal chemicals, these principles also apply to organic chemicals in the environment and to the design of toxicity experiments (Loomis, 1974; also Chapter 4). Patty (1958) discussed the influence of oil and water solubility and of the coefficient of distribution of a vapour between blood and alveolar air on the rates of equilibrium saturation and desaturation of the body during inhalation experiments.

Particle size, shape, and density are of obvious importance in studying the inhalation toxicities of aerosols, as they are important factors in the determination of the site of deposition and the rates and mechanisms of clearance from the respiratory tract (Hatch & Gross, 1964; also Chapter 6). Furthermore, the particle size of substances given orally as suspensions can also markedly influence their toxicity (Boyd, 1971). If critical judgements based on the relative toxicities of the same or different substances, administered orally in suspension, are to be made, it is necessary to ensure uniformity of particle size.

Vapour pressure of a chemical substance is important in the practical consideration of the likelihood of exposure of man through inhalation, and the design of experimental inhalation toxicity studies will be influenced by the ease with which a solid or liquid vaporizes under controlled conditions. However, a high vapour pressure may produce technical problems if the objective of the test is to determine toxicity by the oral route of administration. Studies by Jones et al. (1971) showed that for a large series of food flavouring agents mixed in laboratory animal diets, the amount of loss from the diet was inversely related to the boiling points of the flavouring agents. Frequent chemical analyses of the diet, as well as frequent preparation of fresh diets and/or restricted feeding periods to limit the time for loss by vaporization are necessary to provide accurate estimates of intake in feeding studies on substances with low boiling points.

Knowledge of reactivity with, or binding to, macromolecules may allow specific design of mechanism experiments, when these macromolecules are essential tissue and cell constituents. Knowledge of the chemical reactivity of a substance may also be of considerable importance in the early planning of feeding studies, if the chemical under test is likely to react with the macromolecules present in the laboratory diet. On the one hand, chemical binding or adsorption on macromolecules in the diet may markedly alter the rate and extent of absorption of the test compound from the gastrointestinal tract; in some cases, biologically reactive groups on the test chemical may be neutralized by dietary constituents. On the other hand, reaction of the test chemical with essential dietary constituents may contribute to nutritional deficiency states, or new and more toxic compounds may be formed. Several examples of these types of reactions have been summarized by Golberg (1967).

2.2.3 Impurities

In the design of toxicity experiments, it is extremely important to consider the chemical purity of the sample to be tested. In certain cases, e.g. food additives and pesticides, the regulations will often provide specifications of purity for the compound in actual use and recommended test protocols may specify that toxicity evaluations are to be conducted with samples that meet these specifications (WHO, 1967). However, there is always the possibility that, when testing the technical product, the biological effects observed may be due to, or modified by, trace contaminants. If the contaminants are unknown or their biological activity unsuspected, toxicity tests may lead to erroneous conclusions concerning the primary chemical in question. In contrast, tests on highly purified samples may not detect the toxic action of contaminants present in samples used commercially. Furthermore, for many chemical substances used in manufacturing or incidentally released into the environment, specifications of purity may not be standardized. Therefore, one of the earliest and most difficult decisions that must be made in the design of a toxicity evaluation programme is the selection of the sample to be studied (technical grade, highly purified, etc.)

Requirements for the purity of the compounds selected for toxicological testing depend on the purpose of the testing as discussed in section 2.1. During the development of a new technological process, it may even be useful to test mixtures of unknown composition. The information so obtained may alert organic chemists in the research laboratory or pilot plant operators to the possible hazards of these unknown mixtures which may vary as procedures develop and improve. However, data obtained from such studies will have a limited value. The determination of health standards requires a compound of a high degree of purity or of highly standardized composition combined with a precise knowledge of various impurities. Only in this way will health standards have a universal value. However, for practical purposes, and for extrapolation to human exposure conditions it may be prudent, when a technical grade product standardized by specifications is used in commerce, to select this grade for toxicity testing and carefully characterize it with respect to the nature and amounts of any impurities present. Scheduled analytical spot checks during the course of the experiment to provide assurance of chemical constancy is also desirable.

When a chemical substance used in commerce is not standardized with respect to specifications for purity, experimental toxicity evaluation on a test sample of high purity would, indeed, seem to be the most rational selection. Data derived from this compound could then be used to characterize, toxicologically, the action of the primary chemical under consideration. When certain quantifiable indices of toxicity have been identified, selected tests with typical samples of commercial products could be conducted and the results compared with the purified product to detect possible differences. Of course, if the impurities represent a significant portion of the product, or if their chemical properties or their chemical analogy to other known substances suggest they may have serious toxic properties, the impurities must be evaluated separately.

An alternative approach is to select a sample of a chemical that most nearly represents the impure product used commercially, subject this to comprehensive toxicity evaluation and then make selected, critical toxicity comparison with purified samples of the primary chemical as well as with the impurities.

Either approach contains uncertainties, and little would be gained by short-term spot checks if the toxic action of the impurity were only detectable after long-term exposure or a latent period. It is in problem situations such as these that some of the chemicophysical principles discussed earlier must be applied at several levels of decision making: the sample to choose for testing; the design of the evaluation protocol; or the decision (or regulation) to produce a purer substance for routine use in commerce.

A recent, most controversial problem arising from the contamination of a primary commercial product involves the apparent teratogenic action of the herbicide (2,4,5-trichlorophenoxy)acetic acid (2,4,5-T) (Panel on Herbicides 1971). It is now known that the first studies to reveal this action were conducted with a sample of the herbicide that contained a rather high concentration (about 30 mg/kg) of the contaminant 2,3,7,8-tetrachloro-dibenzo-4-dioxin which is formed during the synthesis of the trichloro-phenol precursor. Tetrachlorodioxin is extremely toxic. For guineapigs, the ratio of the LD_{50} for 2,4,5-T to the LD_{50} of the dioxin is about 630 000. In female rats, the acute oral LD_{50} for dioxin is about 1/10 000 of the oral LD_{50} for 2,4,5-T. The daily dose of dioxin in pregnant rats that produced fetal toxicity was only about one four-hundredth of the maternal LD_{50} of dioxin or about one four-millionth of the single-dose oral LD_{50} of 2,4,5-T for female rats. Thus, even if the concentration of dioxin as a contaminant of 2,4,5-T is kept below 0.5 mg/kg, the major concern for the toxicity of 2,4,5-T should apparently still be directed towards the contaminant rather than towards the herbicide itself (at least insofar as effects on reproduction are concerned).

This kind of problem is not new. Twenty-five years ago, marked differences in the toxicity of different samples of the insecticide parathion were traced to contamination with small quantities of the oxygen analogue and the phosphorothiolate isomer, which are much more potent anticholi-nesterases and more acutely toxic than the parent insecticide (Diggle & Gage, 1951).

2.3 Probable Routes of Exposure

2.3.1 General considerations •

Many chemicals will become distributed in various environmental media or will be used for different purposes, and substantially different populations may be at risk. Thus, it may be necessary to obtain extensive test data by different routes of exposure. The choice of route for practical purposes is generally dictated by: (a) the likely route by which man will be exposed; and (b) whether the chemical will produce local injury at the site of exposure. The second question will often be resolved by acute or short-term studies on animals dosed by oral, inhalation, dermal, and possibly ocular routes. Details of test procedures are included in subsequent chapters. Although it is usually wise to conduct experiments using the route through which man will be exposed, other more convenient routes may be chosen for many of the tests if it is determined that the major toxic effects of a chemical are systemic, occurring only after absorption and distribution in the body. Data on blood and tissue levels should be obtained by several routes of exposure including those that are considered primarily experimental; with this information, it may be possible to relate toxic effects to blood or tissue concentrations of the test chemical and its metabolites. Such information greatly facilitates comparison of experiments using different routes and may either confirm or deny the validity of extrapolating data, obtained experimentally by one route, to the evaluation of potential toxicity by another perhaps more realistic route of exposure.

2.3.2 Specific variables related to route of exposure

2.3.2.1 *Rate of absorption*

As a general rule, one can predict that for the usual routes by which man may be exposed, absorption of chemicals will be most rapid when given by inhalation, less rapid when given by gavage, and slowest with dermal application. This order may, however, be modified depending upon various physicochemical properties of the substance under test in relation to the microenvironment of the absorbing surface (Klassen, 1975; Loomis, 1974). The rate of absorption will be one determinant of the rate of onset of signs of acute poisoning. If the rates of detoxification and excretion or of injury repair exceed the limiting rate at which a chemical is absorbed, it is possible that toxic signs observed by one route of administration will not be detectable by another route for which absorption is slower (Casarett, 1975; Murphy, 1975). Comparative absorption-distribution kinetics by different routes would determine such a possibility.

2.3.2.2 *Site of action*

Specific tests should be conducted to evaluate effects related to local reactions with specific receptors present in the organ of absorption. These may be morphological tests to detect evidence of irritation, inflammation, or oedema, or they may be functional to detect biochemical or reflex action or bronchoconstriction. In addition, the route of exposure may determine the organ or physiological system in which effects will be first observed or detected at lowest doses. For example, pesticides, which are direct inhibitors of acetylcholinesterase, when given in sufficient doses by any route, will produce a characteristic toxic syndrome involving essentially all organs or structures innervated by cholinergic nerves. However, at low doses, only specific organs may be involved. If such compounds are applied to the skin, local sweating and fasciculations may occur in the absence of signs of systemic poisoning. Exposure by inhalation may result in bronchoconstriction, exposure by ingestion may cause gastrointestinal upset before, or at lower doses than, generalized systemic effects (Henderson & Haggard, 1943; Holmstedt, 1959).

2.3.2.3 *Biotransformation*

The route of exposure may determine the likelihood and type of biotransformation before the chemical contacts the specific sites of action. Thus, when chemicals are administered by the oral (or intraperitoneal) routes, they will be absorbed and transported first through the portal circulation to the liver (Lukas et al., 1971). For example, if, with low oral or dietary doses, the capacity of the liver to detoxify the compounds exceeds the rate of absorption, an effective injurious concentration may never reach critical sites of action in other tissues. Absorption of the same quantity through the lung or skin, which generally have less detoxifying capacities, may result in toxic action. It is now known that the lung, skin, and intestinal mucosa, although generally less active than the liver, also have the capacity for biotransformation of foreign organic chemicals (Alvares et al., 1973; Fouts, 1972; Lake et al., 1973; Wattenberg, 1972). Although knowledge is incomplete with regard to the tissue distribution of both activating and detoxifying enzyme systems, it is likely that their relative distribution will determine, to some extent, the specific tissues that will be most affected by low doses of some compounds, when given by different routes of exposure.

2.3.2.4 *Species*

The relative susceptibility of different species to the action of chemicals may differ depending upon the route of exposure. When administering compounds by the oral route, such factors as vomiting reflex (absent in rats) and/or differences in type and distribution of microflora that may detoxify (or activate) the test compound can influence the interpretation of the results (Williams, 1972). The rates of penetration of compounds through the skin and the acute dermal toxicities of various compounds differ markedly among species and not always in a predictable manner (McCreesh, 1965).

Many of the problems encountered in dermal toxicity testing and suggestions for further research have been discussed by Barnes (1968). Roe (1968) discussed various problems encountered in the design and interpretation of inhalation toxicity studies related to species differences in the anatomy of the respiratory tree. Enzootic lung infections are an additional problem in the use of some species of animals for long-term inhalation studies.

2.3.2.5 *Unintended route*

Interpretation of results and measurement of actual dose-response relationships can be made difficult, because appreciable oral ingestion may occur with inhalation or dermal exposures. Animals exposed by either of these routes may ingest the material as a result of preening, unless dermal applications are covered or made inaccessible to licking or unless special exposure chambers (e.g. head only) are used for inhalation exposures (see Chapter 6). In addition, in particle inhalation experiments, the physiological protective mechanisms of clearance by mucous transport of the particles out of the respiratory tree (Hatch & Gross, 1964) with subsequent swallowing may result in gastrointestinal exposure. Some degree of lung exposure to volatile compounds administered in the diet or by dermal application is also likely.

2.3.3 Special tests related to route

When exposure to a compound is most likely to occur by inhalation, it is useful to know the effect of variations in ventilation rates, since this will be a common variable among an exposed human population under different conditions of activity. This may be accomplished by the use of exercise wheels or treadmills.

When dermal exposure is the likely route, it will be useful to conduct some tests to determine the effect of different solvents on penetration of the test compound through the skin. Studies of the influence of factors such as sweating, abrasions, or the presence of detergents on dermal absorption and toxicity will also aid in estimating toxicities under conditions likely to be experienced by man (see Chapter 11, Part 2).

Interpretation and implications of toxicity data obtained with oral exposures can be enhanced by examination of the influence of fasting, dietary variations, and, particularly, administration by gavage versus inclusion in the diet or drinking water. These factors are discussed in more detail in subsequent chapters, but it should be stressed that quite different results and interpretations may ensue if the same daily dose is given rapidly by gavage or gradually in the diet. Interpretation of such experiments is greatly aided, if the design includes comparative absorption and distribution kinetics.

2.4 Selection and Care of Animals

2.4.1 General considerations

The selection and care of laboratory animals to be used in toxicity tests is especially important in determining the success of the experiment itself, the extrapolation of the data to man, and the cost of the evaluation programme. In order to provide data on a sufficient number of animals for valid statistical analyses, it has become common practice to use small laboratory rodents for most large-scale toxicity test programmes. Dogs or nonhuman primates are frequently included in some of the studies, and studies on at least one nonrodent species are often required by the test protocols recommended by regulatory and advisory agencies. Recommendations (with appropriate references for detailed information) concerning the selection and care of laboratory animals to be used in the usual broad scale toxicity evaluation studies are included in Chapter 3. The selection of animals to be used in various special test procedures is discussed in subsequent chapters.

Animals and animal care practices should be selected to provide a scientifically sound and reproducible experiment; however, some of the variables that contribute to nonuniformity may actually be exploited, in special studies, to obtain data that may be useful in extrapolation to nonuniform human populations. For example, if the inherent toxicity of an air pollutant is to be characterized, the occurrence of chronic lung infections should be avoided. On the other hand, specially designed experiments to test the influence of air pollutants on the susceptibility of animals to lung infections have provided a sensitive procedure for measuring the adverse effects of air pollutants on the physiological protective mechanisms that confer resistance to respiratory infections (Ehrlich, 1966). Epidemiologists could certainly use such information in the design of studies on human populations exposed to air pollutants and to infectious microorganisms present in the environment.

The choice of animals and the environment in which they are used in toxicity studies will ultimately be determined (as for any other decisions relating to experimental design) by the nature of the questions asked or the hypotheses formulated. Controlled introduction of additional variables may be desired for special studies. The important principle is that appropriate control conditions should be included in such studies to allow comparisons with results obtained under more conventional procedures.

2.4.2 Animal variables

The objective of most experimental toxicity studies is to predict the adverse effects of chemicals in man. Therefore, in addition to uniformity of response, the guiding principle for the selection of appropriate test species is that the test animals should resemble man as closely as possible with respect to absorption, distribution, metabolic transformation, excretion, and effect at site(s) of action of chemicals. Both male and female animals should be tested and the test protocol should encompass exposures of animals at both ends of the age spectrum (see Chapter 3).

It is generally recommended that random-bred rather than highly inbred strains of animals be used in broad-scale toxicity testing, at least until the action of the chemical is well characterized (Food & Drug Administration, 1970). In more specialized toxicity tests, it may be desirable to use inbred strains, for example, when animal models are needed that represent a genetic variation in human population, or when hypotheses on the mechanism of action are tested.

2.4.2.1 *Selection of species*

The Food Protection Committee (1970) indicated that sensitivity, convenience, and similarity in metabolism to man are the prime factors to be considered in the selection of animal species for toxicity testing. In the absence of information to the contrary, it is generally recommended that data obtained from the most sensitive species should be used as the basis for the extrapolation of test information to man.

There is now ample evidence of wide quantitative variations among species in their rates of biotransformation of foreign compounds (Committee on Problems of Drug Safety, 1969; Parke & Williams, 1969; Williams, 1967). Since many organic chemicals are subject to biotransformation at several reactive groups in the molecule, it is important to identify and quantify the biotransformation and distribution pathways of a chemical in man and in several laboratory animal species as early as possible in toxicity evaluation studies. It seems axiomatic that for costly chronic studies on experimental animals, the species that is most representative of man with respect to the metabolism of the test chemical should be chosen. Often, the only information concerning the metabolism and distribution of the test compound in man may be derived from limited studies on individuals accidentally or occupationally exposed to uncontrolled or unknown doses.

In vitro studies of metabolism using animal tissues and human tissues obtained at autopsy or biopsy could help in comparisons of similarities or differences in metabolism between man and laboratory animals. Although this approach cannot, in itself, provide information that may be obtained in studies on intact animals, it can, coupled with knowledge of the physicochemical properties of the compound and the kinetics of enzymatic biotransformation reactions in tissues of various species, provide a logical basis for selection of species for long-term toxicity tests. Decisions based on comparative human and experimental animal metabolism data should take into account information concerning several pathways of metabolism. This will help to ensure the inclusion of data on quantitatively minor pathways of metabolism that may result in products of major toxicological importance. These considerations of variation in biotransformation can also be applied to intraspecies variations related to age, sex, and strain (Benke & Murphy, 1973; Jori et al., 1971a; MacLeod et al., 1972; Parke & Williams, 1969).

Anatomical and morphological variations can also determine the selection of species. This source of variation is likely to be of particular importance in inhalation toxicity studies (Roe, 1968). Tyler & Gillespie (1969) compared anatomical characteristics of the lungs of human beings with several laboratory and domestic animal species when considering appropriate animal models for human emphysema. They grouped anatomically similar species into four classes: (a) cattle, sheep, and swine; (b) dogs, cats, and rhesus monkeys; (c) rabbits, rats, and guineapigs; and (d) horses and man. From their studies on horses, they concluded that the pathophysiology and the morphological characteristics of emphysema in horses closely resembled the disease in man and that the horse could be a particularly suitable laboratory animal for studies of this disease. Obviously, in the usual toxicity studies on air pollutants, the costs of using horses would be prohibitive. The reactivity of a chemical at primary target sites must also be considered as a potential variable contributing to species differences in toxicity. The acute toxicity of certain organophosphorous insecticides in representative mammalian, avian, and fish species appeared to be more readily related to species differences in the reactivity of the target enzyme (acetylcholinesterase (3.1.1.7)) than to differences in hepatic biotransformation rates (Murphy et al., 1968).

In the absence of specific knowledge of comparative metabolism and sites of action, it is appropriate to apply the principle that quantitative and qualitative similarity of response in several mammalian laboratory species enhances the confidence that man will respond similarly. Tests on several species seem equally as useful for predicting effects in a heterogenous human population as the selection of test species based on the results of limited studies of metabolism in a very few individual human subjects, who may or may not be representative of a broad cross-section of the human population at risk. Of course, any quantitative information on the disposition and action of chemicals in man is useful, as it adds to the accumulation of knowledge from which more specific guidelines for species selection may be derived in the future.

2.4.2.2   Animal models representing special populations at risk

Because many chemicals in the environment are widely dispersed, all segments of the human population may sustain some exposure. For this reason, it may be useful to design special experiments to evaluate toxicity in animal models that represent potentially hypersusceptible segments of the human population. The very young and the aged represent such segments generally, because in the very young, natural protective mechanisms such as metabolic detoxification systems may be incompletely developed and in the aged, cell repair processes may be less active than in younger individuals. Evaluation of the toxicity of chemicals in animal models of commonly occurring human diseases may be of value. Thus, for example, epidemiological studies suggest that individuals suffering from coronary artery disease may be particularly susceptible to carbon monoxide, the severity of signs and symptoms in patients suffering from cardiorespiratory disease appears to be aggravated by air pollution, and asthmatic patients appear to have a higher frequency of attacks during periods of high oxidant air pollution (Heimann, 1967). Few attempts have been made to evaluate experimentally the interactions between exposure to toxic chemicals and model disease conditions. Taylor & Drew (1975) reported that an inbred strain of cardiomyopathic hamsters was more susceptible to acute toxicity and cardiac arrhythmias produced by inhaled trichlorofluoromethane than were random-bred hamsters that were not cardiomyopathic. Easton & Murphy (1967) suggested that their observation of greater mortality and respiratory distress in ozone-preexposed than in air-exposed guineapigs given histamine injections or inhalation exposures might be analogous to the apparent increase in frequency and severity of asthmatic attacks reported for peak periods of photochemical air pollution.

Problems of standardization of disease conditions add another dimension to toxicity studies. However, it seems that animal disease models should be given more consideration in toxicity evaluations that are intended to provide the basis for the safe use of chemicals to which large human populations are exposed. Jones (1969) summarized reference sources for animal models of a large number of specific human diseases. Several papers in a series of symposia proceedings published by the US National Academy of Sciences provide discussion and references to (among other topics) animal models for commonly occurring disease states of the lungs (Tyler & Gillespie, 1969), the cerebrovascular system (Luginbuhl & Detweiler, 1968), the heart (Jobe, 1968), the kidney (Lerner & Dixon, 1968), atherosclerosis (Clarkson et al., 1970), diabetes (Hackel et al., 1968), and chronic degenerative diseases (Abinanti, 1971). Since gut microflora are changed in certain gastrointestinal diseases in man, modifications of the quality and distribution of microflora in experimental animals might be a useful model for special tests

(Williams, 1972). There are at least three possible applications of these disease models to toxicity studies: (*a*) evaluation of the susceptibility of diseased tissues to chemicals known to exert their action on that tissue; (*b*) influence of the disease state on the metabolism and distribution of chemicals that may act on the diseased tissue or at other sites; and (*c*) research on the mechanism of action of toxic chemicals using specific modification of receptor function or biochemistry.

2.4.3 Cyclic variations in function or response

Many physiological variables undergo cyclic peaks and troughs of activity (Altman & Dittmer, 1966) some of which are diurnal (24-h) and others of longer duration. These rhythms may be completely under intrinsic control or they may be partly or largely regulated by environmental variables such as light and temperature. Boyd (1972) considers most diurnal variations in susceptibility to drug toxicity to be mainly related to eating and sleeping habits. Since rats are nocturnal feeders, the greater quantity of food in the stomach early in the morning compared with the afternoon may alter the acute toxicity of chemicals given intragastrically. Attempts to standardize this variable have led to recommendations that acute toxicity tests by intragastric administration should be conducted on animals that have fasted overnight (Food & Drug Administration, 1959). Intragastric LD_{50} values are generally lower in rats fasted overnight compared with those fed *ad libitum*; however, the differences are usually only of the order of two- to three-fold (Boyd, 1972; Loomis, 1974). The influence of fasting may, in some cases, be related to rates of absorption from the gut in the presence or absence of food but this cannot account for all such variations. A striking example has been reported by Jaeger et al. (1975) in which acute toxicity and liver injury in rats exposed through inhalation to several halogenated olefins were enhanced 10- to 20-fold by overnight fasting. A diurnal cycle of susceptibility of rats to the toxicity of inhaled vinylidene chloride appeared to be related to the diurnal cycle of liver glutathione concentrations (Jaeger et al., 1973) which may be secondary to a diurnal cycle in feeding activities. The duration of pentobarbital anaesthesia in mice under usual laboratory housing conditions exhibited a diurnal cycle with the longest duration at 14h00 and the shortest (40–60% of that at 14h00) duration at 02h00 (Davis, 1962). The amplitude of the cycle was considerably reduced, when animals were caged individually as opposed to group caging, and constant light abolished the cycle. That circadian variation in the action of certain organic chemicals may be related to circadian variation in their biotransformation is suggested by the work of Jori et al. (1971b).

Beuthin & Bousquet (1970) reported seasonal or circannual rhythms for drug action and biotransformation rates in rats. The induction of increased drug metabolism by phenobarbital also exhibited a seasonal variation. Basal levels of hexobarbital metabolism were highest during the winter months and lowest in summer, whereas the opposite cycle for induction of hexobarbital oxidase by phenobarbital was observed. It should be noted that studies of seasonal variations in the metabolism or toxic action of chemicals must be carefully controlled with respect to environmental variables that might produce similar variations in response (see 2.4.4). Boyd (1972) suggests that seasonal variations in susceptibility may be related to the hibernation reaction or to weather conditions in the geographical area concerned.

Circadian variation in adrenocortical activity in rats was investigated by Szot & Murphy (1971) in animals exposed acutely or subacutely to the pesticides parathion and DDT. Although the degree of stimulation of corticosterone secretion after single doses of parathion varied depending upon the phase of the cycle at the time of administration, feeding parathion or DDT in the diet at rather high concentrations did not change the phase or the amplitude of the natural adrenocortical rhythm or alter the stimulation of corticosterone secretion produced by irritant stress.

In rodents, locomotor activity is greatest at night and Boyd (1972) suggests that depression of activity is best demonstrated at night or in rats starved for 3 days when their daytime activity is as great as at night time. However, a more convenient approach may be to reverse the lighting schedule, a procedure used successfully for measuring the effects of various inhaled air pollutants on locomotor activity in mice (Murphy, 1964).

The time of day at which biochemical or other tests are conducted in control and experimental animals may influence the reproducibility of the test data, if the biological variables under test display rhythmic variation. An investigator may exploit these rhythmic variations to advantage in special studies of factors that influence susceptibility to chemical injury. However, if the aim is a broad scale characterization of the toxicity of a chemical, the choice may be to carefully standardize times of administration of chemicals and of animal sampling to minimize both known and unrecognized circadian variations as much as possible.

2.4.4 Environmental variables

There are numerous possible variations in the environment in which experimental animals are housed or tested that can influence their response to toxic chemicals. General considerations of these variables are discussed by several authors (Boyd, 1972; Doull, 1972, 1975; Hurni, 1970; Morrison, 1968). Unless the purpose of the experiment is to use these variables to predict possible alterations in effects in man exposed to chemicals under similar environmental variations, it is generally possible to minimize their influence on the toxicity of chemicals by adopting good principles of animal care. Reference sources are available to provide guidelines for proper housing, diets, cage size requirements, etc. (DHEW, 1972; Universities Federation for Animal Welfare, 1972).

Only brief comments will be made on some of the major environmental variables that affect toxicity experiments or that can be used for predicting mechanisms or possible implications to man.

2.4.4.1 *Temperature*

Major variations from the recommended environmental temperatures and relative humidities can contribute not only to the impairment of general health and increased susceptibility to infection of the animals, but also to variation in their response to toxic chemicals.

The mechanisms of interactions between environmental and body temperatures and drugs or toxic agents have been reviewed by Doull (1972) and by Cremer & Bligh (1969). Since absorption, distribution, metabolic transformation, excretion, and reactivity with receptor sites depend on various temperature-dependent chemical reactions, it might be expected that the toxicity of chemicals would be readily influenced by temperature. However, since toxicity studies are usually conducted with homotherms, only minor changes in core body temperature occur with moderate changes in environmental temperatures. By the same token, changes in environmental temperature will elicit homeostatic changes in various physiological or biochemical systems. These may then alter some of the physiological variables (e.g. ventilation, circulation, body water, intermediary metabolism) that are rate-limiting determinants of the absorption, deposition, and action of toxic chemicals. Furthermore, toxic chemicals may exert their action by disruption of the thermoregulatory mechanism as suggested for cholinesterase inhibitors (Meeter & Wolthuis, 1968). Exposure to toxic chemicals can also mimic the actions of extremes in environmental temperature or other physical stressors (Murphy, 1969; Szot & Murphy, 1970). Thus, fluctuations in environmental temperatures can lead to functional changes that might be mistakenly attributed to the action of the chemical or they may actually alter the toxicity. If interference with physiological thermoregulatory mechanisms is a likely action of the chemical, careful control of environmental temperatures is necessary to ensure reproducibility of measurements of this action.

2.4.4.2 *Caging*

The type of cage, grouping, bedding, and other factors related to caging can markedly influence the toxicity of some chemicals and drugs (Boyd, 1972; Doull, 1972; Hurni, 1970). The acute toxicity of 4-[1-hydroxy-2-[(1-methylethyl)amino]ethyl]-1,2-benzenediol (isoproterenol) was markedly greater in rats caged singly for more than three weeks than in rats caged in groups (Hatch et al., 1965). Winter & Flataker (1962) reported that grouped rats held in "closed" (sheet metal on four sides and bottom) cages were more resistant to the acute toxicity of morphine and 1-[2-(4-amino-phenyl)ethyl]-4-phenyl-4-piperidine carboxylic acid ethyl ester (anileridine) than rats held in "open" (wire mesh) cages. These differences were attributed to mechanical factors that prevented depressed rats from maintaining an open airway in the wire mesh cages. Altered toxicity of chemicals related to caging effects are generally purely experimental variables and can be controlled by good practices of laboratory animal housing.

2.4.4.3 *Diet and nutritional status*

Dietary variables can influence the toxicity of chemicals in several ways. The toxicities of several pesticides were enhanced to different degrees in rats given low protein diets (Boyd, 1969). Protein-deficient diets protected rats against the acute hepatotoxicity of carbon tetrachloride and *N*-methyl-*N*-nitrosomethanamine (dimethylnitrosamine) (although the number of kidney tumours after a single dose of the latter increased), while the acute toxicity of chloroform was unchanged and the acute toxicity of aflatoxins was markedly enhanced (McLean & McLean, 1969). These effects could be explained, at least in part, by the reduction of activity of hepatic mixed-function oxidases that generally results from feeding low-protein diets. Whether or not a compound's toxicity is increased or decreased in such circumstances will depend upon whether microsomal biotransformation leads to the formation of more or less toxic metabolites. Numerous other examples of macro and micronutrient deficiencies, which alter the activity of the drug-metabolizing enzyme systems and the toxicity of chemicals, have been reviewed by Campbell & Hayes (1974). Intestinal and pulmonary aryl hydrocarbon hydroxylase activity is modified by diet. Of particular interest is the observation that changing rats from a commercial, natural diet to a balanced, purified diet resulted in an almost total loss of activity of this enzyme system in these tissues (Wattenberg, 1972). Flavonoid compounds, present as natural constituents of alfalfa meal (and other plants), may account for the apparent induction of aryl hydrocarbon hydroxylase by natural diets. The trace mineral content of diets can also influence the metabolism, distribution, and action of toxic chemicals (Moffitt & Murphy, 1974).

The results of toxicity experiments can be markedly influenced if care is not taken to ensure constancy of diets free from residues of contaminating chemicals. However, since nutritional imbalances are widespread in the human populations, controlled variation of experimental diets to simulate major human deficiency states (e.g. kwashiokor resulting from protein deficiency) is an important area for research in toxicology and should, perhaps, be included in standard toxicity evaluations of select groups of chemicals.

2.5 Statistical Considerations

Although various protocols for toxicity testing recommend specific numbers of animals to be used for various acute and chronic tests (see Chapter 3), a useful guiding principle is that sufficient animals should be used to allow statistically valid conclusions concerning differences in the response of test animals compared to controls and to provide a base for statistical extrapolations to larger population samples. Statistical procedures allow the experimenter to make (a) descriptions of sets of data or population characteristics, and (b) statements of probability of events. Various procedures provide for both enumerative data, or yes-no type characteristics, and measurement data, or graded effects or characteristics. Some procedures (t-test, F-test) are restricted to observations that have specific frequency distributions, while others (signed rank test, rank run test) are free of any assumptions about distribution (i.e. nonparametric). Standard texts should be consulted for the application of biostatistics to the design and analyses of experiments. In practice, it is highly advisable to involve a statistician in the experimental design as well as in the analysis.

The number of animals required to make statistically valid conclusions regarding the differences between experimental and control animals will depend upon the degree of confidence desired and the magnitude of the possible sources of variation in the experiment. The second consideration will depend upon the uniformity of the test animals with respect to the biological system or systems under test. This, in turn, will depend upon both genetic and environmental factors. The reproducibility of the bioassay and chemical procedures used in the tests will be another source of variation. A further source of variation in toxicity testing is related to the constancy and stability of the test chemical. Finally, there are the variables introduced by the investigators (often the most difficult to control), beginning with the care and attention given to accurate dosing throughout the various steps of the experiment. Attempts must be made to minimize all these sources of variation as far as possible, without sacrificing any important aspect of the experiment.

When testing whether or not two sets of data may both be valid samples from the same population with normal frequency distribution (i.e. null hypothesis) or whether the control group is not significantly different from the treatment group, statisticians describe the appropriate sample size in terms of the desired "power" of the test. Two types of decision errors exist. One is that a significant difference between groups is stated to exist when, in fact, there is no difference. This is called the type I error and the experimenter must state what probabilities (α) for this error he will accept; most commonly a probability of 0.05 is used, but an experimenter may sometimes require a probability as low as 0.01, or any other he chooses. The second type of decision error is that no significant difference between groups is stated to exist when, in fact, the groups are different. This is called the type II error, and $1-\beta$ (the probability that one will not make this error) is the power of the test. The power is directly related to the sample size and the ratio of "differences between true means of the samples" to "differences between experimental error of the means of the samples". Once this ratio is fixed, the power increases solely as a function of sample size. The experimental error (pooled variance) can be estimated from previous experiments or a pilot study. The acceptable magnitude of the differences between true means of the samples is at the discretion of the experimenter; he must use expert judgment and should have a reasonable rationale; it will usually be the smallest value that is considered to be of practical importance.

Another important statistical consideration is related to the selection of the valid number of sampling units. This may be particularly true in considering quantal (all-none, yes-no) effects that may be multiple occurrences within a single test animal, as, for example, in reproduction and carcinogenesis studies where, respectively, there may be a number of affected offspring or a number of tumours resulting from the treatment of a single animal. The selection of the appropriate unit, either the number of animals exposed or the number of occurrences of an effect, can determine the statistical significance of an observed effect. Weil (1970) suggests that in reproduction studies the number of maternal animals (or litters) and not the number of affected fetuses or offspring is the valid sampling unit, and that in carcinogenesis studies the number of tumour-bearing animals should be the sampling unit and not the total number of tumours. Furthermore, in carcinogenesis studies, animals risk death from factors other than the tumours; in some cases, animals may have died before they had time to develop a tumour; in other cases, information from some animals may be lost from the study because of unexpected death and autolysis of tissues preventing tumour identification. An adjusted tumour incidence may be estimated by the life-table techniques in such experiments (McKinney et al., 1968).

Another problem may be associated with gross or histopathological examination where, because of cost and time considerations, only tissues of a fraction of the total number of animals exposed are subjected to complete examination. This will reduce the likelihood that statistically valid conclusions can be drawn from the data on occurrence of lesions. In practice, reasonable compromises are usually necessary. Irrespective of the statistical methods of analysis used in both the design and interpretation of results of toxicity tests on chemicals, they cannot replace careful experimentation and comprehensive knowledge of the underlying biological mechanisms of the various steps between exposure to a chemical and injury.

2.6 Nature of Effects

2.6.1 Reversible and irreversible effects

Reversible effects are characterized by the fact that the deviation from normal structure or function induced by a chemical will return to within normal limits (controls) following cessation of exposure. With irreversible effects, the deviation persists or may progress, even after exposure ceases. This might be further qualified by time limits, that is, the time required for return to normality after exposure should be a reasonable fraction of the remaining lifetime of a young animal for it to be considered reversible. Reversibility may also be qualified by the normal lifetime of a specific cell or macromolecule that serves as the end-point for the effect. For example, cholinesterase-inhibiting insecticides are generally considered irreversible inhibitors if the rate of reversal of inhibition corresponds approximately to the time required for synthesis and replacement of the enzyme, a process with different rates in different tissues. Certain effects of toxic chemicals are unmistakably irreversible, including the production of terata, or malignant tumours, production of mutations in offspring of exposed animals, certain chronic neurological diseases, production of true cirrhosis, or emphysema. These are rather gross manifestations of certain specific chemical-cell interactions, and, either at the level of the first affected molecule or at intervening points leading to these manifestations, there are probably reversible effects. Understanding these effects and determining the critical dose that produces them will make it possible to predict truly adverse effects more rapidly.

The rate of reversibility of an effect will depend upon the rate of cellular injury and the rate at which this injury is repaired (Casarett, 1975). The rate of injury will depend upon the concentration and duration or frequency with which a test chemical contacts responsive tissue constituents. It is, thus, dose and dose-rate dependent. The rate of repair is determined intrinsically and may involve several cell processes. It may vary between different tissues and probably between different species and strains. From a practical standpoint, it is generally impossible to measure the specific processes involved in injury and repair in a standard toxicity evaluation study. However, it is important to make measurements of the reversibility of effects in early, acute and subacute studies. Thus, the time required for a process to return to normal after single doses (which produce various degrees of injury) will provide a guideline for the selection of doses to be used in subsequent acute or chronic studies. The predictive value of such information will depend upon the persistence of the chemical in the test organism. If the chemical produces an effect and then is rapidly detoxified or excreted, it may be possible to predict, with reasonable accuracy, doses or exposure schedules that would not produce cumulative effects. The manner of exposure and possible actions other than the one being measured would, of course, be important in drawing such conclusions. For example, rapid reversibility after a single dose might not be indicative of the rate of reversal with a repeated dosing if the first dose, in addition to the measured effect, also altered either the repair processes or the processes responsible for detoxification of the chemical. An example of an apparent self-inhibition of detoxification is the insecticide malathion which is rapidly hydrolysed by carboxylesterases. These are, in turn, inhibited by metabolites or contaminants of malathion (Murphy, 1967). Repeated exposure studies are necessary to evaluate such possibilities; thus, the design of short-term feeding or inhalation studies should include extra groups of animals that can be removed from exposure either at the end of the experiment or, preferably, at selected intervals for measurements of rate of reversal of any observed effect.

If the chemical persists or accumulates in the organism, measurements and interpretation of rates of reversal of effects are more complicated. For this reason, it is useful to have kinetic data on absorption and disposition to correspond with data on rates of production and reversal of effects. Further discussion of these and related principles is provided by Hayes (1972) in relation to his proposal that determination of "chronicity factors" (1-dose LD_{50} (mg/kg) $\div$ 90-dose LD_{50} (mg/kg/day) in diet i.e. the ratio of single dose LD_{50} to the daily dose given in diet for 90 days which results in 50% mortality at that time) is useful in predicting candidate chemicals requiring long-term studies. The use of such predictive methods must also take into consideration potential for other effects that could never be detected in a subacute study (e.g. tumorigenesis).

2.6.2   Functional versus morphological changes

Toxic effects are often classed as functional or morphological in nature. There has been a traditional attitude that changes in gross or microscopic structure are more serious than functional changes. Indeed, altered structure often seems to have taken on the implication of irreversibility while altered function is often considered a reversible effect. This conclusion, of course, depends on the level of understanding of mechanisms of injury, rates and mechanisms of repair, and causal associations between related functional and morphological changes. Furthermore, whether the change is regarded as functional or morphological may depend on the manner of detection. For example, accumulation of fat in a cell observed through a microscope will most often be considered a structural change, but, if the same cells or tissues were assayed for triglyceride content, the increased triglyceride would probably be classified as a functional or biochemical change. The introduction of enzyme histochemistry and electron microscopy into toxicity evaluation studies makes the distinction between morphological and functional effects even less clear. It may therefore be inappropriate to attempt to make these distinctions.

Rowe et al. (1959) reviewed data from studies on a large number of chemicals repeatedly administered to animals over periods ranging from one month to two years, and summarized the frequency with which a certain effect was found and the frequency with which it was the only effect found. The effects were considered on: mortality; food intake; body weight; organ weights; the histopathology of virtually every major organ; haematology; blood urea nitrogen; clinical urinalyses; central nervous system (most probably gross behaviour); gross pathology; and cholinesterase activity. The authors found that if growth, liver weight, kidney weight, liver pathology, and kidney pathology had been studied, the lowest dose level that caused any effect would have been detected in 96% of the studies. Changes in food intake, central nervous system depression, excessive mortality, increased lung weight, testicular injury, haematological changes, and cholinesterase depression were the most sensitive effects in one or more of the remaining 4% of cases. The reader should consult the original reference for details but it is important to note that of the commonly used criteria of effects, liver and kidney micropathology were quite sensitive indices.

There are, of course, well-known examples where functional changes are the only manifestations of toxicity. Many of the organophosphate and carbamate insecticides inhibit cholinesterase (3.1.1.8) activity and produce signs and symptoms (even death) that can be characterized as purely functional without the production of morphological lesions, detectable by conventional techniques. Similarly, irritant air pollutants can often cause bronchoconstriction and respiratory distress, without any accompanying morphological changes. Both the functional cholinergic signs and symptoms produced by the anticholinesterase insecticides and the bronchoconstriction produced by irritants provide means of early detection at low levels of exposure. Although these effects are reversible, they are no less important during the period of exposure than certain kinds of morphological effects. On the other hand, certain kinds of "functional" changes, e.g. increased level of plasma transaminase activity, usually reflect some type of structural change in cells that allow these enzymes to "leak" into plasma (Cornish 1971).

It is not possible, with present knowledge, to conclude that either functional or morphological changes represent the most sensitive, the earliest, or the most serious effects of toxic chemicals. Since maintenance of both integrated function and integrated structure ultimately depends on chemical reactions among cell constituents, it is logical to conclude that specific biochemical changes are the first and most sensitive effects. Unfortunately, with relatively few exceptions, the specific biochemical receptors for toxic chemicals are unknown. The more information that can be obtained with respect to time- and dose-relationships for functional and morphological effects, the more predictive the tests will become. This requires an approach to toxicity studies in which proof of a mechanism will require an integrated biochemical, physiological, and morphological approach. Dawkins & Rees (1959) provide a useful short treatise on an integrated biochemical-pathological approach to studies of several toxic chemicals. Although advances in both biochemistry and pathology now allow even more precise studies than those outlined by these authors, the general principles which they develop are still applicable.

2.7 Dynamic Aspects of Predictive Toxicology

2.7.1 Traditional versus new techniques

The objective of any toxicity test programme is prediction: prediction of biological disposition from physicochemical constants, prediction of altered cell or organ system function from reaction with macromolecules, prediction of irreversible consequences of reversible changes, prediction of implications of selected measurable variables to overall health and survival of the test organisms, prediction of effects in individuals of one species from tests conducted in another, and finally predictions of incidence in large populations from tests on small samples. All of these predictions must be related quantitatively to a dose and dose-rate or schedule that can ultimately e related to probable amounts used, the manner of use or the occurrence of the chemicals in the environment.

Generally, traditional approaches to toxicity evaluation have not attempted to make predictions far removed from the final application or interpretation of the data. Thus, as outlined in Chapter 3, test organisms are exposed to a range of doses and their health status is examined by biochemical, physiological, or pathological procedures analogous to those used in clinical medicine. When this approach has been comprehensive, judicious application of the data usually appears to have been successful in preventing chemically-induced disease. Abandoning this approach in favour of new, different, or short-cut methods cannot be advocated without thorough verification of their validity. On the other hand, serious consideration must be given to the application of some short-term ways of predicting toxicity in order to provide a practical means of evaluating the many chemicals already in the environment and those new compounds that are continuously being added to the environment and have not been subjected to traditional tests. Preceding sections have discussed some possibilities, the following sections contain brief comments and examples for consideration in selecting tests.

2.7.2 Toxicity of chemical analogues

Although it may be possible to predict the toxicity of individual compounds in a homologous series from detailed knowledge of some members of the series, some special exceptions should be noted. A classical example involves the series of fluorine-substituted aliphatic alcohols and acids, in which high acute toxicity alternates with odd and even numbers of carbon atoms, the latter being the most toxic (Pattison, 1959). The odd number of total carbon atoms confers high toxicity in a homologous series of fluoronitriles, however. This demonstrates the possibility that detailed information concerning only a few members of a homologous series might fail to predict the toxicity of another member of the series.

Recently, Johnstone et al. (1974) examined a number of biochemical effects in a series of isomerically pure compounds for their potency as liver enzyme inducers. Potency for this effect increased with increasing chlorination that was related to differences in biotransformation and excretion rates; however, there were also striking differences in the potency of positional isomers in the lower chlorinated biphenyls.

The mechanism of the toxic action of organophosphorus insecticides was known to be the inhibition of acetylcholinesterase even before they were introduced into use 30 years ago. However, quantitative prediction of their acute toxicity from *in vitro* tests of their relative potency as anticholinesterases is still inadequate because of incomplete knowledge of the dynamic relationships between several pathways of metabolism which yield both more and less potent metabolites (Murphy, 1975). Nevertheless, these compounds have been subjected to a great deal of research on both their physicochemical and biological properties which should be applicable to predictions of their relative environmental persistence, interaction with other compounds, and, ultimately, to the design of safe molecules (Eto, 1974).

Using model ecosystems, Lu & Metcalf (1975) studied bioaccumulation, biodegradability, and comparative detoxification mechanisms in several benzene derivatives with widely-varying physicochemical constants and biological activities. They concluded that biological disposition and action could be predicted by the basic molecular properties of water solubility, the partition coefficient for lipid/water, and reactivity as determined by electron density.

Johnson (1975) recently reviewed the problems encountered in the pursuit of the mechanism of delayed peripheral neuropathy produced by some organophosphorus esters. The structure-activity relationships identified in this research may be considered as a model of thorough investigation that began as a problem in retrospective toxicology and led to promising developments applicable to prospective toxicology. Some interesting aspects of this problem are: the particular usefulness of a non-mammalian species, the hen, as a predictor of a toxic action that occurs in man; the concept of primary metabolic effects on central neurons as a precursor to pathological change detected in peripheral nerve fibres; and the difficulties of detecting a specific critical esterase inhibition that represented only a small percentage of the total esterase activity. Production of peripheral neuropathy appears to be characteristic of organophosphorus esters which may not only phosphorylate the specific "neurotoxic esterase" but are also capable of dealkylation (or aging) following phosphorylation. Although the steps between this primary phosphorylating-aging process and the eventual manifestation of peripheral neuropathy are still unclear, it appears that it may be possible to predict probable occurrence of a delayed, chronic disease from studies of the primary chemical-macromolecular interaction of neurotoxic esterase inhibition that occurs immediately following exposure.

2.7.3 Relation between site of metabolism and site of injury

Although for many years it was thought that the biotransformation of organic chemicals represented detoxification mechanisms, it is now apparent that numerous compounds are enzymatically converted to intrinsically more active compounds *in vivo* (Fouts, 1972; Murphy, 1975;

Parke, 1968). The liver is generally the most active tissue in catalysing these "activation" reactions, but it is not always the most susceptible target tissue as, for example, in the case of activation of phosphorothioate insecticides to phosphate insecticides. This may be explained, in part, by the presence of detoxifying enzymes or reactive but noncritical binding sites in the liver that may prevent the phosphates from escaping to inhibit cholinesterase in nerve target tissues. The brain tissue has only a small fraction of the liver's capacity to activate phosphorothioates, but because the activation occurs in the same tissue as the critical target site, activation in the brain may be the most important in determining toxicity.

Recently, the characteristic hepatotoxicity of several chemicals has been related to their enzymatic conversion to highly reactive derivatives that covalently bind to essential liver cell constituents at, or near, the site of activation (Brodie et al., 1971). A similar possibility may explain the bronchiolar neurosis produced in rats and mice by bromobenzene and other aromatic hydrocarbons (Reid et al., 1973).

The detailed study of the metabolism, storage, or binding and distribution of foreign chemicals in the lung is a relatively recent activity and has focused largely on therapeutic chemicals (Bend et al., 1973; Brown, 1974; Orton et al., 1973). Because inhalation is a common route of exposure to a wide variety of air contaminants in industrial and community environments, future toxicity studies would benefit by the inclusion of metabolic studies concerning rates of absorption from, and local actions in the lung. Witschi (1975) has reviewed biochemical approaches that may be used in the evaluation of toxic injury to the lung.

Since the intensity and duration of the toxic action of a chemical depends on the concentration of the active form at critical receptor sites of action, kinetic aspects of absorption, distribution, and excretion (as well as biotransformation) will influence the specific sites of action. This topic is discussed in detail in Chapter 4 but it is worthy of note that Dedrick (1973) developed several useful kinetic models that might be applied in predicting species differences or similarities in response.

2.7.4 *In vitro* test systems

Where appropriate, studies in experimental animals should be supplemented by isolated perfused organ, tissue slice or extract, and tissue culture techniques. Where possible, attempts should be made to compare the tissues of human subjects available from autopsy or therapeutic biopsies, with those of other species in their response to toxic chemicals (Worden, 1974). When the mechanism(s) of toxicity have been elucidated and the target organ(s) identified, specific species comparisons and dose-response relationships can be studied by these *in vitro* techniques.

Knowledge of a specific enzyme or biological macromolecule that serves as a target for reaction with toxic chemicals may provide a means for screening and predicting relative potencies or specific actions of chemicals in intact organisms. However, as pointed out previously for the organophosphorus insecticides, biotransformations and membrane barriers to the distribution of chemicals in intact animals will often invalidate conclusions drawn from *in vitro* assays. This problem may be partly overcome by incorporating enzymic biotransformation systems with the target macromolecule (or organism) in the *in vitro* test system. Such an approach is used for screening for potential mutagens in microorganism test systems (Malling & Frantz, 1973) and has been applied to studies of the biochemical actions of pesticides (Chow & Murphy, 1975; Cohen & Murphy, 1974). A major problem in the use of *in vitro* test systems for predicting toxicity is the difficulty of quantitatively relating concentrations in the simplified *in vitro* systems to action in complex intact organisms. With adequate correlative data in both *in vitro* and *in vivo* systems this may become possible, but such information is generally lacking at present. For the most part, therefore, *in vitro* model test systems are qualitative predictors rather than quantitative. This need not decrease their usefulness, however, as long as this limitation is recognized in the interpretation of results.

In general, *in vitro* test systems have been useful in qualitatively predicting acute actions. However, as discussed earlier, neurotoxic esterase inhibition provides promise for predicting delayed chronic neuropathy produced by certain organophosphate compounds. Major research efforts are now being devoted to *in vitro* test systems for the prediction of mutagenesis and carcinogenesis. These are discussed in detail in Chapter 7. There is general recognition of the value of these test systems (Council of Environmental Mutagen Society, 1975; Food & Drug Administration, 1970; Food Protection Committee, 1970) as screening procedures, but much less agreement as to the priority that they should have in the conduct and interpretation of toxicity evaluations.

When it is possible to obtain comparisons between exposures of organs or tissues of experimental animals and humans to toxic chemicals, such comparisons will provide useful baseline data for the future extrapolation of data from intact animal studies to man. Culture systems of human cells may also be useful as comparative systems. The difficulties of maintaining some human cell lines are well documented, but primary cultures of differentiated mammary and liver epithelia have been established and maintained (Buehring, 1972; Lasfargues & Moore, 1971; Potter, 1972). Human lymphocytes have also been used *in vitro* (Kellermann et al., 1973).

It may be possible to use these isolated systems to determine the susceptibility to toxic chemicals of different cell types in different organs and to determine the reversibility of adverse effects in these cell lines and organs. Of particular usefulness would be the determination of dose-response curves for many tissues and their interspecies comparison. Such information could be used to predict target cells and organs with a high degree of susceptibility or resistance. However, as mentioned earlier, the usefulness of the data may be limited if the cells, tissues, or organs are incapable of metabolizing the chemical to a toxic form in the intact animal. Such a biotransformation may even occur in a different tissue or organ from the one under test *in vitro*. To overcome this problem, biotransformation systems from animal or human tissues (e.g. microsomal activating systems) are often added with the chemical to the isolated culture systems.

One problem with these methods is the uncertainty that all the steps of metabolism are equally duplicated, that is, in addition to activation of a chemical there should also be an opportunity for the chemical to be detoxified or conjugated and eliminated. Some of these detoxification steps require different coenzymes or metabolites, and the enzyme systems may not be limited to microsome fractions or liver tissue. However, as long as it is realized that these *in vitro* test systems may exaggerate the situation that occurs *in vivo* they can prove useful, especially for tests where only very small quantities of material are available, as might be the case with some impurities or metabolites.

In summary, short-term, *in vitro* tests both for carcinogenicity and other forms of toxicity show great promise (Golberg, 1974), and although no single test is likely to be reliable, appropriate combinations may provide valuable information concerning the fundamental toxicity of environmental chemicals. This would currently provide a useful adjunct to long-term studies in animal populations, and may develop further in the future to provide the more reliable method of assessment. Such tests will require much development and will take years to validate and perhaps even longer to win public confidence with regard to their reliability.

ABINANTI, R. R. (1971) Chronic and degenerative diseases of man: the value of natural and experimentally induced diseases of animals. In: *Animal models for biomedical research IV, Proceedings of a Symposium*, Washington DC, National Academy of Sciences, pp. 31–46.

ALTMAN, P. L. & DITTMER, D. S., ed. (1966) *Environmental biology*, Bethesda, MD, Federation of American Societies for Experimental Biology, pp. 565–608.

ALVARES, A. P., LEIGH, S., KAPPAS, A., LEVIN, W., & CONNEY, A. H. Induction of aryl hydrocarbon hydroxylase in human skin. *Drug Metabol. Disposition*, 1: 386–390.

BARNES, J. M. (1968) Percutaneous toxicity. In: Boyland, E. & Goulding, R., ed. *Modern trends in toxicology*, London, Butterworths, pp. 18–38.

BEND, J. R., HOOK, G. E., & GRAM, T. E. (1973) Characterization of lung microsomes as related to drug metabolism. *Drug Metabol. Disposition*, 1: 358–367.

BENKE, G. M. & MURPHY, S. D. (1975) The influence of age on the toxicity and metabolism of methyl parathion and parathion in male and female rats. *Toxicol. appl. Pharmacol.*, 31: 254–269.

BEUTHIN, P. K. & BOUSQUET, W. F. (1970) Long-term variation in basal and phenobarbital-stimulated oxidative drug metabolism in the rat. *Biochem. Pharmacol.*, 19: 620–625.

BOYD, E. M. (1969) Dietary protein and pesticide toxicity in male weanling rats. *Bull. World Health Org.*, 40: 801–805.

BOYD, E. M. (1972) *Predictive toxicometrics*, Baltimore, Williams & Wilkins, 408 pp.

BRODIE, B. B., CHO, A. K., KRISHNA, G., & REID, W. D. (1971) Drug metabolism in man: past, present and future. *Ann. NY Acad. Sci.*, 179: 5–18.

BROWN, E. A. B. (1974) The localization, metabolism and effects of drugs and toxicants in lung. *Drug Metabol. Rev.*, 3: 33–87.

BUEHRING, G. C. (1972) Culture of human mammary epithelial cells: keeping abreast with a new method. *J. Natl Cancer Inst.*, 49: 1433–1434.

CAMPBELL, T. & HAYES, J. R. (1974) Role of nutrition in the drug-metabolizing enzyme system. *Pharmacol. Rev.*, 26: 171–197.

CASARETT, L. J. (1975) Toxicologic evaluation. In: Casarett, L. J. & Doull, J., ed. *Toxicology—the basic science of poisons*, New York, Macmillan, pp. 11–25.

CLARKSON, T. B., PRICHARD, R. W., BULLOCK, B. C., LEHNER, N. D. M., LOFLAND, H. B. & CLAIR, R. W. St. (1970) Animal models for atherosclerosis. In: *Animal models for biomedical research III. Proceedings of a Symposium*, Washington DC, National Academy of Sciences, pp. 22–41.

CHOW, A. Y. K. & MURPHY, S. D. (1975) Production of a methemoglobin-forming metabolite of 3,4-dichloroaniline by liver *in vitro*. *Bull. environ. Contam. Toxicol.*, 13: 9–13.

COHEN, S. D. & MURPHY, S. D. (1974) A simplified bioassay for organophosphate detoxification and interactions. *Toxicol. appl. Pharmacol.*, 27: 537–550.

COMMITTEE ON PROBLEMS OF DRUG SAFETY (1969) Application of metabolic data to the evaluation of drugs: report prepared by the Committee on Problems of Drug Safety of the NAS/NRC Drug Research Board. *Clin. Pharmacol. Therap.*, 10: 607–634.

CORNISH, H. H. (1971) Problems posed by observations of serum enzyme changes in toxicology. *CRC Crit. Rev. Toxicol.*, 1: 1–132.

COUNCIL OF EUROPE (1973) Guide to the testing and toxicological evaluation of flavouring substances. In: *Natural flavouring substances, their sources and added artificial flavouring substances*, Strasbourg, Council of Europe, pp. 403–410.

COUNCIL OF ENVIRONMENTAL MUTAGEN SOCIETY (1975) Environmental mutagenic hazards. *Science*, 187: 503–514.

CREMER, J. E. & BLIGH, J. (1969) Body-temperature and response to drugs. *Brit. med. Bull.*, 25(3): 299–306.

CROSBY, D. G. (1972) Environmental photooxidation pf pesticides. In: *Proceedings of a* conference on degradation of synthetic organic molecules in the biosphere, San Francisco, June 1971, Washington DC, National Academy of Sciences, pp. 260–278.

DAVIS, W. M. (1962) Day-night periodicity in pentobarbital response of mice and the influence of socio-physiological conditions. *Experientia (Basel)*, **18**: 235–237.

DAWKINS, M. J. R. & REES, K. R. (1959) *A biochemical approach to pathology*, London, Edward Arnold, 128 pp.

DEDRICK, R. L. (1973) Animal scale-up. *J. Pharmacokin. & Biopharm.*, **1**: 435–461.

DHEW (1972) *Guide for the care and use of laboratory animals* (prepared by Committee on Revision of the Guide for Laboratory Animals and Care, ILAR, NRC). Washington DC, US Gov. Print. Office (DHEW Publ. No. (NIH) 72.23).

DIGGLE, W. M. & GAGE, J. C. (1951) Cholinesterase inhibition *in vivo* by *O,O*-diethyl *O-p*-nitrophenyl thiophosphate (Parathion E 605). *Biochem. J.*, **49**: 491–494.

DILLINGHAM, E. O., MAST, R. W., BASS, G. E., & AUTIAN, J. (1973) Toxicity of methyl- and halogen substituted alcohols in tissue culture relative to structure-activity models and acute toxicity in mice. *J. Pharm. Sci.*, **62**: 22–30.

DOULL, J. (1972) The effect of physical environmental factors on drug response. In: Hayes, W. J., ed. *Essays in toxicology*, New York, Academic Press, Vol. 3, pp. 37–63.

DOULL, J. (1973) Factors influencing toxicity. In: Casarett, L. J. & Doull, J., ed. *Toxicology—the basic science of poisons*, New York, Macmillan, pp. 133–147.

EASTON, R. E. & MURPHY, S. D. (1967) Experimental ozone pre-exposure and histamine: effect on the acute toxicity and respiratory function effects of histamine in guinea pigs. *Arch. environ. Health*, **15**: 160–166.

EHRLICH, R. (1966) Effect of nitrogen dioxide on resistance to respiratory infection. *Bact. Rev.*, **30**: 604–614.

ETO, M. (1974) *Organophosphorus pesticides: organic and biological chemistry*. Cleveland, OH, CRC Press, pp. 387 (57–78).

FOOD & DRUG ADMINISTRATION (1959) *Appraisal of the safety of chemicals in foods, drugs and cosmetics*. Austin, Texas, Association of Food & Drug Officials of the USA, pp. 107.

FOOD & DRUG ADMINISTRATION (1970) Report on reproduction studies in the safety evaluation of food additives and pesticide residues (Report of panel on reproduction of the FDA Advisory Committee on Protocols for Safety Evaluation). *Toxicol. appl. Pharmacol.*, **16**: 264–269.

FOOD PROTECTION COMMITTEE (1970) *Evaluating the safety of food chemicals*, Washington, DC, National Academy of Sciences, 55 pp.

FOUTS, J. R. (1972) Some studies and comments on hepatic and extrahepatic microsomal toxication-detoxification system. *Environ. Health Perspect.*, Experimental Issue No. 2, Oct. pp. 55–66.

GOLBERG, L. (1967) The amelioration of food (The Milroy Lectures). *J. Roy. Coll. Phys.*, **1** (4): 385–426.

GOLBERG, L. (1974) Short-term predictive tests. *Proc. Eur. Soc. Drug Toxicity*, **15**: 178–191.

HACKEL, D. B., MIKAT, E., LEBOVITZ, H., & SCHMIDT-NIELSEN, K. (1968) Animal models for diabetes mellitus with special reference to the sand rat (*Prommomys obesus*). In: *Animal models for biomedical research: Proceedings of a Symposium*, Washington, DC, National Academy of Sciences, pp. 14–20.

HANSCH, C. & DUNN, W. J. (1972) Linear relationships between lipophilic character and biological activity of drugs. *J. pharm. Sc.*, **61**: 1–18.

HATCH, A., BALEZO, T., WIBERG, G. S., & GRICE, H. C. (1965) The importance of avoiding mental suffering in laboratory animals. *Anim. Welfare Inst. Rep.*, Vol. 14, No. 3.

HATCH, T. F. & GROSS, P. (1964) *Pulmonary deposition and retention of inhaled aerosols*, New York, Academic Press, 184 pp.

HAYES, W. J. (1972) Tests for detecting and measuring long-term toxicity. In: Hayes, W. J., ed. *Essays in toxicology*, New York, Academic Press, Vol. 3, pp. 65–77.

HEIMANN, H. (1967) Status of air pollution health research. *Arch. environ. Health*. **14**: 488–503.

91

HENDERSON, Y. & HAGGARD, H. W. (1943) *Noxious gases and the principles of respiration influencing their action*, New York, Reinhold, 287 pp.

HOLMSTEDT, B. (1959) Pharmacology of organophosphorus cholinesterase inhibitors. *Pharmacol. Rev.*, **11**: 567–688.

HURNI, H. (1970) The provision of laboratory animals. In: Paget, G. E., ed. *Methods in toxicology*, Philadelphia, F. A. Davis, pp. 11–48.

JAEGER, R. J., CONOLLY, R. B., & MURPHY, S. D. (1973) Diurnal variation of hepatic glutathione concentration and its correlation with 1,1-dichloroethylene inhalation toxicity in rats. *Res. Commun. Chem. Pathol. Pharmacol.*, **6**: 465–471

JAEGER, R. J., CONOLLY, R. B., & MURPHY, S. D. (1975) Short-term inhalation toxicity of halogenated hydrocarbons. *Arch. environ. Health*, **30**: 26–31.

JOBE, C. L. (1968) Selection and development of animal models of myocardial infarction. In: *Proceedings of a Symposium on Animal Models for Biomedial Research*, Washington, DC, National Academy of Sciences, pp. 101–108.

JOHNSON, M. K. (1975) The delayed neuropathy caused by some organophosphorus esters: mechanism and challenge. *CRC Crit. Rev. Toxicol.*, **3**: 289–316.

JOHNSTONE, G. J., ECOBICHON, D. J., & HUTZINGER, O. (1974) The influence of pure polychlorinated biphenyl compounds on hepatic function in the rat. *Toxicol. appl. Pharmacol.*, **28**: 66–81.

JONES, T. C. (1969) Mammalian and avian models of disease in man. *Fed. Proc.*, **28** (1): 162–169.

JONES, W. I., ROBACK, L. A., & TAYLOR, J. M. (1971) The loss of food flavours from laboratory animal diets. II. Effect of laboratory environment. *J. Assoc. Offic. Anal. Chem.*, **54**: 42–46.

JORI, A., PUGLIATTI, C., & PESCADOR, R. (1971a) Rat strain differences in the activity of hepatic microsomal enzymes. *Biochem. Pharmacol.*, **20**: 2695–2701.

JORI, A., SALLE, E., & SANTINI, V. (1971b) Daily rhythmic variation and liver drug metabolism in rats. *Biochem. Pharmacol.*, **20**: 2965–2969.

KLASSEN, C. D. (1975) Absorption, distribution and excretion of toxicants. In: Casarett, J. L. & Doull, J., ed. *The basic science of poisons*, New York, Macmillan, pp. 26–44.

KELLERMAN, G., LUYTEN-KELLERMAN, M. L., & SHAW, C. R. (1973) Genetic variation of aryl hydrocarbon hydroxylase in human lymphocytes. *Am. J. Hum. Genet.*, **25**: 327–331.

LA DU, B. N., MANDEL, G., & WAY, E. L., ed. (1971) *Fundamentals of drug metabolism and drug disposition*, Baltimore, Williams & Wilkins, 615 pp.

LAKE, B. G., HOPKINS, R., CHAKRABORTY, J., BRIDGES, J. W., & PARKE, V. W. (1973) The influence of some hepatic enzyme inducers on extrahepatic drug metabolism. *Drug Metabol. Disposition*, **1**: 342–349.

LASFARGUES, E. Y. & MOORE, D. H. (1971) A method for the continuous cultivation of mammary epithelium. *In Vitro*, **7**: 21–25.

LERNER, R. A. & DIXON, F. J. (1968) Experimental and human glomerulonephritis associated with antiglomerular basement membrane antibodies. In: *Proceedings of a Symposium on Animal Models for Biomedical Research*, Washington, DC, National Academy of Sciences, pp. 109–130.

LJUBLINA, E. I. & FILOV, V. A. (1975) Chemical structure, physical and chemical properties and biological activity. In: *Methods used in the USSR for establishing biologically safe levels of toxic substances*, Geneva, WHO, pp. 19–44.

LOOMIS, T. A. (1974) *Essentials of toxicology*, 2nd ed., Philadelphia, Lea & Febiger, 233 pp.

LU, P. Y. & METCALF, R. (1975) Environmental fate and biodegradability of benzene derivatives as studied in a model aquatic ecosystem. *Environ. Health Perspect.*, **10**: 269–284.

LUGINBUHL, H. & DETWEILER, D. K. (1968) Animal models for the study of cerebro-vascular disease. In: *Proceedings of a Symposium on Animal Models for Biomedial Research*, Washington DC, National Academy of Sciences, pp. 35–41.

LUKAS, G., BRINDLE, S., & GREENGARD, P. (1971) The route of absorption of intraperitoneally administered compounds. *J. Pharmacol. exp. Therap.*, **178**: 562–566.

McLeod, S. M., Renton, K. W., & Eade, N. R. (1972) Development of hepatic microsomal drug-oxidizing enzymes in immature male and female rats. *J. Pharmacol. exp. Therap.*, **183:** 489–498.

Malling, H. V. & Frantz, C. N. (1973) *In vitro* vs *in vivo* metabolic activation of mutagens. *Environ. Health Perspect.*, **6:** 71–82.

McCreesh, A. H. (1965) Percutaneous toxicity. *Toxicol. appl. Pharmacol.*, **7:** 20–26.

McKinney, G. R., Weikel, J. H., Webb, W. K., & Dick, R. J. (1968) Use of life-table technique to estimate effects of certain steroids on probability of tumour formation in a long-term study in rats. *Toxicol. appl. Pharmacol.*, **12:** 68–79.

McLean, A. E. M. & McLean, E. K. (1969) Diet and toxicity. *Brit. med. Bull.*, **25:** 278–281.

Meeter, E. & Wolthuis, O. L. (1968) The effects of cholinesterase inhibitors on the body temperature of the rat. *Environ. J. Pharmacol.*, **4:** 18–24.

Moffitt, A. E. & Murphy, S. D. (1974) Effect of excess and deficient copper intake on hepatic microsomal metabolism and toxicity of foreign chemicals. In: Hemphill, D. D., ed. *Trace substances in environmental health*, Columbia, MO, University of Missouri Press, Vol. VII, pp. 205–210.

Morrison, J. K. (1968) The purpose and value of LD_{50} determinations. In: Boyland, E. & Goulding, R., ed. *Modern trends in toxicology*, Appleton-Century-Crofts, pp. 1–17.

Murphy, S. D. (1964) A review of effects on animals of exposure to auto exhaust and some of its components. *Air Pollut. Control J.*, **14:** 303–308.

Murphy, S. D. (1967) Malathion inhibition of esterases as a determinant of malathion toxicity. *J. Pharmacol. exp. Therap.*, **156:** 352–365.

Murphy, S. D. (1969) Some relationships between effects of insecticides and other stress conditions. *Ann. NY Acad. Sci.*, **160:** 366–377.

Murphy, S. D. (1975) Pesticides. In: Casarett, L. J. & Doull, J., ed. *Toxicology: the basic science of poisons*, New York, Macmillan, pp. 408–453.

Murphy, S. D., Lauwerys, R. R., & Cheeven, K. L. (1968) Comparative anticholinesterase action of organophosphorus insecticides in vertebrates. *Toxicol. appl. Pharmacol.*, **12:** 22–35.

Orton, J. C., Anderson, M. W., Pickett, R. D., Eling, T. E., & Fouts, J. R. (1973) Xenobiotic accumulation and metabolism by isolated perfused rabbit lungs. *J. Pharmacol. exp. therap.*, **186:** 482–497.

Panel on Herbicides (1971) *Report on 2,4,5-T*, Washington, DC, US Govt Print. Office, 68 pp.

Parke, D. V. (1968) *The biochemistry of foreign compounds*. Oxford, Pergamon Press, 269 pp.

Parke, D. V. & Williams, R. T. (1969) Metabolism of toxic substances. *Brit. med. Bull.*, **25:** 256–262.

Pattison. F. L. M. (1959) *Toxic aliphatic fluorine compounds*, Amsterdam, Elsevier, 227 pp. (Elsevier Monographs).

Patty, F. A. (1958) *Industrial hygiene and toxicology*, 2nd ed., New York, Interscience, Vol. 1, 153 pp.

Potter, V. R. (1972) Workshop on liver cell culture. *Cancer Res.*, **32:** 1998–2000.

Reid, W. D., Hett, K. F., Hik, J. M., & Krishna, G. (1973) Metabolism and binding of aromatic hydrocarbons in the lung. *Am. Rev. Resp. Dis.*, **107:** 539–551.

Roe, F. J. C. (1968) Inhalation tests. In: Boyland, E. & Goulding, R., ed. *Modern trends in toxicology*, London, Butterworths, pp. 39–74.

Rowe, V. K., Wolf, M. A., Neil, C. S., & Smith, H. F. (1959) The toxicological basis of threshold limit values: 2. Pathological and biochemical criteria. *Am. Ind. Hyg. Assoc. J.*, **20:** 346–349.

Smyth, H. F. (1959) The toxicological basis of threshold limit values: 1. Experience with threshold limit values based on animal data. *Am. Ind. Hyg. Assoc. J.*, **20:** 341–345.

Szot, R. J. & Murphy, S. D. (1970) Phenobarbital and dexamethasone inhibition of the adrenocortical response of rats to toxic chemicals and other stresses. *Toxicol. appl. Pharmacol.*, **17:** 761–773.

SZOT, J. R. & MURPHY, S. D. (1971) Relationships between cyclic variations in adrenocortical secretary activity in rats and the adrenocortical response to toxic chemical stress. *Environ. Res.*, **4:** 530–538.

TAYLOR, G. J. & DREW, R. T. (1975) Cardiomyopathy predisposes hamsters to trichlorofluoromethane toxicity. *Toxicol. appl. Pharmacol.*, **32:** 177–183.

TYLER, W. S. & GILLESPIE, J. R. (1969) Structural and functional alterations in horses with emphysema. In: *Proceedings of a Symposium on Animal Models for Biomedical Research*, Washington, DC, National Academy of Sciences, Vol. II, pp. 38–51.

UNIVERSITIES FEDERATION FOR ANIMAL WELFARE (1972) *Handbook on the care and management of laboratory animals*, 4th ed., Baltimore, Williams & Wilkins, 624 pp.

WATTENBERG, L. (1972) Dietary modification of intestinal and pulmonary aryl hydrocarbon hydroxylase activity. *Toxicol. appl. Pharmacol.*, **23:** 741–748.

WEIL, C. S. (1970) Selection of the valid numbers of sampling units and a consideration of their combination in toxicological studies in involving reproduction, teratogenesis and carcinogenesis. *Food Cosmet. Toxicol.*, **8:** 177–182.

WHO (1967) WHO Technical Report Series, No. 348. (Procedures for investigating intentional and unintentional food additives: Report of a WHO Scientific Group) 25 pp.

WILLIAMS, R. T. (1967) Comparative patterns of drug metabolism. In: Proceedings of an International Symposium on Comparative Pharmacology. *Fed. Proc.*, **26** (4): 1029–1046.

WILLIAMS, R. T. (1972) Toxicological implications of biotransformation by intestinal microflora. *Toxicol. appl. Pharmacol.*, **23:** 769–781.

WINTER, C. A. & FLATAKER, L. (1962) Cage design as a factor influencing acute toxicity of respiratory depressant drugs in rats. *Toxicol. appl. Pharmacol.*, **4:** 650–655.

WITSCHI, H. (1975) Exploitable biochemical approaches for the evaluation of toxic lung damage. *Essays in Toxicol.*, **6:** 125–191.

WORDEN, A. N. (1974) Toxicology and the environment. *Toxicol.*, **1:** 3–27.

ZBINDEN, G. (1973) *Progress in toxicology: special topics*, New York, Springer-Verlag, 88 pp.

3. ACUTE, SUBACUTE, AND CHRONIC TOXICITY TESTS

3.1 Introduction

The primary objective of toxicological testing is to determine the effects of chemicals on biological systems and to obtain data on the dose-response characteristics of the chemical. These data may provide information on the degree of hazard to man and the environment associated with a potential exposure related to a specific use of this chemical. Elucidation of the metabolic behaviour of the chemical in test animals increases confidence in defining the hazard (see Chapter 4). The degree of confidence with which hazard may be estimated depends on the quality of the toxicological data. Selection of the most appropriate test procedures coupled with strict adherence to accepted experimental practices and astute observation are of paramount importance in experimental toxicology.

3.2 General Nature of Test Procedures

Several types of toxicity testing procedures have been developed. These include acute, subacute, and chronic studies. The major difference between these tests is the dose employed and the length of exposure to the chemical agent, but other differences in intent and nature do exist and will be discussed. All of the tests share some common characteristics. Each requires that groups of healthy animals, housed under suitable conditions, be exposed to graded doses of the test chemical. Rats, mice, guineapigs, rabbits, and hamsters are commonly used for this purpose, but in some cases it may be necessary to use dogs, swine, nonhuman primates, or other species. As a rule, a control group is given the dosing vehicle or is sham treated. Following treatment, the animals are closely observed for signs of toxicity. Laboratory procedures designed to measure biological effects are carried out on the treated and control animals. Detailed records are maintained on each animal. Following completion of the test, all animals, including controls, are subjected to a pathological examination. Data should be analysed by appropriate statistical procedures.

3.2.1 Housing, diet, and clinical examination of test animals

Animals should be healthy, genetically stable, and adequately identified as to colony source. The controls and treated animals should be of the same strain and species, age, and weight range, and be supplied from the same source. Before starting the experiment, the health status of all animals should be determined and monitored for some time. During this time, a small randomly selected number of animals from each shipment should be sacrificed and examined for disease, parasites, and other specific pathogens. During the quarantine period, animals may be caged together according to the weight-space specifications. Acceptable standards for the housing and care of experimental animals have been published (DHEW, 1972; Canadian Council on Animal Care, 1973; Sontag et al., 1975).

During toxicity studies, rodents should be housed singly or in pairs in stainless steel or plastic shoe-box cages while nonrodents should be housed in suitable runs. The animals should be randomly allotted to the cages and treatment regimes should be randomly applied (Cox, 1958). Rodents should be allowed free access to food and water. Nonrodents should be fed meal and given water *ad libitum*. The diet fed to the animals should meet all of their nutritional requirements (National Academy of Sciences, 1975) and should be free of toxic chemical impurities that might influence the outcome of the test. Periodic analysis of the diet to ensure its nutrient composition should be undertaken since nutritional status may affect the nature of toxic responses (Arcos, 1968). Although commercially available diets of recognized quality are suitable for most subacute studies, semipurified diets may be preferred because the nutrient and nonnutrient components of the diet may be altered readily, where necessary (Munro et al., 1974; Newberne, 1968).

Careful clinical observation of test animals is the most neglected area in experimental toxicology. Few investigators are aware or recognize that the skills required of a good medical diagnostician are also required in assessing or diagnosing the toxic state or condition of an animal. In toxicity studies, many animals may be lost for evaluation because of death from intercurrent disease and subsequent autolysis. With concerned, reliable staff, these losses can be greatly reduced if a conscientious effort is made to recognize early clinical signs of disease in the test animal. Ideally, each animal on test should be looked upon as an individual patient. In this way, there is an awareness of the idiosyncrasies of the animal and departures from the normal will be more easily recognized. Once a routine of careful clinical assessment has been established, it is possible either to treat diseased test animals or, if necessary, sacrifice them. In the latter case, the tissues are available for histological examination. Otherwise, chronic disease effects might render the tissues useless for the assessment of effects due to test substances.

Detailed clinical examinations should be conducted weekly on the test animals by competent, laboratory animal technicians under the supervision of a veterinarian skilled in laboratory animal medicine (Health and Welfare,

Canada, 1973). These should include general observation of the animals for overt signs of toxicity, quality of hair, coat, general condition of the eyes, mouth, teeth, nose, and ears (Leclair & Willard, 1970; Loomis, 1968). Assessment of cardiac and respiratory function should be conducted by auscultation. If neurological effects are anticipated, a detailed neurological examination should be conducted. In larger species, this can be done by skilled personnel using the methods of Charbonneau (1974), McGrath (1960), and Mowbray & Cadell (1962). Examination of the eyes using opthalmoscopic and slit-lamp techniques (Marzulli, 1968) may assist in detecting ocular toxicity. The external and internal structures should be carefully palpated and any tissue masses should be noted. Detailed records of clinical evaluation should be maintained and should be accessible to the attendant pathologist.

3.3 Acute Toxicity Tests

3.3.1 Underlying principles

Acute toxicity has been defined as the adverse effects occurring within a short time of administration of single dose or multiple doses given within 24 h (Hagan, 1959). When data are unavailable concerning the toxicity of the test agent, acute toxicity studies are indicated to identify the relative toxicity of the compound, to investigate its mode of action and its specific toxic effect, and to determine the existence of species differences.

The most frequently used acute toxicity test involves determination of the median lethal dose (LD_{50}) of the compound. The LD_{50} has been defined as "a statistically derived expression of a single dose of a material that can be expected to kill 50% of the animals" (Gehring, 1973). The basic protocol for the determination of the LD_{50} is well established and consists of treating groups of animals with a mathematically-related series of doses in order to determine the dose that kills 50% of the group and the dose-response function. The LD_{50}, being a calculated value, is always accompanied by some estimation of the error of the value, such as the confidence limits. The most commonly used methods for calculation of the LD_{50} are the graphic method of Litchfield & Wilcoxon (1947), the logarithmic probit graph paper method of Miller & Tainter (1944), and the method of moving averages of Thompson (1947) and Weil (1952). A comparative review of these and other methods was published by Armitage & Allen (1950). Death which occurs after the first 24 h is more likely to be due to delayed toxic effects, which may be direct or indirect. Signs occurring after the first 24-h period may give some indication of the effect that the chemical may have at lower levels, when administered for longer time periods.

3.3.2 Experimental design

3.3.2.1 *Selection of species*

The extent of species variation in toxicity testing has been well documented in the reviews of Brodie (1964) and Rumke (1964). The usefulness of determining species variability in order to assess the applicability of toxicity data to man has been discussed by Hagan (1959). Litchfield (1962) has postulated that if the toxicity of a compound is the same in several species, there would appear to be an increased likelihood that man would react in a similar manner.

The mouse, rat and dog are the most commonly used species for acute toxicity testing. Both the rat and mouse should be used, as marked differences in the LD_{50} between these two species are not uncommon (Morrison et al., 1968).

The LD_{50} determination should be conducted in both male and female animals, as differences in the LD_{50} between sexes have been well documented (Hurst, 1958; Rumke, 1964) and are probably related, in part, to differences in hepatic metabolism (Conney et al., 1965).

Acute toxicity may vary substantially with the age of the test animal (Dieke & Richter, 1945; Lu et al., 1965; Scott et al., 1965; Yeary & Benish, 1965), and animals of various ages should be used in LD_{50} determinations. The effect of the age of the animal on the LD_{50} is well documented and may be related to different levels of drug metabolizing enzymes, absence of sex hormonal influences, or an altered sensitivity of the central nervous system (Fouts & Hart, 1965; Jondorf et al., 1959; Setnika & Magistretti, 1964).

The animals should be derived from previously untreated healthy females. Weinberg et al. (1966) have demonstrated an effect of treatment of dams during gestation with various compounds on the acute oral toxicity in the newborn.

Furthermore, the animals should not have been previously used for other studies, nor should there be a history of recent exposure to anthelminthics or any other drug treatment.

The number of animals used should be sufficient for statistical analysis and will depend on the method used for the calculation of the LD_{50}. Usually 8–10 rodents (4–6 animals of each sex) are used per dose group (Leclair & Willard, 1970). Diechmann & LeBlanc (1943) described a method using a total of 6 animals, while other methods involved the use of 4–5 animals per dose group (Horn, 1956; Litchfield & Wilcoxon, 1947; Thompson, 1947).

3.3.2.2 *Selection of doses*

The doses are selected to provide data for estimating the LD_{50} and to obtain information on the slope of the dose-response curve. At least four doses, selected in logarithmic progression, should be used (Weil, 1952).

In general, however, the doses can be arrived at only by experimentation. The initial dose may be such that no effect is manifested in the animals. In subsequent groups of animals, the dose should be increased by a constant multiple until the dose of the compound administered is sufficiently high that all of the animals in the group die. Under these conditions, data can be obtained that can be plotted to give a dose-response curve and from which the LD_{50} value may be calculated.

3.3.2.3 *Method of administration*

Generally, the chemical should be administered by the route by which man would be exposed. If the route is oral, the compound should be administered by gavage rather than mixed in the diet. In some cases, the administration of the chemical along with the diet has been shown to increase its toxicity compared with gavage dosing (Bein, 1963; Worden & Harper, 1963), but, in general, the oral toxicity of a compound is greatest when it is administered by gavage to animals that have fasted (Griffith, 1964). Griffith (1964) has demonstrated the effect of the type and concentration of the vehicle on the LD_{50} value. The amount of the liquid or carrier administered should be appropriate and the carrier should not, in itself, be toxic to the animal.

In certain cases, even though the route of human exposure would be oral, acute dermal, eye, and inhalation studies may be indicated to assess the hazard to personnel handling the compound in the laboratory.

3.3.2.4 *Postmortem examination*

In general, all animals dying during the observation period and all surviving animals should be autopsied by a qualified pathologist (Leclair & Willard, 1970). The autopsy should include gross and histopathological examination of all organs.

If death is almost instantaneous and due to a pharmacological or physical effect, i.e. massive gastrointestinal haemorrhage or acute respiratory collapse, detailed histopathological examination of all organs may not be indicated.

3.3.3 Repeated high-dose studies

Because of the inherent limitations of the LD_{50} in predicting long-term toxicity, a short but intensive study or a series of such studies may be indicated before commencing subacute tests. The purpose of such studies is to define more precisely the doses to be used in subacute tests and to elucidate more fully the organ systems affected. The design of these repeated high-dose studies may vary but consists, essentially, of repeated daily administration of a mathematically-related series of doses to groups of animals for 5–21 days.

One type of repeated-dose study (Sonntag et al., 1975) consists of treating groups of five young adult animals of each sex at each of five dose levels, the upper level being the one that is estimated to produce no more than 10% lethality following a single dose, the remaining doses being fractions of this dose.

A seven-day feeding study described by Weil et al. (1969) consisted of treating five rodents of each sex at each of three or four dose levels for seven days. Criteria of effects were mortality, body weight gain, relative liver and kidney weights, and feed consumption. This study showed that the results of the seven-day feeding test were of significantly greater value in predicting dose levels for the 90-day toxicity test than the LD_{50} values.

Daily observations, as described in section 3.1.3, should be conducted and weekly body weight and food consumption (if the animals are caged individually) monitored. For some test agents, especially those with delayed toxicity or cumulative effects, other measurements, such as organ function, body burden, absorption, and excretion of the compound may be indicated. Animals should be necropsied and the tissues should be examined for gross pathological changes and studied histopathologically, if indicated.

3.4 Subacute and Chronic Toxicity Tests

3.4.1 Underlying principles

The subacute toxicity test generally involves daily or frequent exposure to the compound over a period up to about 90 days. It provides information on the major toxic effects of the test compound and the target organs affected (Barnes, 1960). The latency of development of the effect as related to dose, the relationship of the blood and tissue levels of the compound to the development of lesions, and the reversibility of the effects may also be studied. Data derived from these studies are used for designing chronic toxicity tests in which animals are exposed to the chemical for longer periods of time.

Man may be exposed for the greater part of his life-time to low levels of a wide variety of environmental chemicals. Usually, the degree of exposure is insufficient to produce overt signs of toxicity; thus, cause-effect relationships cannot be easily established. Epidemiological studies may assist in this respect, but, because man is exposed simultaneously to several chemicals, it is difficult to establish unequivocally the degree of hazard associated with any one chemical. Acute and subacute toxicity tests are of limited value in predicting chronic toxic effects because: (*a*) chemicals may produce different toxic responses when administered repeatedly over a period; and (*b*) during the aging process, factors such as altered tissue sensitivity, changing metabolic and physiological capability, and spontaneous disease may influence the degree and nature of toxic responses. In addition, several important diseases such as heart disease, chronic renal failure, and neoplasia are associated with advancing age. These are multicausal in nature and thought to be due, in part, to the presence of chemical substances, both natural and synthetic, in the environment (WHO, 1972). Chronic toxicity tests, in which animals are exposed for their entire lifetime to environmental chemicals, have provided useful means of identifying those substances of greatest public health concern. The tests are usually conducted with the aim of establishing "no-observed-adverse-effect levels" that may be used in setting acceptable daily intakes (ADIs), tolerance limits for chemicals in food or water, or threshold limit values in the case of occupational exposure. Since chronic toxicity testing is expensive and requires specialized facilities and personnel, great care must be taken in the design, execution, and interpretation of the results of such studies.

3.4.2 Experimental design

3.4.2.1 *Selection of species and duration of studies*

In the subacute studies, if the compound has produced evidence of toxicity in man and if sufficient toxicological and metabolic information is available, it is often possible to select an appropriate species on the basis of these data. For compounds about to be put on the market about which little is known toxicologically, the recommendations of the World Health Organization (WHO, 1958) and competent national agencies (Friedman, 1969; Leclair / & Willard 1970; National Academy of Sciences, 1975) should be followed in selecting appropriate test species. As a minimum recommendation, subacute studies should be undertaken in two species, one rodent and one nonrodent. Traditionally, the rat and dog are selected for subacute toxicity testing because of their availability and the large amount of background information available on them. When rats are used, the test should be initiated just after weaning so that observations may be made during the period of most rapid growth. A conventional strain should be selected, so that the results in control and treated animals can be compared with known literature values, and both sexes should be tested to ascertain the influence of the sex hormones on the toxic response. At least 10 animals of each sex should be included in each dose group and the experiment should continue for 10% of the animals' lifetime or about 3 months. If it is desired to study the pathogenesis and reversibility of induced lesions or biochemokinetics, it is recommended that observations be made at 3-week intervals during exposure and last up to 3 months following termination of exposure.

In chronic toxicity testing, it is usual to expose the animals to the chemical for the greater part of the life span. A wide variety of animal species have been used in this type of work, although in most cases rodents are the animals of choice, since large numbers can be used to aid in the statistical interpretation of the results. Larger animals should also be used (e.g. dog and monkey) for such species have the advantage that larger samples of blood can be obtained on a routine basis.

If the objective of the test is to study the carcinogenic potential of a compound, the rat, mouse, or hamster is usually chosen because of its shorter lifetime and the fact that large numbers may be used to increase the sensitivity of the test.

When data on the metabolic fate of the test chemical in man is not available, the species showing the greatest sensitivity in subacute studies should be selected as the test species, provided the species does not react atypically to the compound due to metabolic peculiarities.

Sufficient numbers of animals should be included in the test to ensure that a statistically valid design is achieved. Based on the incidence of effects observed in subacute studies and the anticipated incidence of chronic effects, the number of animals that should be used can be calculated (Snedecor & Cochran, 1967).

Since it is usually the intention in chronic toxicity studies to expose animals over the major portion of their life span, it is essential to commence exposure early in life.

3.4.2.2   *Selection of doses*

Guidance on the selection of doses for subacute studies may be obtained from the results of acute and repeated high-dose studies. For compounds having a tendency to bioaccumulation, selection of doses is particularly difficult. Kinetic studies may assist in establishing acceptable dose levels since the half-time $(t_{1/2})$ for elimination (Chapter 4) may provide guidance on the degree of bioaccumulation that could be anticipated. To establish the nature of the toxic reaction, the highest dose should provide a distinct toxic effect while the lowest dose should not produce any detectable toxic reaction (Leclair & Willard, 1970). To obtain maximum information on the dose-response characteristics of the compound, at least two intermediate doses should be included.

Information from subacute toxicity tests is of value in the selection of appropriate dose levels, when commencing chronic toxicity studies. In general, however, it is highly desirable to establish the chemobiokinetic behaviour (Chapter 4) of the test compound and if possible its major metabolites in the test species prior to undertaking a chronic toxicity test. Particular attention should be given to evidence for dose-dependent detoxification. Studies of this nature will provide information on the degree to which the chemical may be expected to accumulate in various body compartments and unexpectedly produce evidence of toxicity. Since it is the object of chronic toxicity tests to establish dose-response patterns and "no-observed-adverse-effect levels", a minimum of three dose levels should be used. The upper dose level should produce some slight evidence of toxicity, but should be compatible with normal physiological function (Leclair & Willard, 1970). The lowest dose level would not be expected to produce evidence of toxicity (Health & Welfare, Canada, 1973).

3.4.2.3 Method of administration

The route of administration in subacute and chronic studies should be that through which man is likely to be exposed. For gases and volatile industrial solvents, inhalation studies are recommended (Magill et al., 1956) (Chapter 6), while for food additives, pesticides, and other chemicals likely to come into contact with food or water, the oral route is recommended (Leclair & Willard, 1970; National Academy of Sciences, 1975). Incorporation of the test chemical into the diet or drinking water is an appropriate means of administration; however, care must be taken to ensure the stability of the chemical in the dosing medium. The concentration of the test chemical in the diet should be determined periodically to ensure uniform dispersion and to aid in the quantification of achieved doses. In some cases, the chemical may be unpalatable and administration by gavage, or, in the case of dogs, by capsules may be necessary.

The diet is the preferred vehicle of administration, but it is absolutely essential that the chemical be present in the diet in an unaltered form; toxicity may be altered by interaction with dietary constituents (Kello & Kostial, 1973). In rodent studies, the compound may be administered in the diet as a fraction of the total diet, or a sufficient quantity of the chemical may be added to the diet to achieve predetermined dose levels (in mg per kg body weight per day). In the latter case, it is necessary to adjust the dietary concentration weekly or biweekly to maintain a constant dose level, since food consumption per unit of body weight decreases as the animal gets older. If, in rodent tests, the concentration of the test compound in the diet is kept constant from weaning to maturity, the actual dose received will be reduced by approximately 2.5 times over the dosing period. This may have profound effects on the severity of the toxic response and may be mistaken for tolerance. In chronic toxicity tests, the chemical should be administered daily over the entire treatment period. As an aid to interpretation of the test, only one lot chemical should be used for the entire test unless the purity of the chemical is definitely assured.

3.4.2.4   *Biochemical organ function tests*

In subacute studies, the use of a species such as the dog instead of a rodent species permits the application of a wider range of biochemical organ function tests because larger samples of blood can be collected on a routine basis. Organ function studies should be undertaken prior to initiation of the test, 3 and 10 days after the start of dosing, at 30-day intervals thereafter throughout the test, and terminally. The tests described for the chronic studies are also applicable in subacute studies.

In the course of chronic toxicity tests, studies should be undertaken to evaluate the functional integrity of various organ systems. Assessment of the urinary system should commence with an examination of the urine. Freshly-voided urine samples should be obtained every one to three months from the test animals and examined for the presence of occult blood, glucose, protein, and bilirubin using simple diagnostic procedures. If positive effects are noted, quantitative methods should be applied as outlined by Bergmeyer (1965). Samples of freshly-voided urine should also be filtered through Millipore filters and the filters stained according to the Papanicolaou method (Frost, 1969) to detect the presence of renal tubular cells or other cell types derived from the urinary system. Urinary calculi and parasite eggs (Chapman, 1969) may be detected by this method. Blood urea-nitrogen levels and other standard tests of kidney function may be applied but they usually lack sufficient sensitivity to detect subtle changes in kidney function.

Several test procedures are available for the assessment of liver function. Most of these methods involve an examination of the serum levels of hepatic enzymes that may be released in the serum folowing liver injury (Czok, 1965; Henley et al., 1966; Zimmerman, 1974). Korsrud et al. (1972) compared the sensitivity of various liver function tests in the rat and noted that serum sorbitol dehydrogenase (1.1.1.14) activity (an enzyme specific to the liver) correlated well with the degree of histological alteration produced by hepatotoxic agents such as carbon tetrachloride, 2,2'-iminobisethanol (diethanolamine), and ethanethioamide (thioacetamide). However, Grice et al. (1971) noted that pathological changes induced by these compounds must be reasonably advanced before elevations are noted in serum glutamic-oxaloacetic transaminase (2.6.1.1), lactate dehydrogenase (1.1.1.27), or lactate dehydrogenase isoenzymes, suggesting that changes in serum enzyme activity may not be as sensitive an indicator of toxicity as pathomorphological examination. Tests of liver function such as serum enzyme activities and various clearance tests were reviewed recently by

Balazs (1975). A complete review of the principles and applications of these tests is given by Cornish (1971) and further discussion of these methods is found in Part II, Chapter 8. Suffice it to say, that a transient increase in the activity of serum enzymes or other organ-derived constituents may result from a transient change in organ homeostasis that produces no lasting toxic effect.

For routine screening of organ function in large animals, Charbonneau et al. (1974) used clinical procedures that can measure the concentration of several serum enzymes and inorganic and other constituents by automated methods. In general, these methods are not sufficiently standardized or reproducible to detect minor alterations in organ function but they do serve as a useful guide to general clinical status.

3.4.2.5 *Physiological measurements*

In subacute studies, it is often possible to detect ensuing pathological events through application of physiological function tests.

In all studies, food consumption and body weight should be recorded weekly in all animals. Weight gain per unit of food consumed should be calculated (Munro et al., 1969). This gives a measure of the efficiency of food use. The daily dose of chemical should be calculated from data on food intake and body weight. Similar measurements of food intake and body weight must be carried out in chronic toxicity tests. If the test chemical is incorporated into the drinking water, water intake must be measured. These measurements should be conducted on a weekly basis during the entire test. The data can be used to estimate the dose of chemical received and are necessary in the establishment of dose-response relationships. Body weight changes serve as a sensitive indication of the general health status of test animals. Any rapid loss in body weight may signal the onset of intoxication or disease. Computerized methods for recording and analysing this type of data are available (Munro et al., 1972).

Under special circumstances, when the target organs of toxicity have been identified during subacute studies, it is appropriate to conduct measurements of the physiological function of organ systems. Procedures such as electrocardiography (Grice et al., 1971), electroencephalography (Flodmark & Steinwall, 1963; Harada et al., 1967; Mann, 1970), electromyography (Chaffin, 1969), nerve conduction studies and measurement of evoked potentials (Barnet et al., 1971; Hrbek et al., 1972) may greatly assist in defining the functional effects of chemicals (Chapter 8). Such tests are expensive to perform and require highly specialized equipment and personnel. They have limited application in routine testing but may be used to define mechanisms of action. It is imperative that the results of such studies be correlated with clinical and pathological findings (Grice, 1972; Osborne & Dent, 1973).

3.4.2.6 *Metabolic studies*

Subacute studies provide an excellent opportunity to undertake metabolic investigations under conditions of repeated exposure that may alter the nature of the metabolites and the rate of metabolic transformation of the test compound. Urine and faeces can be collected and examined for the presence of metabolites and, by undertaking serial sacrifices at three-week intervals, the kinetics of accumulation of the compound in various body compartments can be evaluated.

To gain an understanding of the metabolic fate of a chemical that may have a long biological half-time, such as hexachlorobenzene (Grant et al., 1975), three extra groups of animals need to be studied for tissue distribution to provide information that is necessary for estimating the potential hazard to man. The principles of these methods are reviewed in Chapter 4. Often it is desirable, in subacute studies, to study the kinetics of the test compound and its metabolites following completion of the dosing period. If extra groups of animals are initially included for this purpose, much valuable additional information on the compound may be obtained.

3.4.2.7 *Haematological information*

In subacute studies involving rodents, haematological studies should be undertaken on randomly selected subgroups of animals prior to initiation of the test, at 30-day intervals, and on all animals terminally. Bone marrow should be examined terminally. Nonrodent test animals should be examined at similar intervals.

In chronic toxicity studies involving rodents, haematological studies of circulating blood cells should be undertaken on randomly selected subgroups of animals prior to initiation of the test, at 3 to 6-month intervals and, on selected animals, terminally. Bone marrow should be examined terminally and, if indicated, at interim times by biopsy.

To assess the clinical state of nonrodents, haematological variables should be examined frequently.

A set of test procedures is necessary for routine haematological screening and the tests must be of sufficient sensitivity and accuracy to be of practical value for use in large numbers of laboratory animals (Cartwright, 1969; Schalm, 1967; Sirridge, 1967). Quantification of blood cells and thorough study of cellular morphology by a haematologist, experienced in small animal medicine, is necessary in the study of haematological disorders. Haematological evaluation of experimental animals is facilitated by the fact that repeated sampling is relatively easy and small amounts of blood are required, and that single-cell systems can be studied to obtain information on cell production, destruction, defects, and dysfunction. For erythroid evaluation, the numbers of circulating erythrocytes must be counted and the haematocrit and haemoglobin concentration measured. As an index of erythropoietic activity in the bone marrow, a reticulocyte count should be carried out. Morphological assessment of erythrocytes is mandatory. The number of circulating leucocytes should be quantified and a differential count and morphological assessment should be made. To evaluate the functional capacity and malignant changes in the blood-forming organs, bone marrow should be examined terminally. From bone marrow smears a differential count and morphological assessment can be carried out. Imprints of lymph nodes or spleen permit a detailed cytological study of normal and abnormal cells present that may be of diagnostic significance.

To assess haemostatic function, it will be necessary to evaluate platelets, coagulation systems, and fibrinolysis. Screening tests include platelet count, clot retraction, one stage prothrombin time, and activated partial thromboplastin time. More specific evaluation may require factor assays, thrombin time, fibrinogen determination, euglobulin clot lysis time, prothrombin consumption time, platelet aggregation, and adhesiveness.

3.4.2.8 *Postmortem examination*

In every toxicity evaluation, all animals should be given a thorough gross autopsy and detailed records kept on each animal. Samples of all organs and supporting structures should be saved for histopathological examination. Detailed autopsy methods are outlined in Chapter 5.

In chronic toxicity testing it is often useful to incorporate interim autopsy dates so that the progression of lesions may be studied. At interim sacrifices and terminally (if sufficient animals are in a healthy state), the major organs should be weighed. Organ weights may serve as a useful index of toxicity; however, care must be taken in the interpretation of the data. Decreased absolute organ weights in treated animals may be merely a reflection of lower body weight and calculation of organ to body weight ratios may increase the usefulness of the data (Feron, 1973).

3.4.2.9 *Controls*

In the evaluation of both subacute and chronic toxicity, special attention must be given to the control animals. The quality of data obtained from the control animals has an important bearing on the interpretation of results from the treated animals. Suitable numbers of control animals of the same age and body weight as the treated animals must be included in the experimental design in a statistically randomized fashion.

Except for treatment with the test chemical, these animals should be handled identically to the test subjects and all measurements conducted on the treated animals must be carried out on the controls with the same precision and frequency. In studies in which the chemical is administered by gavage, the control animals should receive the suspending vehicle in an amount equivalent to the treated animals. The incidence of spontaneous lesions or of other changes in control animals must be carefully noted and the interpretation of data obtained from treated animals must include an appreciation of the role that spontaneous disease processes may play in the manifestation of chemical toxicity. It is particularly important, in studies with rodents, to have detailed information on the incidence of neoplastic diseases, since some species and strains (Sher, 1972) may have a high background incidence of certain tumours which tends to reduce longevity and decrease the chance of observing chronic toxic effects. In addition, the chemical under test may alter the incidence of spontaneous tumours and other diseases or may induce new tumours, and this possibility must be taken into consideration in the evaluation of the chronic toxicity of chemicals. In all cases, responses attributable to the test compound must be compared with background observations in controls. For this reason, the quality of the toxicological data rests heavily on the adequacy of the control values (Weil & Carpenter, 1969).

3.4.3 Alternative approaches in chronic toxicity

3.4.3.1 *Perinatal exposure*

The majority of chemicals to which man may be exposed are present in air, food, or water for his entire lifetime. Recently, there has been an attempt to duplicate the human situation in the chronic toxicity test by exposing the test animals during the neonatal period as well as throughout life (Friedman, 1969). In this approach, groups of weaning animals (usually rodents) are exposed to the test chemical until they reach sexual maturity. They are then mated, within dose groups, and the treatment is continued during pregnancy and lactation. Following weaning, the offspring are transferred to their parents' diet and exposed for the balance of their lifetime to the test chemical. The details of this test procedure have been outlined in a recent Canadian Government publication (Health & Welfare, Canada, 1973) and by Epstein (1969). It is not known yet whether this technique increases the sensitivity of the chronic toxicity test, but it is known that exposure to carcinogens in the perinatal period will often increase the incidence and decrease the latent period of carcinogenesis (Tomatis & Mohr, ed., 1973).

Further study of this method is required to evaluate its usefulness fully. It should be pointed out, however, that this procedure adds considerably to the cost and length of the chronic toxicity test.

3.4.3.2 *Use of nonrodent species*

In chronic toxicity studies with nonrodent species such as nonhuman primates, dogs, or cats, it is often not feasible to expose the animals to the test compound for their entire lifespan, even though they may be the species of choice. Under such conditions, careful examination of the kinetic and metabolic behaviour of the test compound in these species may substitute, to some extent, for the decreased treatment period (provided the anticipated endpoint is not carcinogenesis). Carefully conducted kinetic studies will assist in establishing when steady-state tissue concentrations of the test chemical and its metabolites have been achieved. If treatment is continued for a substantial period after the establishment of steady-state kinetics without any increase in the degree of toxic effects observed clinically, or during interim sacrifice, this may partially substitute for a lifetime study and provide increased assurance for those having to make regulatory decisions If this approach is not feasible, it may be possible to test human metabolites in rodent species (Health & Welfare, Canada, 1973).

3.5   Evaluation and Interpretation of the Results of Toxicity Tests

The evaluation and interpretation of toxicity studies starts with a clear definition of experimental objectives. The design of the experiment should be such that the objectives can be reasonably achieved. Well designed and carefully executed experiments add greatly to the ease with which results can be evaluated and interpreted and also to confidence in the experimental data.

The primary usefulness of the LD_{50} determination is to obtain some idea of the magnitude of the acute toxic dose (Frazer & Sharratt, 1969) and information concerning the type of toxic effects of the chemical. Such information includes whether death is immediate or delayed, whether recovery from a near lethal dose is rapid or complete or both, or whether the cause of death is narcosis with respiratory failure, lung oedema, or liver necrosis.

However, the LD_{50} provides little information for the assessment of the hazard from compounds to which the human population is exposed for extended periods of time. Although it has been suggested that compounds that do not show adverse effects when given in doses of 3–5 g per kg body weight are essentially non-toxic (National Academy of Sciences, 1975), there are numerous examples in the literature of compounds with LD_{50}

values greater than 5 g per kg which produce toxic effects, when given in low doses for extended periods of time (Frazer & Sharratt, 1968). If the main object of an acute toxicity test is not to establish a value for the LD_{50} with precision, but to learn something about the way in which the chemical acts as a poison, as suggested by Paget & Barnes (1964), this can best be accomplished by tests involving repeated daily administration to a few animals for a period of 5–21 days. The information provided by the LD_{50} regarding the effects of acute exposure to toxic compounds may be useful as a guide for selecting doses for such studies.

The primary objective of subacute and chronic toxicity studies is to determine the nature and severity of toxic effects and the "no-observed-adverse-effect" dose level. These data may then be used in the establishment of acceptable levels of exposure for man.

Data on group weight gain or body weight change should be plotted against time, and differences between groups should be evaluated statistically. Changes in body weight with time are best evaluated statistically using trend analysis procedures (Armitage, 1955). Food (and water) consumption data should be handled in a similar fashion. Reduced body weight or weight gain in otherwise healthy treated animals may be due to reduced food intake owing to its unpalatability or to a specific toxic effect of the chemical resulting in reduced efficiency of food use. Using data on the dietary concentration of the test chemical, food consumption, and body weight, the mean daily dose of chemical received (in mg/kg body weight/day or similar units) should be calculated. Automated data processing procedures to accomplish this are available (Munro et al., 1972).

Data on organ weights should be evaluated and interpreted with great care. Increased relative (to body or brain weight) organ weights may also result from adaptation to stress phenomena or from metabolic overloading of biochemical pathways or physiological processes. Increased liver weight, for example, may result from a stimulation of *de novo* protein synthesis in the smooth endoplasmic reticulum (SER). This results in a morphologically detectable increase in SER. The biochemical counterpart of this increase is an increased ability of the liver to metabolize certain foreign substances, sometimes including the test compound and endogenous substrates, due to a stimulation in the activity of hepatic mixed function oxidases (Staubli et al., 1969). These adaptative changes may manifest themselves clinically as tolerance. Often these changes are reversible upon cessation of dosing and do not produce lasting toxicological effects but the implications of chronically elevated levels of these enzymes is not known. Certain enzyme inducers may cause impairment of liver function and produce pathological and biochemical changes (Feuer et al., 1965).

Data on biochemical and haematological effects should be tabulated and compared with control values using statistical procedures (Johnson, 1950). Any observed effects should be correlated with clinical and pathological findings. A biochemical or haematological change such as reduction in liver glycogen or an alteration in white cell count may not be indicative of a toxic effect, but an adaptation to a stress situation (National Academy of Sciences, 1975). In general, changes in homeostasis must be carefully evaluated since reversible shifts do not necessarily imply a toxic effect in the absence of other toxic manifestations.

Changes in the functional state of physiological or neurological processes, such as an alteration in the electrocardiogram or abnormal behaviour, may result from pharmacological or pathological effects of the test compound. Changes in functional state must be closely correlated with their morphological counterpart in order to evaluate their toxicological importance properly (Grice, 1972).

The cornerstone of experimental toxicology is the pathological examination. Usually, decisions regarding the safety of a compound are based on this evidence. All pathological findings in test animals should be graded carefully and their incidence tabulated (see Chapter 5). Spontaneous lesions in control animals should also be noted and compared to the observations in control animals in previous experiments or in the literature (Peck, 1974) to ensure that the incidence and nature of the lesions is representative of the strain. Pathological data should be analysed rigorously using appropriate statistical methods (Fleiss, 1973) and spurious observations apparently unrelated to treatment should be identified. Lesions that are dose-related should be studied in detail and correlated with gross pathological findings, clinical observations, and other variables (Grice, 1972).

It is not uncommon in chronic toxicity testing to find pathological or other changes that occur in low incidence and that are not dose-related but occur only in treated animals. Such reactions may be idiosyncratic in nature or may be due to the hypersensitivity of certain animals. Nevertheless, they deserve special attention since they may be indicative of a hitherto unsuspected toxic effect. The clinical history and other data from such animals should be reviewed with great care and an attempt should be made to determine the reason for the observed effects. Toxic effects that occur in extremely low incidence present special problems in interpretation. There is no substitute for experience in this respect and the prudent investigator will consult the knowledgeable experts in this field (Zbinden, 1973).

ARCOS, J. C. (1968) *Chemical induction of cancer.* Vol. 1, New York, Academic Press.

ARMITAGE, P. & ALLEN, I. (1950) Methods of estimating the LD_{50} in quantal response data. *J. Hyg. (Lond.),* **48:** 298–322.

ARMITAGE, P. (1955) Tests for linear trends in proportions and frequencies. *Biometrics,* **11:** 375–385.

BALAZS, T. (1975) Toxic effects of chemicals in the liver. *FDA By-lines,* **5:** 291–303.

BARNES, J. M. (1960) Toxicity testing. In: Schilling, R. S. F., ed. *Modern trends in occupational health,* London, Butterworths & Co., pp. 20–32.

BARNET, A. B., OHRICH, E. S., & SHANKS, B. L. (1971) EEG evoked responses to repetitive auditory stimulation in normal Down's-syndrome infants. *Dev. Med. Child. Neurol.,* **13:** 321–329.

BEIN, H. J. (1963) Rational and irrational numbers in toxicology. *Proc. Euro. Soc. Study Drug Toxicity,* **2:** 15–26.

BERGMEYER, H. U. (1965) *Methods of enzymatic analysis.* New York, Academic Press.

BRODIE, B. B. (1964) [The difficulties of transposing experimental results obtained in animals to man.]. *Actual. pharmacol.,* **17:** 1–23 (in French).

CANADIAN COUNCIL ON ANIMAL CARE (1973) *Care of experimental animals—a guide for Canada.*

CARTWRIGHT, G. E. (1969) *Diagnostic laboratory hematology,* 4th ed. New York, Grune & Stratton.

CHAFFIN, D. B. (1969) Surface electromyography frequency analysis as a diagnostic tool. *J. occup. Med.,* **11:** 109–115.

CHAPMAN, W. H. (1969) Infection with *Trichosomomoides crassicauda* as a factor in the induction of bladder tumours in rats fed 2-acetylaminofluorene. *Invest. Urol.,* **7:** 154–159.

CHARBONNEAU, S. M., MUNRO, I. C., NERA, E. A., WILLES, R. F., KUIPER-GOODMAN, T., IVERSON, F., MOODIE, C. A., STOLZ, D. R., ARMSTRONG, F. A. J., UTHE, J. F., & GRICE, H. C. (1974) Subacute toxicity of methylmercury in the adult cat. *Toxicol. appl. Pharmacol.,* **27:** 569–581.

CONNEY, A. H., SCHNEIDERMAN, K., JACOBSON, M., & KUNTZMAN, R. (1965) Drug-induced changes in steroid metabolism. *Ann. NY Acad. Sci.,* **123:** 98–109.

CORNISH, H. H. (1971) Problems posed by observations of serum enzyme changes in toxicology. *CRC Crit. Rev. Toxicol.,* **1:** 1–32.

COX, D. R. (1958) *Planning of experiments,* New York, John Wiley, Chapter 5.

CZOK, R. (1965) The behaviour of plasma enzymes in toxicological experiments. *Proc. Eur. Soc. Study Drug Toxicity,* **5:** 68–83.

DHEW (1972) *Guide for the care and use of laboratory animals* (prepared by Committee for the Revision of the Guide for Laboratory Animal Facilities and Care, Institute of Laboratory Animal Resources). Washington DC, Govt Printing Office (DHEW Publ. No. (NIH) 73–23).

DIECHMANN, W. B. & LEBLANC, T. J. (1943) Determination of the approximate lethal dose with about six animals. *J. ind. Hyg. Toxicol.,* **25:** 415–417.

DIEKE, S. H. & RICHTER, C. P. (1945) Acute toxicity of thiourea to rats in relation to age, diet, strain and species variation. *J. Pharmacol. exp. Ther.,* **83:** 195–202.

EPSTEIN, S. (1969) A catch-all toxicological screen. *Experientia (Basle),* **25:** 617.

FERON, V. J. (1973) An evaluation of the criterion "organ weight" under conditions of growth retardation. *Food Cosmet. Toxicol.* **11:** 85–94.

FEUER, G., GOLBERG, L., & LE PELLEY, J. R. (1965) Liver response tests. I. Exploratory studies on glucose 6-phosphatase and other liver enzymes. *Food Cosmet. Toxicol.,* **3:** 235–249.

FLEISS, J. L. (1973) *Statistical methods for rates and proportions.* New York, John Wiley (Wiley Series in Probability and Mathematical Statistics).

FLODMARK, S. & STEINWALL, O. (1963) Differentiated effects on certain blood brain barrier phenomena and on the EEG produced by means of intracarotidly applied mercuric dichloride. *Acta. Physiol. Scand.,* **57:** 446–453.

FOUTS, J. R. & HART, L. G. (1965) Hepatic drug metabolism during the perinatal period. *Ann. NY Acad. Sci.,* **123:** 245–251.

FRAZER, A. C. & SHARRATT, M. (1969) The value and limitations of animal studies in the prediction of effects in man. In: *The use of animals in toxicological studies—UFAW Symposium, England, 1968,* Potters Bar, England, 41 pp.

FRIEDMAN, L. (1969) Symposium on the evaluation of the safety of food additives and chemical residues. II. The role of the laboratory animal study of intermediate duration for evaluation of safety. *Toxicol. appl. Pharmacol.,* **16:** 498–506.

FROST, J. K. (1969) *Manual for the tenth postgraduate institute for pathologists in clinical cytopathology.* Baltimore, MD, Johns Hopkins Hospital.

GEHRING, P. J., ROWE, V. K., & MCCOLLISTER, S. B. (1973) Toxicology: cost-time. *Food Cosmet. Toxicol.,* **11:** 1097–1110.

GRANT, D. L., HATINA, G. V., & MUNRO, I. C. (1975) Hexachlorobenzene accumulation and decline of tissue residues and relationship to some toxicity criteria in rats. *Environ. Qual. Saf.,* Supplement Vol. III, pp. 562–568.

GRICE, H. C. (1972) The changing role of pathology in modern safety evaluation. *CRC Crit. Rev. Toxicol.,* **1:** 119–152.

GRICE, H. C., BARTH, M. L., CORNISH, H. H., FOSTER, G. V., & GRAY, R. H. (1971) Experimental cobalt cardiomyopathy: correlation between electrocardiography and pathology. *Cardiol. Res.,* **4:** 452–456.

GRIFFITH, J. F. (1964) Inter-laboratory variations in the determination of acute oral LD_{50}. *Toxicol. appl. Pharmacol.,* **6:** 726–730.

HAGAN, J. M. (1959) Acute toxicity. In: *Appraisal of the safety of chemicals in food, drugs and cosmetics,* Assoc. Food & Drug Officials of USA, pp. 17–25.

HARADA, Y., MIYAMOTO, Y., NONAKA, I., OHTA, S., & NINOMIYA, T. (1967) Electro-encephalographic studies on Minamata Disease in children. *Dev. Med. Child Neurol.,* **10:** 257–258.

HEALTH & WELFARE, CANADA (1970) *Guide for the preparation of submissions for food additives.* Ottawa, Health & Welfare.

HEALTH & WELFARE, CANADA (1973) *The testing of chemicals for carcinogenicity, mutagenicity and teratogenicity.* Ottawa, Health & Welfare.

HENLEY, K. S., SCHMIDT, E., & SCHMIDT, W. (1966) *Enzymes in serum, their use in diagnosis.* Springfield, IL, Thomas.

HORN, H. J. (1956) Simplified LD_{50} (or ED_{50}) calculations. *Biometrics,* **12:** 311–321.

HRBEK, A., KARLBERG, P., KJELLMER, J., & OLSSON, T. (1972) Evoked EEG responses in newborns with asphyxia and IRDs. *Pediatr. Res.,* **6:** 61.

HURST, E. W. (1958) Sexual differences in the toxicity and therapeutic action of chemical substances. In: Walpole, A. L. & Spinks, A., ed. *The evaluation of drug toxicity,* London, Churchill, pp. 12–25.

JOHNSON, L. P. V. (1950) *An introduction to applied biometrics.* Minneapolis, Burgers Publ., Co.

JONDORF, W. R., MAICKEL, R. P., & BRODIE, B. B. (1959) Instability of newborn mice and guinea pigs to metabolize drugs. *Biochem. Pharmacol.,* **1:** 352–354.

KELLO, D. & KOSTIAL, K. (1973) The effect of milk diets on lead metabolism in rats. *Environ. Res.,* **6:** 355–360.

KORSRUD, G. O., GRICE, H. C., & McLAUGHLAN, J. U. (1972) Sensitivity of several serum enzymes in detecting carbon tetrachloride—including liver damage in rats. *Toxicol. appl. Pharmacol.,* **22:** 474–483.

LECLAIR, J. M. & WILLARD, J. W. (1970) *Guide for the preparation of submissions on tolerances for incidental contaminants and agricultural chemicals in food.* Ottawa, Canada, Food & Drug Directorate, Dept of National Health & Welfare.

LITCHFIELD, J. T. (1962) Evaluation of the safety of new drugs by means of tests in animals.

113

Clin. Pharmacol. & Therap., **3:** 665–672.

LITCHFIELD, J. T. & WILCOXON, F. A. (1947) A simplified method of evaluating dose-effect experiments. *J. Pharm. exp. Ther.,* **95:** 99–113.

LOOMIS, T. A. (1968) *Essentials of toxicology.* Philadelphia, Lea & Febiger.

LU, F. J., JESSUP, D. C., & LAVALLEE, A. (1965) Toxicity of pesticides in young versus adult rats. *Food Cosmet. Toxicol.,* **3:** 591–596.

MAGILL, P. I., HOLDEN, F. R., & ACKLEY, C. (1956) *Air Pollution Handbook.* New York, McGraw-Hill.

MANN, L. I. (1970) Developmental aspects and the effect of carbon dioxide tension on fetal cephalic metabolism and electroencephalogram. *Exp. Neurol.,* **26:** 148–159.

MARZULLI, F. N. (1968) Ocular side effects of drugs. *Food Cosmet. Toxicol.,* **6:** 221–223.

McGRATH, J. T. (1960) *Neurological examination of the dog with clinicopathological observation.* 2nd ed. Philadelphia, Lea & Febiger.

MILLER, L. C. & TAINTER, M. L. (1944) Estimation of the ED_{50} and its error by means of log-probit graph paper. *Proc. Soc. Exp. Biol. Med. NY,* **57:** 261–264.

MORRISON, J. K., QUINTON, R. M., & REINERT, H. (1968) The purpose and value of LD_{50} determinations. In: Boyland, E. & Goulding, R., ed. *Modern trends in toxicology.* London, Butterworths, pp. 1–17.

MOWBRAY, J. B. & CADELL, T. E. (1962) Early behaviour patterns in rhesus monkeys. *J. Comp. Physiol. Psychol.,* **55:** 350–357.

MUNRO, I. C., MIDDLETON, E. J., & GRICE, H. C. (1969) Biochemical and pathological changes in rats fed brominated cottonseed oil for 80 days. *Food Cosmet. Toxicol.,* **7:** 25–33.

MUNRO, I. C., CHARBONNEAU, S. M., & WILLES, R. F. (1972) An automated data acquisition and computer-based computation system for application to toxicological studies in laboratory animals. *Lab. Anim. Sci.,* **22:** 753–756.

MUNRO, I. C., MOODIE, C. A., KREWSKI, D., & GRICE, H. C. (1974) Carcinogenicity study of commercial saccharin in the rat. *Toxicol. appl. Pharmacol.,* **32:** 513–526.

NATIONAL ACADEMY OF SCIENCES (1975) *Principles for evaluating chemicals in the environment.* Washington, DC, National Academy of Sciences.

NEWBERNE, P., ROGERS, A. E., & WOGAN, G. N. (1968) Hepatorenal lesions in rats fed a low lipotrope diet and exposed to aflatoxin. *J. Nutr.,* **94:** 331–343.

OSBORNE, B. E. & DENT, N. J. (1973) Electrocardiography and blood chemistry in the detection of myocardial lesions in dogs. *Food Cosmet. Toxicol.,* **11:** 265–276.

PAGET, G. E. & BARNES, J. M. (1964) Toxicity tests. In: Laurence, D. R. & Bacharach, A. L., ed. *Evaluation of drug activities: Pharmacometrics,* London, New York, Academic Press, Vol. 1, pp. 135–166.

PECK, H. M. (1974) Design of experiments to detect carcinogenic effects of drugs. In: *CRC Carcinogenesis testing of chemicals,* Cleveland, OH, CRC Press, pp. 1–13.

RUMKE, CHR. L. (1964) Some limitations of animal tests. In: Laurence, D. R. & Bacharach, A. L., ed. *Evaluation of drug activities: Pharmacometrics,* London, New York, Academic Press, Vol. 1, pp. 125–133.

SCHALM, O. W. (1967) *Veterinary haematology,* 2nd ed. Philadelphia, Lea & Febiger.

SCOTT, W. J., JOHNSTON, J. W., JOHNSTON, C. D., & BELILES, R. P. (1966) Comparative acute toxicities of isoproterenol and metraproterenol. *Toxicol. appl. Pharmacol.,* **8:** 353.

SETNIKAR, I. & MAGISTRETTI, M. J. (1964) The toxicity of central nervous system stimulants in rats of different ages. *Proc. Eur. Soc. Drug Toxicity,* **4:** 132–139.

SHER, S. P. (1972) Mammary tumours in control rats: literature tabulation. *Toxicol. appl. Pharmacol.,* **22:** 562–588.

SIRRIDGE, M. S. (1967) *Laboratory evaluation of haemostasis.* Philadelphia, Lea & Febiger.

SNEDECOR, J. W. & COCHRAN, W. G. (1967) *Statistical methods* 6th ed., Ames, IA, Iowa State University Press, pp. 111–114, 221–223.

SONTAG, J. M., PAGE, N. P., & SAFFIOTTI, U. (1975) *Guidelines for carcinogen bioassay in small rodents.* Bethesda, MD, National Cancer Institute.

STAUBLI, W., HESS, R., & WEIBEL, E. R. (1969) Correlated morphometric and biochemical studies on the liver cell. II. Effects of phenobarbital on rat hepatocytes. *J. cell. Biol.*, **42:** 92–112.

THOMPSON, W. (1947) Use of moving averages and interpolation to estimate median effective dose. *Bac. Rev.*, **11:** 115–141.

TOMATIS, L. & MOHR, U., ed. (1973) *Transplacental carcinogenesis,* IARC Sci. Publ. No. 4, 181 pp.

WEIL, C. S. (1952) Relationship between short- and long-term feeding studies in designing an effective toxicity test. *Agric. Food Chem.*, **11:** 486–491.

WEIL, C. S., WOODSIDE, M. D., BERNARD, J. R., & CARPENTER, C. P. (1969) Relationship between single peroral, one-week and ninety-day feeding studies. *Toxicol. appl. Pharmacol.*, **14:** 426–431.

WEIL, C. S., & CARPENTER, C. P. (1969) Abnormal values in control groups during repeated-dose toxicological studies. *Toxicol. appl. Pharmacol.*, **14:** 335–339.

WEINBERG, M. S., GOLDHAMEN, R. E., & CARSON, S. (1966) Acute oral toxicity of various drugs in newborn rats after treatment of the dam during gestation. *Toxicol. appl. Pharmacol.*, **9:** 234–239.

WORDEN, A. N. & HARPER, K. H. (1963) Oral toxicity as influenced by method of administration. *Proc. Eur. Soc. Study Drug Toxicity,* **2:** 15–26.

WHO (1958) WHO Technical Report Series No. 144. (Procedures for the testing of intentional food additives to establish their safety for use—2nd report of the joint FAO/WHO Expert Committee on Food Additives), 19 pp.

WHO (1972) *Health hazards of the human environment,* Geneva, WHO, 387 pp.

YEARLY, R. A. & BENISH, R. A. (1965) A comparison of the acute toxicities of drugs in newborn and adult rats. *Toxicol. appl. Pharmacol.*, **7:** 504.

ZBINDEN, G. (1973) *Progress in toxicology: special topics.* Vol. 1. New York, Springer-Verlag.

ZIMMERMAN, H. J. (1974) Serum enzyme measurement in experimental hepatotoxicity. *Israel J. med. Sci.*, **10:** 328–332.

4. CHEMOBIOKINETICS AND METABOLISM

4.1 Introduction

The objective of chemobiokinetic studies is to obtain data that allow reliable assessment of the hazard of environmental chemicals to man. Since effects are related to the amounts or concentrations of a chemical in tissues and cells, it is imperative to elucidate the dynamics of the toxicant at the target site. It should be emphasized that the toxicant may be either the parent chemical or a metabolite or degradation product formed from it. Thus, the qualitative identification of the degradation products of a chemical together with a quantitative characterization of their fate, as well as the fate of the parent chemical, as a function of time, are inextricably associated in a proper chemobiokinetic evaluation. In the context of this chapter, the word "chemobiokinetics" has been used in place of "pharmacokinetics" because too often the latter implies restriction of this scientific discipline to drugs. The term chemobiokinetics is proposed to emphasize its importance in evaluating the biological effects of all chemicals.

4.2 Absorption

4.2.1 General principles

Absorption of a chemical into the body can take place, potentially, by all routes of exposure. In assessing the toxicity and, ultimately, the hazard of a chemical, the oral, dermal, and inhalation routes of exposure are of primary importance. Following absorption, the chemical is distributed by the blood to the various tissues. Therefore, the rate of absorption is frequently estimated by determining the concentration of the chemical in the plasma as a function of time following exposure.

The route of administration can greatly influence the rate at which a foreign chemical enters the body. Upon ingestion, the gastric contents and pH of the stomach can influence the rate of absorption of the chemical. In the small intestine, food may either enhance or delay absorption. Indeed, the environment of the gastrointestinal tract (pH, food, bacteria) may change the parent chemical into another chemical. The inhalation route allows a chemical to pass rapidly into the blood without encountering drastic changes in pH, food, or microflora. The skin effectively retards the absorption of many chemicals; however, it should not be considered as an absolute barrier. Some chemicals readily penetrate intact skin and a minor abrasion of the skin may greatly enhance the absorption of many chemicals.

In order that a chemical may be absorbed into the bloodstream, it must cross one or more semipermeable membranes, such as the gastrointestinal epithelium, the lining of the respiratory tract, or the epidermis of the skin. Membranes are essentially lipoproteins with aqueous pores through which water-soluble molecules can pass. The pore size varies from 4 Å (intestinal epithelium and mast cells) to 30 Å (capillaries), allowing the passage of molecules with molecular weights less than 100–200 to approximately 60 000, respectively. Most membranes have an electrical potential that may effectively preclude the ready penetration of charged chemical species. Thus it is obvious that the absorption of a chemical depends on its physico-chemical properties, molecular size, shape, degree of ionization, and lipid solubility. For a more thorough discussion, the reader is referred to Davson & Danielli (1952) and Schanker (1962a).

Three mechanisms have been proposed to explain how a chemical passes across a cell membrane: (*a*) passive diffusion through the membrane, (*b*) filtration through membranous pores, and (*c*) specialized transport systems that carry water-soluble and large molecules across the membrane by means of a "carrier".

Passive diffusion is considered to be the principal mechanism by which chemicals can cross cell membranes. The rate of passive diffusion of a molecule is proportional to the concentration gradient across the membrane, the membrane thickness, the area available for diffusion, and the diffusion constant, in accordance with Fick's Law (La Du et al., 1972). The rate of passage is related directly to the lipid solubility (Brodie, 1964). However, since absorption requires passage through an aqueous- as well as a lipo-phase, the absorption of a chemical with an extremely low solubility in water may be impeded in spite of a high lipid-to-water partition coefficient. The passive diffusion also depends on the extent of the ionization and the lipid solubility of the ionized and nonionized species (Brodie, 1964).

Filtration is a process by which a chemical passes through the aqueous pores in the membrane, and is governed by the size and shape of the molecule. The bulk flow of water across the membrane produced by an osmotic gradient or hydrostatic pressure can act as a carrier for chemicals.

Specialized transport processes are needed to explain the transport and kinetic behaviour of large, lipid insoluble molecules and ions. Two types of carrier-mediated transport systems have been recognized: active transport and facilitated diffusion. The carrier in both systems is some component of the membrane that combines with the chemical and assists its passage across the membrane. It has a limited capacity and when it is saturated, the rate of transfer is no longer dependent on the concentration of the chemical and assumes zero order kinetics. Structure, conformation, size, and charge

117

are important in determining the affinity of a molecule for a carrier site, and competition for carrier site will occur.

Active transport is a carrier-mediated transport system which moves a molecule across a membrane against a concentration gradient, or, if the molecule is an ion, against an electrochemical gradient. It requires the expenditure of metabolic energy and can be inhibited by poisons that interfere with cell metabolism. Active transport plays an important role in the renal and biliary excretion of chemicals.

Facilitated diffusion is a carrier transport mechanism by which a water-soluble molecule (i.e. glucose) is transported through a membrane down a concentration gradient. No apparent energy is required and metabolic poisons will not inhibit this process. The difference between facilitated diffusion and active transport is that the latter moves molecules against a concentration gradient, whereas the former does not. For more complete discussion of membrane transport, refer to La Du et al. (1972) and Goldstein et al. (1974).

Another active process, pinocytosis, has been implicated as a mechanism for transferring large molecules and particles into cells. In this process, the membrane engulfs the material and pinches off an envelope containing the material within the cell.

4.2.2 Absorption from the lungs

The pulmonary epithelial lining is very thin, possesses a large surface area, and is highly vascular. Thus, absorption of foreign chemicals can take place at a very rapid rate. Most rapidly absorbed are gases and aerosols with small particle size and a high lipid-to-water partition coefficient. In most inhalation studies, absorption may occur by routes other than the lungs and the investigator should be aware of this in the interpretation of data.

A more complete discussion of the inhalation of chemicals is presented in Chapter 6.

4.2.3 Absorption from the skin

The structure of the skin enables rapid penetration of lipid-soluble compounds through the epidermis, a lipoprotein barrier, whereas the highly porous dermis is permeable to both lipid- and water-soluble substances (Katz & Poulsen, 1971). Factors which govern penetration through the skin are hydration, pH, temperature, blood supply, and metabolism as well as vehicle-skin interactions. Abrasion of the skin may enhance absorption greatly. For a more complete discussion of the principles for absorption through the skin and experimental methods, refer to Part II, Chapter 11.

4.2.4 Gastrointestinal absorption

The gastrointestinal tract is one of the most important routes of absorption of foreign compounds (Schanker, 1971). Chemicals can be absorbed along any section of the gastrointestinal tract, but because of the large surface area and rich blood supply, absorption is favoured from the small intestines. In most parts, the movement of a chemical across the epithelial lining of the gastrointestinal tract is by diffusion and carrier transport mechanisms are involved to a lesser degree.

Although therapeutic amounts of drugs may be absorbed from the buccal mucosa (Beckett & Hossie, 1971), absorption of environmental chemicals from the mouth is minimal compared with that from the stomach and intestine. Chemicals absorbed from the mouth are not exposed to the gastrointestinal digestive juices and drug-metabolizing enzymes. Furthermore, since they are not transported by the hepatic portal system directly to the liver, their normally rapid metabolism may be precluded, thus prolonging their effect.

The stomach is a significant site of absorption by passive diffusion of many acid, and neutral, foreign compounds (Schanker et al., 1957). Due to the acidity of the stomach, weak acids will exist in the diffusible, nonionized, lipid-soluble form, whereas weak bases will be highly ionized and therefore not generally absorbable.

Absorption from the small intestine is similar in principle to that from the stomach (passive diffusion), except that the pH of the intestinal contents (pH 6.6) may alter the fraction of the chemical in the nonionized form favouring the absorption of both weakly-acid and weakly-alkaline chemicals. The aqueous pore size, 4 Å, limits absorption by filtration to molecules having a molecular weight of less than 100–200. Rarely, an environmental chemical may be absorbed from the intestinal tract by an active transport system that is normally involved in the absorption of nutrients, e.g. sugars and amino acids (Schanker, 1963).

Many factors can affect the absorption of foreign compounds from the gastrointestinal tract (Brodie, 1964; Levine, 1970; Place & Benson, 1971; Prescott, 1975): (a) increased gastric emptying can decrease gastric absorption and increase intestinal absorption; (b) increased intestinal peristalsis generally inhibits intestinal absorption; (c) gastric acid, intestinal digestive juices, and gut microflora can all degrade chemicals to other absorbable or nonabsorbable chemical species; (d) food in the gastrointestinal tract can impair absorption by producing a nonabsorbable complex, by decreasing gastric emptying (especially fats), and by reducing, mixing, or altering pH; (e) normal digestion produces increased gastrointestinal blood flow which will enhance absorption; (f) absorption of a solid will be impaired if dissolution in the gastrointestinal tract does not take place. The practice of administering chemicals admixed with the diet must take these factors into account, especially the possible reaction of the chemical with dietary constituents.

4.3 Distribution

Once absorbed, the distribution of a chemical is determined by the relative plasma concentration, the rate of blood flow through various organs and tissues, the rate by which the chemical penetrates cell membranes, and the binding sites that are immediately available in the plasma and tissues. After the initial distribution phase, the rate by which a chemical penetrates cell membranes and the available sites for binding are the predominating factors influencing the final distribution of a chemical in the body.

When the plasma concentration of a chemical is high and the cell membranes do not provide significant barriers to diffusion, distribution is mainly to organs with high blood flow, e.g. brain, liver, and kidney. A classic example of distribution and redistribution is thiopental, a highly lipid-soluble chemical that, after administration, is first distributed to the brain and subsequently to muscle and body fat which have poor blood flow (Price et al., 1960). Lipid-soluble, foreign compounds tend to be distributed and localized in adipose tissue (Mark, 1971), in accordance with their lipid-to-water partition coefficients, e.g. the chlorinated hydrocarbon pesticides, dieldrin, DDT, and DDE (Rodomski et al., 1968) and polychlorinated biphenyls (PCBs) (Allen et al., 1974). Distribution of chemicals into organs and tissues is influenced by membraneous barriers in the same way as absorption (see 4.2). For a more detailed treatment, see Quastel (1965). The capillary membrane, unlike other body or cell membranes, is freely permeable to foreign compounds of a molecular weight of 60 000 or less, whether lipid-soluble or not (Pappenheimer, 1953; Renkin, 1964); generally chemicals pass these membranes readily, except in the brain, testicles, and the eye (Gehring & Buerge, 1969).

The movement of foreign chemicals to the brain represents a unique example that cannot be explained by the physicochemical properties of the chemical and the tissue distribution. Many chemicals fail to penetrate into the brain tissue or cerebrospinal fluid as readily as into other tissues (Brodie & Hogben, 1957). The boundary between blood and brain consists of several membranes; those of the blood capillary wall, the glial cells closely surrounding the capillary, and the membrane of the neurons or nerve cells. The so-called "blood-brain barrier" is located at the capillary wall-glial cell region. The capillary walls in the brain tend to be more like cell membranes than capillary membranes. Therefore, ionized substances and large water-soluble molecules such as proteins are almost entirely excluded from passage (Rall, 1971). The chief mode of exit of both lipid-soluble and polar compounds is by filtration across the arachnoid villi. The method for studying the movement of chemicals into and from the brain has been discussed by Rall (1971).

The red blood cell has unusual permeability in that organic anions penetrate much more readily than cations. This may be explained by the presence of positively charged membrane pores that will accept anions but repel cations (Schanker et al., 1957).

4.4 Binding

A major factor, that can affect the distribution of a chemical, is its affinity to bind to proteins and other macromolecules of the body. Foreign chemicals have been shown to bind reversibly to such substrates as albumen, globulins, haemoglobin, mucopolysaccharides, nucleoproteins, and phospholipids (Shore et al., 1957). For a survey of the biological implications of the protein binding of chemicals, the reader is referred to Gillette (1973a).

Once a chemical is bound to a body constituent, it is temporarily localized. This localization modifies the initial pattern of distribution and affects the rates of absorption, metabolism, and elimination of the chemical from the body.

4.4.1 Plasma-protein binding

Most chemicals show some degree of binding to plasma proteins, the most important fraction of which is albumen. Albumen at pH = 7.3 contains a net negative charge; however, cationic groups must be accessible because albumen has been shown to bind anions as well as cations. Although the plasma proteins show an appreciable capacity for binding many chemicals, this is limited, making it important to understand such binding as a function of the concentration of the chemical.

Since plasma proteins possess a limited number of binding sites and the sites are somewhat nonspecific, two chemicals with an affinity for the same binding site will compete with one another for binding. The plasma proteins of various laboratory animals and man show differences in the degree and nature of binding. This is due to differences in the total concentrations and relative proportions of the various plasma proteins as well as the composition and conformation of albumens (Gillette, 1973b).

4.4.2 Tissue binding

The binding of chemicals to tissue constituents also contributes to the localization of a chemical. Certain chemicals show a much greater affinity for tissue than for plasma proteins, and in some instances the affinity for tissue is quite specific. For example, polycyclic aromatic compounds have been shown to have particular affinity for the melanin in the eye (Potts, 1964).

Some metals and several chemicals and organic anions are bound to proteins (Y and Z proteins or ligandins) in the liver (Levi et al., 1969). These proteins may play a key role in the transfer of organic anions from plasma to liver (Levi et al., 1969; Reyes et al., 1971), and they also bind corticosteroids and azo-dye carcinogens (Litwack et al., 1971). For further details concerning the nature and effects of binding of chemicals by proteins and for methods of study, see Chignell (1971), Gillette (1975), Keen (1971) and Settle et al. (1971).

Many inorganic ions, particularly metals, as well as tetracycline, are concentrated in various tissues and organs, particularly in bones and teeth (Foreman, 1971). A convenient method for studying the accumulation of chemicals in organs and tissue is autoradiography (Roth, 1971). Valuable measurements may also be obtained with classical chemical and radio-chemical techniques which have the added advantage of being quantitative.

4.5 Excretion

Chemicals are excreted as the parent chemical, as metabolites, or as conjugates of the parent chemical or its metabolites. The principal routes of excretion are the urine and bile, and to a lesser degree expired air, sweat, saliva, milk, and secretions of the gastrointestinal tract.

4.5.1 Renal excretion

The kidneys are the most important route of excretion of foreign compounds (Weiner, 1971). The three mechanisms of renal excretion are: glomerular filtration, active tubular transport, and passive tubular transport. Only compounds of high molecular weight or those bound tightly to plasma proteins escape glomerular filtration and the resulting filtrate contains approximately the same concentration of foreign compounds as that found in the plasma in an unbound state.

Water and endogenous substrates are reabsorbed from the glomerular filtrate as it passes down the tubule. In the tubule, lipid-soluble, unionized chemicals pass in either direction by passive diffusion. Thus, lipid-soluble chemicals may be reabsorbed by the tubule, prolonging their retention in the body. Ionic chemicals, such as conjugates and other metabolites, are poorly reabsorbed and pass directly out of the body in the urine.

Active transport takes place in the proximal tubule of the kidney. There are two distinct active transport processes. One process is specific for organic anions and the other specific for organic cations. Chemicals transported by the same transport process compete with each other, and the excretion rate of one compound can be reduced by the administration of the other. The active transport process can be saturated as the concentration of the chemical in the plasma is increased. When the active tubular secretion is saturated, that is, when an increase in the concentration of the chemical in the plasma is no longer accompanied by a proportional increase in the concentration of the chemical in the urine, the concentration in the plasma is referred to as the renal-plasma threshold.

The anionic secretory process is responsible for the excretion of metabolites formed through conjugation of the parent chemical or its degradation products with various endogenous substrates such as glycine, sulfate, or glucuronic acid. These relatively polar, lipid-insoluble metabolites are poorly reabsorbed from the tubules and more readily excreted.

4.5.2 Biliary excretion

Biliary excretion is a major route for the excretion of foreign chemicals (Smith, 1971a, 1973). It is has been demonstrated (Brauer, 1959; Schanker, 1962b; Sperber, 1963; Williams, 1965) that compounds with high polarity, anionic and cationic conjugates of compounds bound to plasma proteins, and compounds with molecular weights greater than 300 are actively transported against a concentration gradient into the bile. It has also been shown that, once these compounds are in the bile, they are not reabsorbed into the blood and are excreted into the gastrointestinal tract (Schanker, 1965). Factors that influence the biliary excretion of foreign chemicals and metabolites are considered to be of two types: (*a*) physicochemical, relating to molecular size, structural features, and polarity; and (*b*) biological, relating to protein binding, renal excretion, metabolism, species, and sex. For a comprehensive and detailed discussion of these subjects, the reader is referred to Smith (1971a, 1973), and Stowe & Plaa (1968).

4.5.3 Enterohepatic circulation

Enterohepatic circulation is the phenomenon that occurs when a compound is excreted via the bile into the gastrointestinal tract, reabsorbed from the gastrointestinal tract and carried via the portal system back to the liver, where it is again excreted via the bile and recycled. Physiologically, enterohepatic circulation is important because it permits reuse of endogenous biliary excretion products. However, when a foreign compound is involved in enterohepatic circulation, it must make its way either to the faeces or to the peripheral blood to be excreted from the body. Thus, enterohepatic circulation of a foreign compound serves to enhance its retention in the body. There are examples in the literature (Gibson & Becker, 1967; Keberle et al., 1962) which demonstrate that the half-life of a compound involved in enterohepatic circulation can be decreased after surgically interrupting the enterohepatic cycle. Administration of a sequestering agent that binds the compound in the gastrointestinal tract would serve the same purpose.

Smith (1973) has described the following factors that can affect the enterohepatic circulation of a compound: (a) the extent and rate of excretion of the compound in the bile; (b) the activity of the gall bladder; (c) the fate of the substance in the small intestine; and (d) the fate of the compound after reabsorption from the gut. Since many foreign chemicals are excreted in the bile as unabsorbable conjugates, the hydrolysis of these conjugates in the intestine may play a key role in enterohepatic circulation. For a thorough discussion of enterohepatic circulation, the reader is referred to Plaa (1975).

4.5.4 Other routes of excretion

In addition to excretion in bile and urine, other routes for the excretion of foreign chemicals and their metabolites should not be overlooked. In accordance with the pH partition theory, organic bases highly ionized at the pH value of gastric juice may be secreted into the stomach (Shore et al., 1957). Similarly, weak acids ionized at neutral pH may be transferred from the plasma to the lumen of the intestine. These chemicals are sequestered by the intestinal contents, augmenting their excretion in the faeces.

Many volatile organic chemicals are excreted readily via exhaled air (see Chapter 6). This route of excretion is common for carbon dioxide, an ultimate end-product of an extensively metabolized organic chemical. For this reason, the quantification of expired radiolabelled carbon dioxide ($^{14}CO_2$) is very important in chemobiokinetic studies using carbon-14-labelled compounds.

Many foreign compounds are excreted, to different degrees, in milk, in either the aqueous or lipid phase (Rasmussen, 1971). Although this route may be of minor importance for the elimination of a chemical from the body, it should be given particular attention in evaluating the hazard of chemicals to man. First, consumption of cow's milk may constitute an important vehicle of exposure. Secondly, the consumption of mother's milk by the newborn may provide very high doses of a chemical that is concentrated in the milk. It should also be noted that the volume of milk consumed by the newborn per unit body weight may, in itself, magnify the dose received by this segment of the population.

Chemicals are also excreted in sweat and saliva. The presence of a chemical in sweat may lead to dermatitis. Although saliva is usually swallowed and thus does not lead to elimination of the agent from the body, recent work has shown that analysis of saliva for the presence of a chemical may preclude the necessity for venepuncture to obtain plasma for analysis.

4.6 Metabolic Transformation

Metabolic transformation or biotransformation are terms that have been used to describe the process which converts a foreign chemical to another derivative (metabolite) in the body. Metabolic transformation has been the subject of several excellent reviews (Conney, 1967; Conney & Burns, 1962; Dahm, 1971; Daly, 1971; Dutton, 1971; Garattini et al., 1975; Gillette, 1971a,b & 1974a,b; Gillette et al., 1974; Kuntzman, 1969; McClean, 1971; Smuckler, 1971; Weisburger & Weisburger, 1971). It usually results in the formation of more polar and water-soluble derivatives of a foreign chemical which can be more readily excreted from the body. Generally, such metabolic transformation of a foreign chemical also results in the formation of a less toxic chemical. However, there are many cases where the metabolites are more toxic than the parent chemicals (McLean, 1971; Miller & Miller, 1971a).

A few compounds resist metabolic transformation. Most strong acids and bases are excreted unchanged. Also the resistance of long-acting nonpolar compounds (barbital, halogenated benzene, etc.), to metabolic transformation might explain their slow elimination from the body.

A metabolic activation is suggested, if a compound is more toxic when given orally than intravenously, if there is a long delay between the administration of a chemical and the onset of its biological effect, or, if there is an increased effect following pretreatment with compounds that induce metabolic transformation (Garattini et al., 1975).

4.6.1 Mechanisms of metabolic transformation

Usually, the metabolic transformation of chemicals takes place to the greatest extent in the liver and is catalysed by enzymes found in the soluble, mitochondrial, and microsomal fractions of the cell. Enzymes metabolizing foreign chemicals are also found, to a lesser degree, in the cells of the gastrointestinal tract, kidney, lung, placenta, and blood (Aitio, 1973; Gillette, 1963; Gram, 1973; Hietanen, 1974; Hietanen & Valinio, 1973; Wattenberg & Leong, 1971; Wattenberg et al., 1962; Witschi, 1975). It must be emphasized that for a particular chemical, or a particular route of administration, other organs may play a more important role in the metabolic transformation of the chemical than the liver. The role of enzymatic reactions carried out by the intestinal flora may be very important and should not be overlooked (Scheline, 1968; Smith, 1971a). Enzyme-catalysed, biochemical transformations can be classified into four main types: (a) oxidations, (b) reductions, (c) hydrolyses and (d) synthetic reactions (see Table 4.1 in Annex to this Chapter).

The metabolic transformation of a chemical can occur via various pathways which can consist of a single reaction or multiple reactions. If the metabolic pathway consists of one reaction it is usually oxidation, reduction, or hydrolysis which tends to increase the polarity of the compound. Multiple-reaction metabolic pathways can consist of a series or any combination of oxidation, reduction, or hydrolysis. The final reaction in a multiple-reaction pathway is usually a conjugation reaction involving the addition of polar endogenous functional groups (D-glucuronic acid, glycine etc.) which usually render the molecule more polar, less lipid-soluble, and therefore more readily excretable. The predominant sequence of reactions or metabolic pathways is determined by many factors such as the dose of the chemical, species, strain, age, sex, and certain environmental variables.

4.6.1.1   Microsomal, mixed-function oxidations

The metabolism of a large variety of foreign compounds involves oxidative processes. Microsomal oxidation refers to reactions catalysed by the enzymes found in the microsomes of the endoplasmic reticulum. These enzymes are sometimes referred to as microsomal, mixed-function oxygenases (mono-oxygenases) (Mason, 1957). The reactions require molecular oxygen and nicotinamide adenine dinucleotide phosphate, reduced form (NADPH). The reduction equivalents from NADPH are used to reduce molecular oxygen so that it can be carried by a cytochrome called P-450 to the compound to be oxygenated. The oxygen is then fixed into the compounds, usually as a hydroxyl group (Estabrook, 1971; Estabrook et al., 1971).

The apparent sequence of events in the course of a mixed function oxidation has been described (Boyd & Smellie, 1972; Estabrook et al., 1972; Gillette, 1971c). The compound (substrate) forms a complex with the oxidized cytochrome P-450; this is reduced either directly by NADPH-cytochrome-c-reductase (1.6.2.4) or indirectly via an unidentified electron carrier. The reduced cytochrome P-450-substrate complex then reacts with oxygen to form an "active oxygen" complex, which decomposes with the formation of the oxidized substrate and oxidized cytochrome P-450. Substantial progress has been made in elucidating this mechanism by the development of a method involving the resolution and reconstitution of the components of the liver microsomal hydroxylating system (Lu & Levin, 1974).

Measurement of mixed-function oxidase activities of liver microsomes *in vitro* has become an important aspect in evaluating the toxicity of chemicals. The mixed-function oxidase system may be either a biotransformation system or a site of action of chemicals. Measurements of the activity of this system can be performed using either a 9000 g supernatant fraction (Henderson & Kersten, 1970; Klinger, 1974) of a liver homogenate prepared in buffered KCl solution, or a microsome fraction sedimented by centrifugation at about 105 000 g (Flynn et al., 1972; Hewick & Fouts, 1970a,b; Liu et al., 1975).

The reaction mixtures consisting of the particle-bound enzymes have to be supplemented with an NADPH-generating system. This may be fulfilled by the addition of NADP and glucose-6-phosphate, if the 9000 g fraction is used, but if washed microsomes are used, glucose-6-phosphate dehydrogenase (1.1.1.49) must also be added.

Isolated tissue cells, tissue cultures, or slices of organs, as well as perfused organs can also be used for metabolic studies.

Because cytochrome P-450 is intimately associated with the metabolism of many foreign chemicals, the following methods and variables have been developed for ascertaining its activity in the tissues of animals used in toxicological investigations.

The method of Omura & Sato (1964a,b) has been used to measure the change in the microsomal content of cytochrome P-450 and cytochrome b_5. This method relies on a spectral shift of the pigment upon exposure to carbon monoxide. An increase in the cytochrome P-450 content can be explained as a consequence of enzyme induction, whereas the decrease of the haem pigment content may be the result of enhanced permeability of microsomal membranes due to the damaging effects of the chemical (Bond & De Matteis, 1969). The concentration of cytochrome P-450 in the liver, however, is not always directly proportional to the activity of the mixed-function oxidases.

Spectral changes of cytochrome P-450, determined in the presence of various substrates, provide information about the binding between the pigment and substrate (Hewick & Fouts, 1970a; Remmer et al., 1966). Compounds may be classified into type I or type II according to their spectral reactions with cytochrome P-450. When type I compounds bind to cytochrome P-450, the characteristic spectral shift, spectral difference, gives a peak at 385–390 nm and a trough at 418–427 nm, whereas with type II compounds, the peak occurs at 425–435 nm and the trough at 390–405 nm. Originally, it was thought that the magnitudes of these spectral shifts, especially type I spectra, could be correlated with microsomal biotransformations (Schenkman et al., 1967). This correlation, however, is not universally applicable (Davies et al., 1969; Gigon et al., 1969; Holtzman et al., 1968). Thus, differences in the magnitude of these spectral changes are difficult to interpret when they are detected in animals treated with a chemical (Gillette et al., 1972). The same is true for the ethylisocyanide difference spectra of cytochrome P-450 which are characterized by two peaks at about 455 nm and 430 nm (Omura & Sato, 1964a).

Determination of the NADPH-cytochrome P-450 reductase activity, the assumed rate limiting step in microsomal oxidations, has proved useful in evaluating the effectiveness of the cytochrome P-450 system prior to the oxygenation step (Fouts & Pohl, 1971; Gigon et al., 1969; Hewick & Fouts, 1970b; Holtzman et al., 1968; Zannoni et al., 1972). Measurement of the NADPH-cytochrome-c-reductase activity may give information about the rate of flow of reducing equivalents from NADPH to cytochrome P-450.

Determination of the rate of enzymatic conversion of a substrate is a most valuable tool in elucidating the metabolic process. For this purpose, however, it is essential to know the pathway for the transformation of the chemical, and analytical methods are essential to quantify the parent chemical and its reaction products. Selected methods for monitoring some compounds and enzymatic reactions are listed in Table 4.2 (see Annex to this Chapter).

There are large variations in the metabolism of foreign chemicals as well as in susceptibility to metabolic inducers depending on the species (Hucker, 1970), strain, age, and sex of animals.

Many variables must be considered as important factors in species differences in the metabolism of foreign chemicals. Among these are differences in binding, either to tissues or to plasma components, such as albumen. Considerable variations in binding have been reported for the same chemical in different species (Borgå et al., 1968; Kurz & Friemel, 1967; Scholtan, 1963; Sturman & Smith, 1967; Witiak & Whitehouse, 1969). More obvious are the concentrations and types of foreign chemical-metabolizing enzymes in each species (Flynn et al., 1972).

4.6.1.2 *Conjugation reactions*

The major conjugation mechanisms are: glucuronide synthesis, "ethereal" sulfate synthesis, glutathione conjugation, glycine conjugation, methylation, acetylation, and thiocyanate synthesis. Glutamine conjugation has also been shown to occur in man and monkey. The conjugates formed by these mechanisms are usually nontoxic, therefore conjugation has also been referred to as a detoxification mechanism.

These conjugations are biosynthetic reactions in which foreign compounds or their metabolites containing suitable groups (hydroxyl, amino, carbonyl, or epoxide) combine with some endogenous substrates to form conjugates (Parke, 1968; Williams, 1967a, 1971). These reactions require ATP as source of energy, coenzymes, and transferases which are usually specific for the formation of conjugates of foreign compounds. The conjugations usually proceed in at least two steps: first, the extramicrosomal synthesis of acylcoenzyme and next the transfer of the acyl moiety to the aglycone, which, in some but not all cases, is localized in the microsomes. Thus, these reactions cannot be considered as transformations, characteristic of microsomes.

In accordance with the coenzymes participating in these reactions, they include:

formation of glucuronides (via uridine diphosphate glucuronic acid, UDPGA);

formation of sulfate esters (via 3-phosphadenosine-5-phosphosulfate, PAPS);

O-, N-, and S-methylation via 5'-[(3-amino-3-carboxypropyl)methylsulfonio]-5'-dioxyadenosine(S-adenosylmethionine);

acetylations (via acetyl coenzyme A);

formation of peptide conjugates (via different acylcoenzyme A derivatives);

formation of glutathione conjugates and mercapturic acids (conjugations with glutathione).

Formation of glucuronides is probably the most important microsomal conjugation mechanism (Dutton, 1971). It occurs in the liver and to a lesser extent in the kidney, gastrointestinal tract, and the skin. Biosynthesis of glucuronides can be measured in intact animals by determining D-glucaric acid (Marsh, 1963) and D-glucuronolactone dehydrogenase (1.1.1.70) (Marselos & Hanninen, 1974), by enhancement of D-glucuronolactone and aldehyde dehydrogenase (1.2.1.3) by inducers of microsomal metabolism (Marselos & Hanninen, 1974), glucuronides (Gregory, 1960; Yuki & Fishman, 1963) and L-ascorbic acid in urine. Elevation in urinary excretion of these compounds may be an indicator of an adaptive acceleration of hepatic glucuronide formation (Notten & Henderson, 1975). It should be emphasized that increased excretion of D-glucaric acid can result from enzyme induction; therefore it cannot be assumed that this occurrence is indicative only of an increased glucuronide formation. Methods for the measurement of glucuronide synthesis in whole organs and tissue cultures, as well as in tissue slices, have been summarized by Dutton (1966). In assays with homogenates and cell fractions the reaction mixtures have to be supplemented with added UDPGA.

UDP-glucuronosyl transferase (2.4.1.17) activity can be determined using 2-aminophenol (Burchell et al., 1972; Dutton & Storey, 1962), 4-nitrophenol (Isselbacher 1956; Zakim & Vessey, 1973), bilirubin (Heirwegh et al., 1972), 7-hydroxy-4-methyl-2H-I-benzopyran-2-one (4-methylumbelliferone) (Aitio, 1973; Arias, 1962) or morphine (Strickland et al., 1974).

In contrast to glucuronide synthesis, the formation of sulfate esters is most probably an extramicrosomal process and is catalysed generally by sulfate-conjugating enzymes in the presence of 3-phosphoadenosine-5-phosphosulfate as a co-enzyme (Roy, 1971). Among the compounds of toxicological interest, phenols are converted by sulfation to esters and excreted in the urine. Aminophenols yield sulfamates. There are specific assays for the determination of sulfotransferase (2.8.2) activity using 4-nitrophenol (Gregory & Lipmann, 1957), or 3-(2-aminoethyl)-1H-indol-5-ol (serotonin) (Hidaka et al., 1967) as acceptors.

The methyltransferases (2.1.1) catalyse O-, N- and S-methylation of several physiologically active compounds and drugs (Axelrod, 1971). They are widely distributed in different organs, but only a small amount of catechol-O-methyltransferase (2.1.1.6) and almost all of the phenol-O-methyltransferase (2.1.1.25) (Axelrod & Daly, 1968) activity is localized in the microsomes of the liver. Only microsomal transferases are induced by benzo(a)pyrene and inhibited by SKF 525A[a]. The methods used for the determination of catechol-O-methyltransferase activity are based on the principle that the enzyme catalyses the transfer of methyl groups to catechols in the presence of S-adenosylmethionine as a methyl donor. The substrates employed include adrenaline (Axelrod & Tomchick, 1958), 3,4-dihydrobenzoic acid (MacCaman, 1965), 3,4-dihydroxybenzeneacetic acid (3,4-dihydrophenylacetic acid) (Assicot & Bohuon, 1969; Broch & Guldberg, 1971) as well as I-(3,4-dihydroxyphenyl)ethanone (3,4-dihydroxyacetophenone) (Borchardt, 1974). The end products of the enzymatic reaction are measured either spectrofluorimetrically (Axelrod & Tomchick, 1958; Borchardt, 1974; Broch & Guldberg, 1971), or radio-

---

[a] Diethyl aminoethanol ester of diphenyl-propyl acetic acid.

metrically using labelled methyl groups in the coenzyme (MacCaman, 1965).

Acetylation reactions of the amino group of foreign compounds are catalysed by acetyltransferases (Weber, 1971). Substrates of these enzyme reactions, localized in the soluble part of the cells, are arylamines, hydrazines, and certain aliphatic amines. Coenzyme A is an essential factor in these acetylations. Acetylation of arylamines has been studied quantitatively, *in vivo*, in human beings and animals (Williams, 1967b).

Methods for the determination of N-acetyltransferase (2.3.1.35) activities *in vitro* summarized by Weber (1971) include colorimetric (Brodie & Axelrod, 1948; Maher et al., 1957; Marshall, 1948; Shulert, 1961; Weber, 1970), spectrophotometric (Jenne & Boyer, 1962; Tabor et al., 1953; Weber & Cohen, 1968; Weber et al., 1968) as well as radiometric procedures (Stotz et al., 1969).

Conjugation of aromatic carboxylic acids (benzoic acid, substituted benzoic acids, and heterocyclic carboxylic acids) with amino acids by means of acetyl coenzyme A and ATP is called peptide conjugation. Glycine is the most generally involved amino acid in this reaction resulting in the formation of N-benzoylglycine (hippuric acid). Indole-3-acetic acid, benzeneacetic acid, as well as 4-aminosalicylic acid, can conjugate with glutamine in man, and several mammals. Determination of hippuric acids (Ogata et al., 1969) enables the quantitative investigation of this conjugation reaction.

Conjugation of glutathione with foreign compounds, catalysed by at least ten different glutathione S-transferases, is an important pathway for the elimination of these compounds (Boyland, 1971). Following the conjugation of foreign compounds with glutathione, the conjugate is most frequently hydrolysed to the cysteine conjugate which is excreted in the urine. Furthermore, the cysteine conjugate may be acetylated and the resulting mercapturic acid excreted. The significance of the mercapturic acid biosynthesis in man, however, is difficult to assess.

Determination of glutathione S-transferase activities are based on spectral change of the substrate (1,2-dichloro-4-nitrobenzene) due to conjugation (Booth et al., 1961), or loss of glutathione content (Boyland & Chasseaud, 1967; Boyland & Williams, 1965; Johnson, 1966) or release of labile groups (Al-Kassab et al., 1963; Boyland & Williams, 1965; Johnson, 1966) as well as on chromatographic separation of the products (Suga et al., 1967). The determination of the activity of γ-glutamyltransferase (2.3.2.2), catalysing one intermediary step of the overall mercapturic acid synthesis may also be informative.

4.6.1.3 *Extramicrosomal metabolic transformations*

Foreign compounds, either transformed by oxidation or initially having characteristic groups (hydroxyl, amino) may resemble normal constituents of physiological metabolism. Thus, they may undergo metabolic transformations similar to those of normal body constituents: oxidation, reduction, deamination, hydrolysis. The enzymes catalysing these reactions are localized in the cytosol or are intrinsic compounds of the mitochondria.

In contrast to the extensive data in the literature on enzyme-chemical interactions (MacMahon, 1971; Zeller, 1971) only a few enzyme activities are commonly used to monitor toxicological events.

The alcohol dehydrogenase (1.1.1.1) of the liver is one of the most important enzymes which catalyses the NAD-mediated oxidation of various aliphatic and aromatic primary and secondary alcohols. Determination of the activity of alcohol dehydrogenase is based on the spectrophotometric measurement of the amount of NAD being reduced in the presence of excess alcohol (Bonnichsen & Brink, 1955).

Among the amine oxidases, monoamine oxidase (1.4.3.4), localized in the mitochondria, regulates the balance of the biogenic amines and probably does not participate in the metabolism of foreign amines to a great degree (Zeller, 1971). However, the fact that a large number of substances (substrates and substrate analogues, alkyl and arylamines, hydrazine derivatives, sulfhydryl reagents, etc.) inhibit this enzyme, enables monoamine oxidase to be used as a tool in studies of the toxicity of these inhibitors.

Monoamine oxidase activity can be measured manometrically (Creasey, 1956) based on oxygen-consumption, by determination of ammonia production (Cotzias & Dole, 1951), spectrophotometrically (Dietrich & Erwin, 1969; Obata et al., 1971; Weissbach et al., 1960), fluorimetrically (Takahashi & Takahara, 1968; Tufvesson, 1970) as well as radiometrically (Otsuka & Kobayashi, 1964).

Hydrolysis by carboxylesterases (ali-esterases or arylesterases) of foreign compounds containing ester groups may be important in assessing their toxicity (La Du & Snady, 1971). Determination of esterase activities using different substrates in the presence of the chemical to be tested can disclose its possible inhibitory potency.

4.6.1.4 *Nonenzymatic reactions*

Although the foregoing sections have discussed enzymatic modifications of chemicals, the investigator should not overlook nonenzymatic, spontaneous reactions between chemicals and natural constituents in the body that lead to the formation of metabolites, e.g. the reaction of an alkylating agent with glutathione.

4.6.2 Species variability

A serious problem facing every research worker using an animal species to study the metabolism of a foreign compound is whether or not the metabolic pathway in the animal is similar to the metabolic pathway in man. The problem is not only important in metabolic studies, but is of utmost importance in using animal toxicity studies to predict toxicological phenomena in man. Conney et al. (1974) illustrated that the use of an animal species that metabolizes a foreign compound in a similar manner to man will give a more precise prediction of the type of toxicological phenomena to be expected in man.

Different animal species have been shown to metabolize foreign compounds at different rates. Quinn et al. (1958) has shown that benzeneamine (aniline) has a metabolic half-time in the mouse of 35 minutes and in the dog of 167 minutes. In the same study it was demonstrated that the metabolic half-time of an antipyrine in the rat was 140 minutes, whereas in man it was 600 minutes.

Considerable species differences in metabolic pathways have also been demonstrated. In the rat, mouse, and dog the carcinogen, N-2-fluoranylacetamide (FAA), is N-hydroxylated to N-hydroxy-FAA which is a more potent carcinogen than FAA. In the guineapig little or no hydroxylation of FAA occurs. In toxicity studies, Miller & Miller (1971b) and Weisburger et al. (1964) demonstrated that the rat, mouse, and dog are susceptible to the carcinogenic activity of FAA, whereas the guineapig is not. Thus, a difference in the metabolic pathways of a foreign compound may greatly influence its toxicity.

Species variability in metabolism has been related to other factors such as species differences in protein binding, and enzyme concentration and type. Hucker (1970) described, in detail, species differences in chemical metabolism and some of the factors responsible for these differences.

4.6.3 Enzyme induction and inhibition

For some time it has been known that chemicals can increase the activity of metabolizing enzyme systems. These chemicals have been termed enzyme "inducers". Inducers exert their action by quantitatively increasing the enzymes and components responsible for the metabolism of foreign compounds. The importance of induction to the toxicologist is two-fold. If metabolism leads to the formation of excretable or nontoxic metabolites, induction will enhance detoxification and excretion of the compound. However, if metabolism leads to the production of a more toxic metabolite, induction will increase the toxicity of a compound.

Many chemicals are known to increase metabolizing enzyme systems. The reviews by Conney (1967), Kuntzman (1969), and Mannering (1968), depict the large number of chemicals which induce metabolizing enzymes and comprehensively review the factors involved in enzyme inductions.

Most inducers give maximum effects rather quickly—within 2–3 days (Fouts, 1970). However, some require 2 weeks or longer (Gillette et al., 1966; Hart & Fouts, 1965; Hoffman et al., 1968, 1970; Kinoshita et al., 1966). Frequently, the degree of induction after obtaining a maximum level may decline despite continuing treatment of the animal with a chemical (Gillette et al., 1966; Hoffman et al., 1968; Kinoshita et al., 1966).

Drug-metabolizing enzymes can also be depressed by foreign chemicals, and these compounds are termed inhibitors. 2-(Diethylamino) ethyl-α-phenyl-α-propyl benzeneacetate hydrochloride (SKF-525A) is the best known of the inhibitors and is used routinely in determining the effect of enzyme inhibition on the metabolism of chemicals.

4.6.4 Metabolic saturation

In vivo saturation of metabolic pathways can play an important role in determining the toxic profile of a chemical. A recent article by Jollow et al. (1974) demonstrated the effect of enzyme saturation on the metabolism and toxicity of bromobenzene. Bromobenzene was first metabolically transformed to an epoxide which is hepatotoxic. After a small nontoxic dose, approximately 75% was converted to the glutathione conjugate and excreted as bromophenylmercapturic acid. After a large toxic dose, only 45% was excreted as the mercapturic acid. It was established that, at the toxic dose, the metabolic conjugation pathway was overwhelmed due to lack of glutathione, which resulted in an increased reaction of the epoxide hepatotoxin with DNA, RNA, and protein.

It is very important to elucidate dose-dependent metabolism to assess the hazard of a chemical. Frequently, the doses of a chemical used to characterize toxicity are many times those encountered in the environment. Toxicity incurred at these large doses may be influenced by relative changes in metabolism and therefore must be interpreted with caution and judgment in assessing the hazard of low doses.

4.7 Experimental Design

Since, for the most part, toxicity is a function of the concentration of the toxicant in the tissues and cells, this information together with its dynamics provides for inter- as well as intra-species extrapolation of the results of toxicological effects.

The overall objectives of a chemobiokinetic study are to determine the amount, rate, and nature of absorption, distribution, metabolism, and excretion of a chemical. The approach to meeting those objectives must be flexible and designed to meet the specific needs of each chemical.

It is difficult to predict, without prior data, an animal species that will metabolize a chemical similarly to man. Usually, initial studies are performed in the rat and one other nonrodent species, such as the dog or monkey, in an attempt to determine species variability. If there are significant differences among species, it is important to determine whether differences in the chemobiokinetic parameters correlate with differences in toxicity or pharmacological activity. Animals should be acclimatized to the environment of the metabolism cage prior to the experiment. Light cycle, temperature, humidity, and time of feeding should be standardized. The physical condition, weight, and food and water consumption of each animal should be monitored and recorded throughout the study.

There are advantages in using radioactively-labelled chemicals in initial studies because of the ease with which radiochemical methods (Chase & Rabinowitz, 1968) can be applied to chemobiokinetic studies. An important advantage of using a radioactively-labelled chemical is that it allows the establishment of the total recovery of the parent chemical and its metabolites, i.e. the mass balance. To obtain this the total radioactivity eliminated via the urine, faeces, and exhaled air as well as that remaining in the carcass following termination of the experiment should be determined. Until a reasonably good recovery is obtained, 90% or greater, one can never be sure whether other chemobiokinetic parameters obtained from the study are accurate. Furthermore, the isolation and ultimate identification of unknown metabolites is greatly enhanced by using radioactively-labelled chemicals.

When using a radiolabelled chemical, the measurement of radioactivity confirms the presence of the radioisotope, not the chemical or its metabolites. In order to determine the identity of the radioactively-labelled compound, the parent chemical and its metabolites, analytical methods such as gas, high-pressure liquid, and thin-layer chromatography and a combination of gas chromatography and mass spectroscopy are frequently employed.

Until it is established that the radioactivity being monitored is from the chemical in question, kinetic parameters apply to the radioactivity only, not to the chemical studied. Difficulties can arise if the radioactive atom does not remain an integral part of the molecule under study. Tritium and carbon-14 are often incorporated into the body pools of normal tissue components (Griffiths, 1968; Rosenblum, 1965). Once the radioactivity is incorporated into these compartments, its clearance depends on their rates of turnover. Therefore, by monitoring radioactivity only, it can be falsely assumed that a compound is being retained in the body.

Another very important reason for differentiating the parent chemical from its metabolite is to assure that toxic effects that may be present are associated with the parent chemical and not a metabolite. Also persistence of a metabolite in the body rather than the parent chemical may constitute the ultimate hazard.

In initial studies, consideration should be given to the administration of the compound by intravenous injection as well as via the route by which man is exposed to the chemical. The intravenous route is used to provide a more definite assessment of the earlier phases of distribution and/or elimination. Also, large variation in rates of absorption will in some cases make the differentiation of the early phases of distribution and elimination difficult. At least two doses should be used. One dose should be equivalent to the dose required to cause signs of toxicity. The second dose should be well below the toxic dose and, if possible, equivalent to anticipated human exposure levels.

Most frequently, kinetic parameters for elimination of a chemical are established by sequential sampling of blood plasma and excreta, following its administration. A preliminary probe study using one or two animals is often needed to establish the time at which samples should be collected, because this will vary with the species and the chemical in question. After collection and until prepared for analysis of the chemical or its metabolites, samples should be stored in a manner that will preclude the breakdown of the chemical or its metabolites. The data required from the initial chemobiokinetic studies can be used to design further studies which may include the following: distribution studies using autoradiography; the isolation and identification of metabolites; studies to determine the chemobiokinetic profile of metabolites; biliary excretion studies; bioconcentration; and *in vitro* metabolism studies. The methods and techniques needed to perform these studies are documented by La Du et al. (1972).

4.8 Chemobiokinetics

Chemobiokinetics aims at quantification of the processes discussed previously in this chapter. Thus, chemobiokinetics provides quantitative information on the absorption, distribution, biotransformation, and excretion of chemicals (including drugs and endogenous substances) as a function of time. Since the classical introduction of this discipline by Teorell (1937a,b), the concepts and methods have been developed extensively, principally for application to the clinical evaluation and/or use of drugs

(Levy & Gibaldi, 1972, 1975; Wagner, 1968, 1971). The reader is also referred to Gehring et al. (1976) who discuss the subject in greater detail.

One difficulty of many toxicologists and biologists on first exposure to chemobiokinetics is the concept of compartments. The body is composed of a large number of organs, tissues, cells, and fluids, any one of which could be referred to morphologically and functionally as a compartment. However, in chemobiokinetics, a compartment refers collectively to those organs, tissues, cells, and fluids for which the rates of uptake and subsequent clearance of a chemical are sufficiently similar to preclude kinetic resolution. The rapidly equilibrating compartment, referred to as the central compartment, may be comprised of all those tissues with a profuse blood supply whereas the slow or peripheral compartment may include tissues with a more limited blood supply, i.e. fat and bone.

4.8.1 One-compartment open model

The simplest chemobiokinetic model is a one-compartment, open model as shown in Fig. 4.1. In using this model, it is assumed that the chemical equilibrates with all tissues to which it is distributed sufficiently rapidly to preclude kinetic differentiation by the techniques being used to characterize its movement in the body. For example, if it requires 30 min for a chemical to attain equilibration in the body after entering the blood stream, and if samples of blood, tissues, and excreta are taken at 30 min intervals, it will appear that the body consists of only one compartment.

Assuming that the rate of elimination of the chemical is proportional to its concentration in the plasma, the concentration in the plasma will be described by apparent first-order kinetics. The rate of change of concentration in the plasma may be expressed in the form of the linear differential equation

$$\frac{dC(t)}{dt} = -k_e C(t) \tag{1}$$

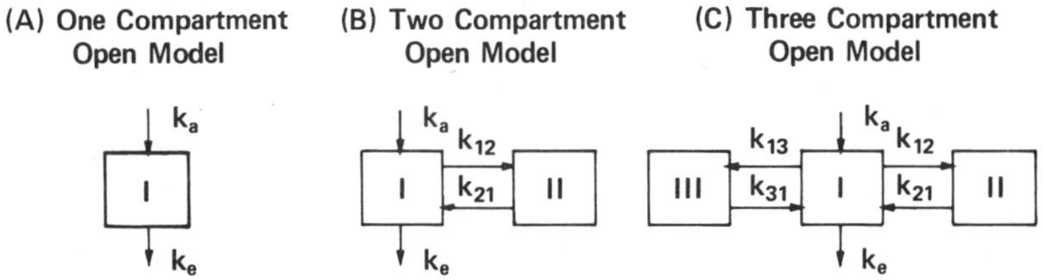

(A) One Compartment Open Model **(B) Two Compartment Open Model** **(C) Three Compartment Open Model**

Fig. 4.1 Schematic representation of a one-compartment (A), two-compartment (B) and three-compartment (C) open model system as routinely used in chemobiokinetic analyses. The rate constants for absorption and elimination are denoted k_a and k_e respectively. The rate constants (k_{12}, k_{21}, k_{13}, k_{31}) represent the transfer from the compartment denoted by the first integer in the subscript to the compartment denoted by the second integer.

where $C(t)$ is the concentration at time t, and k_e is the rate constant for elimination. Solution of this differential equation with initial condition $C(t) = C(0)$ at time zero gives

$$C(t) = C(0) \exp(-k_e t) \qquad \text{(exponential form)} \qquad (2)$$

or,

$$\left. \begin{array}{l} \ln C(t) = -k_e t + \ln C(0) \\ \log C(t) = -k_e t/2.303 + \log C(0) \end{array} \right\} \text{(logarithmic form)} \qquad \begin{array}{l} (3) \\ (4) \end{array}$$

In these equations, $C(0)$ is the concentration of the chemical in the plasma at time zero. A plot of $C(t)$ versus time on semilogarithmic paper will yield a straight line (Fig. 4.2) with slope $-k_e$ and intercept $C(0)$.

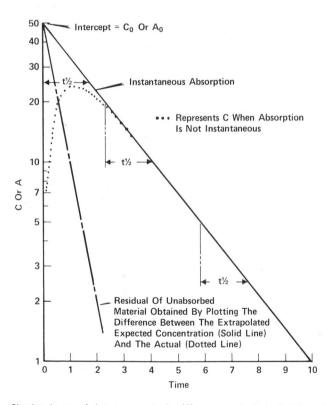

Fig. 4.2   Simulated curve of plasma concentration (C) or amount in the body (A) as a function of time following instantaneous absorption (intravenous injection: solid line) or delayed absorption (oral, subcutaneous administration: dotted line). The half-time of elimination is $t_{1/2}$. The residuals (dash-dot line) indicate the rate of absorption (k_a) in the case of delayed absorption following oral or subcutaneous administration.

Having determined k_e, which is measured in units of reciprocal time, the time required to reduce the plasma concentration by one-half is estimated; this time is referred to as the $t_{1/2}$ or half-time. It can be determined from the equation

$$t_{1/2} = \frac{\ln 2}{k_e} = \frac{0.693}{k_e} \qquad (5)$$

When the chemical is not absorbed instantaneously, the mathematics needed to describe the concentration in plasma as a function of time become somewhat more complicated. Assuming apparent first-order absorption as well as elimination, the concentration $C(t)$ in plasma is given by the expression

$$C(t) = \frac{f \cdot D_0 \cdot k_a}{V_d(k_a - k_e)} \{\exp(-k_e t) - \exp(-k_a t)\} \qquad (6)$$

In this expression, the terms not previously mentioned are D_0, the dose; f, the fraction of dose absorbed; V_d, the apparent volume of distribution; and k_a, the apparent first-order absorption rate constant.

The elimination rate constant, k_e, is determined as described previously using that portion of the solid line representing the plasma concentration after absorption is essentially complete. In Fig. 4.2, this occurs when the dotted line blends into the solid line. The rate constant for absorption, k_a, may be estimated by projecting the solid line backward to the origin. The difference between the experimentally-determined values used to characterize the dotted line are subtracted from those predicted by the backward projection at corresponding times. Subsequently, the values obtained by this "curve stripping" procedure are plotted producing a curve like the dash-dash line in Fig. 4.2. Using this procedure, the $t_{1/2}$ for absorption and k_a are determined.

The volume of distribution, V_d, is a term used to describe the apparent volume to which a chemical is distributed when it is assumed that the affinity of the plasma and all tissues is equivalent. An analogy is placing a known amount of a dye in a liquid contained in a system of unknown volume. After the concentration of the dye has attained a constant value, the volume of the system can be determined by dividing the dose, D_0, by the concentration to give the volume of distribution, V_d.

In the plasma, the concentration of the chemical declines because of elimination as well as distribution to tissues. Therefore, to estimate V_d, it is necessary to project the elimination phase of the curve back to the origin. The value obtained at the time zero intercept by this projection is divided into D_0 to obtain the volume of distribution, V_d, in ml/kg.

The value of V_d provides some important information about the distribution of the chemical in the body. As the distribution to the tissues increases, for whatever reason, physicochemical affinity, active transport into cells, V_d increases. If the distribution of a chemical in the human body is limited to plasma, extracellular fluid, or total body water, the respective values of V_d will be approximately 40, 170, and 580 ml/kg. If a chemical has a high affinity for a particular tissue, for example, the affinity of a lipophilic chemical for fat, V_d may exceed significantly 1000 mg/kg. When the volume of distribution is known, the amount of chemical in the body at any time t, $A(t)$, can be calculated from the equation

$$A(t) = C(t)V_d \tag{7}$$

Until now, concepts relating only to the concentration of the chemical in the plasma have been discussed.

However, these concepts are equally applicable to other tissues or, for that matter, to excreta, expired air, or urine. In the case of urine, the concentrating power of the kidney must be accounted for to normalize the data. If the affinity of the chemical for the various tissues and excreta is equivalent and if rapid equilibration is assumed, the concentration curves will be superimposable. However, this would be an unusual occurrence. Because of the differences in affinity, it is more likely that a family of parallel concentration curves will be obtained. It is emphasized that these curves will be parallel only after an apparent steady state has been achieved between the tissues.

In addition to concentration, the same concepts apply if one desires to characterize the total amount of chemical in the body, $A(t)$, as a function of time following exposure. For example, if a dose D_0 is ingested and apparent first-order kinetics is assumed, the amount of the chemical in the body is given by the expression

$$A(t) = D_0 \exp{(-k_e t)} \tag{8}$$

Using equation (7), equation (8) can be shown to be equivalent to

$$C(t) = C(0) \exp{(-k_e t)} \tag{9}$$

Logarithmic transformation of equations (8) or (9) may be used to obtain curves like those in Fig. 4.2. The dotted curve would apply if the chemical were applied to the skin and subsequently absorbed.

One caution must be emphasized in resolving the kinetics of the amount of an agent in the body. Usually, it is not adequate to determine the amount of the agent excreted and calculate the amount remaining in the body by subtracting the cumulative amount excreted from the original dose. This can be done if, and only if, the agent is metabolically transformed to a very limited degree and, essentially, all of the original dose is recovered. This seldom happens.

To circumvent the problem just described, the amount of the chemical excreted over designated time intervals is determined until a significant amount can no longer be detected. Assume that the rate of excretion is proportional to the amount of chemical in the body, $A(t)$. Let $B(t)$ be the cumulative amount excreted to time t after administration. Then

$$\frac{dA(t)}{dt} = -k_e A(t) \tag{10}$$

or,

$$A(t) = D_0 \exp(-k_e t) \tag{11}$$

And

$$\frac{dB(t)}{dt} = k_{ex} A(t) \tag{12}$$

$$\frac{dB(t)}{dt} = \frac{k_{ex}}{k_e} D_0 \exp(-k_e t) \tag{13}$$

or,

$$B(t) = D_0 \frac{k_{ex}}{k_e} \{1 - \exp(-k_e t)\} \tag{14}$$

In these equations, k_e represents the apparent first-order overall elimination rate constant and k_{ex} is the rate constant for excretion via the route being analysed. If E_i is the amount excreted in the ith time interval of duration Δ_t then

$$E_i = B(t_i) - B(t_i - \Delta t) \tag{15}$$

where $B(t_i)$ is the amount excreted between administration and t_i, the time at the end of the ith time interval.

In terms of the dose administered D_0, and the rate constant k_e,

$$E_i = D_0 \frac{k_{ex}}{k_e} \exp(-k_e t_i) \{\exp(k_e \Delta t) - 1\} \tag{16}$$

the logarithmic form of which is

$$\ln E_i = -k_e t_i + \ln \left\{ D_0 \frac{k_{ex}}{k_e} [\exp(k_e \Delta t) - 1] \right\} \tag{17}$$

A semilogarithmic plot of E_i versus t_i will give a straight line with slope $-k_e$. The above expression can be modified to accommodate unequal time intervals, but in doing so graphic insights are lost.

In using excretion data to resolve kinetic parameters, it is desirable to keep the collection intervals as short as practical. Ideally, the collection intervals should be shorter than the $t_{1/2}$ for elimination of the chemical; otherwise resolution of a biphasic excretion pattern may be precluded. Biphasic refers to two kinetically distinct excretion phases. For a volatile chemical excreted to some degree by exhalation, determination of the chemical exhaled as a function of time may be particularly useful for resolving its biochemokinetics.

As already stated, the excretion rate of a chemical by one route of excretion may be different from its overall rate of elimination. This is true because the agent may be eliminated by other routes and/or metabolically transformed. The following scheme may be used to depict a chemical that is eliminated by a metabolic pathway as well as by excretion in the urine and exhalation:

$$C \begin{array}{l} \nearrow k_u \quad \text{excretion in urine} \\ \!\!\!\!- k_r \quad \text{excretion via exhalation} \\ \searrow k_{mx} \quad \text{metabolic transformation to compound y} \end{array}$$

In this case, the overall elimination constant will be $k_e = k_u + k_r + k_{mx}$.

The various metabolic transformation and excretion rates may be estimated using the following equations:

$$k_u = U_\infty (k_e/D_0) \tag{18}$$

$$k_r = R_\infty (k_e/D_0) \tag{19}$$

$$k_{mx} = X_\infty (k_e/D_0) \tag{20}$$

U_∞ and R_∞ are the total amounts of the parent chemical excreted in urine and expired air. X_∞ is the total amount of metabolite, X, recovered from excreta. For excretion of the chemical in the urine, the differential equation is:

$$\frac{dU}{dt} = k_u D_0 \exp(-k_e t) \tag{21}$$

The solution of the equation (21) yields

$$U_\infty = k_u D_0/k_e \tag{22}$$

and

$$k_u = U_\infty k_e / D_0 \tag{23}$$

142

When the urinary excretion of a chemical is determined, it is frequently desirable to determine its renal clearance in order to ascertain whether the chemical is actively secreted, reabsorbed, or only passively filtered by the kidney in the excretion process. Renal clearance is defined as the urinary excretion rate, $\Delta U/\Delta t$, divided by the plasma concentration, C:

$$R_c = (\Delta U/\Delta t)/C \qquad (24)$$

If the plasma concentration is changing during the urinary collection interval, the concentration at the midpoint of the interval is used frequently. It may also be shown using equations (9), (21), and (24) that

$$R_c = k_u V_d \qquad (25)$$

which precludes the necessity of knowing the plasma concentration. Renal clearance values for inulin measure excretion via glomerular filtration. For man, the normal value is 125 ± 15 ml/min (Pitts, 1963). If the renal clearance of a chemical exceeds this value in man, it constitutes evidence that the chemical is actively secreted. If it is less, it indicates the chemical is actively reabsorbed. If the compound is bound to a significant degree to protein, it may be necessary to determine and use the concentration of unbound chemical in plasma in order to obtain a realistic value for renal clearance.

4.8.2 Two-compartment/multicompartment open systems

Rapidly equilibrating compartments in which the chemical has reached equilibrium with plasma before the first blood samples are taken will appear kinetically as one compartment, but a "deep" or more slowly equilibrating compartment will give rise to a plasma concentration curve that appears biphasic. The model used to describe this system is a two-compartment open model (Fig. 4.1). The central and the "shallow" or rapidly equilibrating compartments are considered as one. The major sites of metabolic transformation and excretion are the liver and the kidneys. Since these organs are perfused with blood, it can be assumed, generally, that they are part of the central compartment and that elimination occurs from the central compartment. Fig. 4.3 is a simulated plasma concentration curve representing a two-compartment system following rapid intravenous administration of a chemical. The chemical has first been rapidly distributed to well-perfused tissues, then more slowly to other tissues comprising the deep compartment.

Assuming all the transfer processes are first order, the system of linear

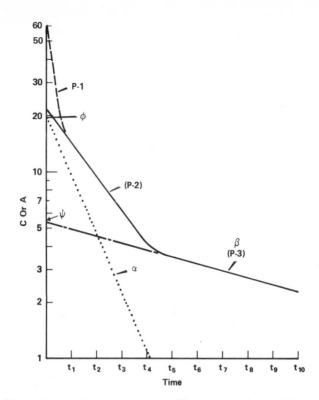

Fig. 4.3 Simulated curve of plasma concentration (C) or amount in the body (A) as a function of time for a material injected intravenously and subsequently eliminated from a rapidly equilibrating, shallow compartment (P-2) and a slowly equilibrating deep compartment (P-3). P-1 represents the initial distribution of the material from the central (blood) compartment to shallow compartment. Alpha (α) and Beta (β) represent the rates of elimination from the shallow and deep compartments with their respective intercepts ϕ and ψ.

differential equations describing the two-compartment model shown in Fig. 4.1 is as follows:

$$\frac{dC(t)}{dt} = -k_{12}C(t) - k_e C(t) + \frac{k_{21}V_D C_D(t)}{V_d} \tag{26}$$

$$\frac{dC_D(t)}{dt} = \frac{k_{12}V_d C(t)}{V_D} - k_{21}C_D(t) \tag{27}$$

where $C(t)$ and $C_D(t)$ are concentrations of the chemical in the central and deep compartments respectively. The apparent volumes of distribution for these compartments are V_d for the central compartment and V_D for the slow exchange compartment. If the apparent volumetric flow rates between the

144

two compartments are the same, i.e. $k_{12}V_d = k_{21}V_D$, the differential equation system can be solved with initial conditions $C(0) = D_0/V_d$ and $C_D(0) = 0$ at time zero to give the following mathematical representation for the solid curve in Fig. 4.3:

$$C(t) = \phi \exp(-\alpha t) + \psi \exp(-\beta t) \qquad (28)$$

β is the slope of the line for the slow phase of elimination and α is the slope for the rapid phase of elimination. The value of β is determined as previously described and a technique called feathering is used to obtain α. This technique constitutes projecting the solid line for the slow phase backward to the origin (dash-dash line) and subtracting the respective projected values from the experimental values used to delineate the rapid phase of clearance. These values are replotted (dotted line). The slope of this line is α. The values for ϕ and ψ are the intercepts at the ordinate for the rapid and slow elimination phases, respectively.

The rate constants k_{12}, k_{21}, and k_e (Fig. 4.1) may be determined as follows:

$$k_{21} = \frac{\phi\beta + \psi\alpha}{\phi + \psi} \qquad (29)$$

$$k_e = \frac{\alpha\beta}{k_{21}} \qquad (30)$$

$$k_{12} = \alpha + \beta - (k_{21} + k_e) \qquad (31)$$

k_{12} is of particular importance because from it the amount of chemical in the deep compartment ($A_D(t)$) is readily calculated from the equation

$$A_D(t) = \frac{k_{12}D_0}{\beta - \alpha} \{\exp(-\alpha t) - \exp(-\beta t)\} \qquad (32)$$

Using this information, toxicologists can ascertain whether there may be correlations between the effect of a chemical and its presence in a deep compartment. Indeed, for the toxicologist, a prominent slow phase for the elimination of a chemical is a red flag suggesting that with repeated administration cumulative toxicity may constitute a problem.

These concepts developed for the plasma concentration of a chemical conforming to a two-compartment open-model system can be extended to describe the amount of the agent in the body or the amount excreted. Also, an absorption component may be added which would give a function involving the sum of three exponential terms:

$$C(t) = \phi \exp(-\alpha t) + \psi \exp(-\beta t) + (\phi + \psi) \exp(-k_a t) \qquad (33)$$

4.8.3 Repeated administration or repeated exposure

The concentration of a chemical in the plasma or tissues or the amount of chemical in the body following repeated administration or exposure is illustrated in Fig. 4.4 for a one-compartment open system. Mathematical

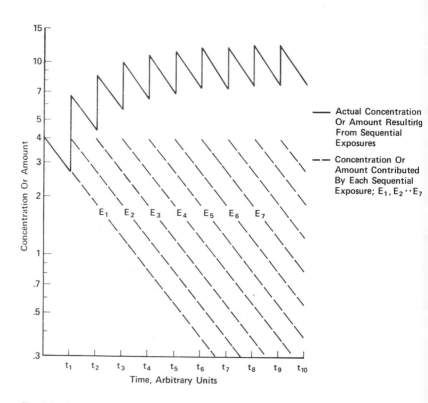

Fig. 4.4 Simulation of the cumulative plasma concentration (C) or amount in the body (A) following repeated administration or exposure.

representation of these concentrations is obtained by addition of the exponential terms for each dose so that the concentration of the chemical at time t following the nth dose is given by

$$C(t)_n = \frac{f D_0}{V_d} \left\{ \frac{1 - \exp(-n k_e \tau)}{1 - \exp(-k_e \tau)} \right\} \exp(-k_e t) \qquad (34)$$

where τ is the interval between doses. After a large number of doses, the term $\exp(-nk_e\tau)$ approaches zero, and the value for the concentration of chemical becomes

$$C(t)_\infty = \frac{fD_0}{V_d}\left\{\frac{\exp(-k_e t)}{1 - \exp(-k_e\tau)}\right\} \qquad (35)$$

Once the plateau concentration is reached, further exposure to the same dose at the same frequency will not result in any further increase in concentration. At the plateau, the maximum concentration which will occur immediately following the last exposure is given by:

$$C(\text{max})_\infty = \frac{fD_0}{V_d}\left\{\frac{1}{1 - \exp(-k_e\tau)}\right\} \qquad (36)$$

The minimum concentration will occur immediately before the next exposure and is given by:

$$C(\text{min})_\infty = \frac{fD_0}{V_d}\left\{\frac{\exp(-k_e\tau)}{1 - \exp(-k_e\tau)}\right\} \qquad (37)$$

The expression defining the average concentration after the plateau has been attained is:

$$C(\text{av})_\infty = \frac{fD_0}{V_d k_e \tau} \qquad (38)$$

If the exposure or the route of administration is such that the first-order rate of absorption, k_a, must be considered, the plasma concentration following n repetitive doses at a dose interval τ is given by:

$$C(t)_n = \frac{fD_0 k_a}{V_d(k_a - k_e)}\left\{\left(\frac{1 - \exp(-nk_e\tau)}{1 - \exp(-k_e\tau)}\right)\exp(-k_e t) - \left(\frac{1 - \exp(-nk_a\tau)}{1 - \exp(-k_a\tau)}\right)\exp(-k_a\tau)\right\}$$

$$(39)$$

The rate constant for absorption, k_a, may be replaced by the rate constant for delivery of a substance being inhaled.

4.8.4 Kinetics of nonlinear or saturable systems

Dose-response curves for an effect arising from the administration of a range of dose levels of a toxic agent usually follow a log-normal distribution. Extrapolation of the logarithmic probability transformation of these curves predicts that some individuals will respond at an infinitesimally small dose, while others will never respond, no matter how large the dose. The assumption inherent in such extrapolation beyond the range of observed data is that the chemobiokinetic profile of the compound in question is independent of the dose level administered.

Assuming dose-independence, a 10-fold increase in the plasma concentration of a chemical will result from a 10-fold increase in the administered dose. However, many metabolic and excretory processes are saturable and, as the dose of chemical begins to overwhelm these processes, it may be expected that there will be a disproportionate increase in toxicity. Therefore, nonlinear chemobiokinetics is of the utmost importance in toxicology.

Many metabolic and active transfer processes as well as some passive protein-binding processes have a finite capacity for reactions with a chemical. The rate of these nonlinear processes can be defined by the Michaelis–Menten equation

$$\frac{-dC(t)}{dt} = \frac{V_m C(t)}{K_m + C(t)} \tag{40}$$

where $C(t)$ represents concentration of the chemical at time t, V_m is the maximum rate of the process, and K_m is the concentration of chemical at which the rate of the process is equal to one-half of V_m. Although this equation has been found useful in delineating *in vivo* nonlinear kinetics, the constants should be referred to as *apparent in vivo* constants, since they are undoubtedly influenced by many other biological processes. Two important limiting cases for this equation are as follows. When the concentration of chemical is much smaller than K_m ($C(t) \ll K_m$) then equation (40) reduces to

$$\frac{-dC(t)}{dt} = \frac{V_m}{K_m} C(t) \tag{41}$$

and the ratio of V_m/K_m will approximate an apparent first-order rate constant. However, when the concentration is much greater than K_m ($C(t) \gg K_m$) then the rate is described by

$$\frac{-dC(t)}{dt} = V_m \tag{42}$$

In this case, the rate is no longer dependent on the prevailing concentration, but has become zero order and thus independent of concentration.

148

Fig. 4.5 displays a typical concentration versus time curve for a chemical the elimination of which follows nonlinear or Michaelis–Menten kinetics. As long as the concentration remains significantly less than K_m, the log-linear portion of the plot is applicable and all the principles of apparent first-order kinetics apply. But, as the concentration approaches and then exceeds K_m, the semi-logarithm plot becomes nonlinear. In this region of zero-order kinetics, the plot will be linear if rectangular coordinates are used.

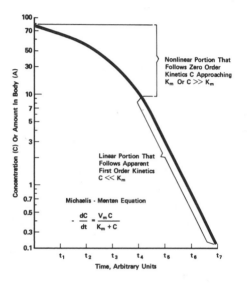

Fig. 4.5   Simulated plasma concentration (C) or amount in the body (A) as a function of time for elimination of a chemical which can be described by the Michaelis–Menten equation. dC/dt is the change in concentration with time. V_m is the maximum rate of the process and K_m is the Michaelis constant.

4.9   Linear and Nonlinear One Compartment Open-model Kinetics of 2,4,5-Trichlorophenoxyacetic acid (2,4,5-T)

To illustrate the use of chemobiokinetics in toxicology, some results obtained from studies with 2,4,5-T are presented below. 2,4,5-T, a herbicide, has been reported to be teratogenic, fetotoxic, and embryotoxic at doses of 100 mg/kg/day during the period of organogenesis (Collins & Williams, 1971; Courtney & Moore, 1971; Courtney et al., 1970; Roll, 1971; Sparschu et al., 1971).

To elucidate the potential hazard of this compound, 5 mg/kg of ^{14}C ring-labelled 2,4,5-T was administered as a single oral dose to rats and dogs

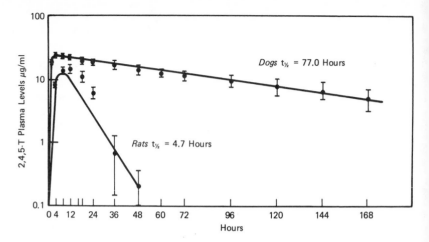

Fig. 4.6   Concentration of ^{14}C-activity expressed as µg equivalents 2,4,5-T/ml plasma in dogs and rats following a single oral dose of ^{14}C-2,4,5-T at 5 mg/kg. Each point represents a mean and S.E.

(Piper et al., 1973). The plasma concentration versus time curves (Fig. 4.6) indicated compliance with a one-compartment open model system having apparent first-order rates of absorption and clearance; the $t_{1/2}$ values for the clearance of 2,4,5-T from the plasma of rats and dogs were 4.7 and 77 h, respectively. For elimination from the body via the urine (Fig. 4.7), the $t_{1/2}$ values were 13.6 and 86.6 h. Since clearance of 2,4,5-T from the plasma of rats was more rapid than its elimination in the urine, the compound may have been actively concentrated in the kidneys prior to excretion in the urine. Also, the much slower elimination by dogs than rats correlates with the higher toxicity in dogs; the single oral LD$_{50}$ is 100 mg/kg and 300 mg/kg for dogs and rats, respectively (Drill & Heratyka, 1953; Rowe & Hymas, 1954).

Another species difference was demonstrated by the fact that virtually all the ^{14}C excreted by the rats was through the urine while approximately 20% of that excreted by dogs was through the faeces. Also, no breakdown products of 2,4,5-T could be detected in the urine of rats given 5 mg/kg, but about 10% of the ^{14}C activity in the urine of dogs was attributable to breakdown products.

If an active secretory process in the kidney was the primary elimination process in rats, then this nonlinear process should be saturable by the administration of higher doses. Figs. 4.8 and 4.9 show that this is the case, since the $t_{1/2}$ for both the clearance of 2,4,5-T from plasma and its urinary elimination increase with increasing dose. At doses of 100 or 200 mg/kg, the process was saturated and the rates of elimination from the plasma and

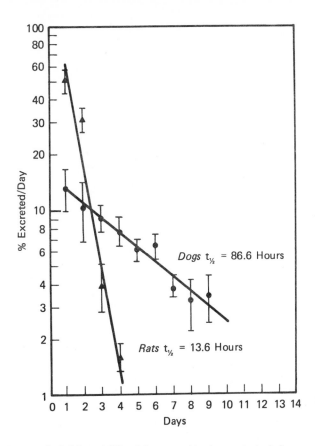

Fig. 4.7   Percent of administered ^{14}C activity excreted by dogs and rats during successive 24-h intervals following a single oral dose of ^{14}C-2,4,5-T at 5 mg/kg. Each point represents a mean and S.E.

from the body were the same. Further evidence of nonlinear kinetics was the fact that a larger percentage of the ^{14}C administered as ^{14}C-2,4,5-T was excreted through the faeces as the dose was increased. Also, degradation products of 2,4,5-T were found in the urine of rats given 100 or 200 mg/kg, but not 5 or 50 mg/kg.

The nonlinear chemobiokinetics of 2,4,5-T were further characterized following intravenous doses in rats of 5 or 100 mg/kg (Sauerhoff et al., 1975). Clearance from the plasma of rats given 100 mg/kg followed classical Michaelis–Menten kinetics (Fig. 4.10). The values for V_m and K_m were calculated to be 16.6 ± 1.82 µg/h/g of plasma and 127.6 ± 25.9 µg/g of plasma, respectively. During the log-linear phase of excretion the $t_{1/2}$ was 5.3 ± 1.2 h.

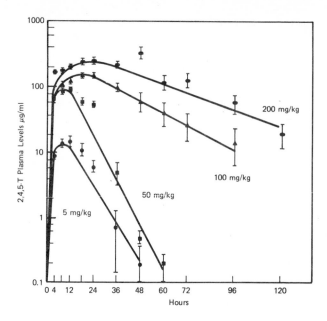

Fig. 4.8 Concentration of ^{14}C activity expressed as μg equivalents 2,4,5-T/ml plasma in rats following a single oral dose of ^{14}C-2,4,5-T at 5, 50, 100 and 200 mg/kg. Each point presents a mean and S.E.

In the experiments of Sauerhoff et al. (1975), the volume of distribution increased from 190 to 235 ml/kg in rats given 5 and 100 mg/kg, respectively. This increase in the volume of distribution indicates that with increasing dose a larger fraction of the dose is distributed into various tissues and cells. Thus, a disproportionate increase in toxicity may be expected. The fate of 2,4,5-T following oral doses of 5 mg/kg has also been investigated in man (Gehring et al., 1973). The elimination of 2,4,5-T from the plasma and in the urine followed apparent first order kinetics with $t_{1/2}$ of 23.1 h (Figs. 4.11, 4.12, 4.13). A comparison of the elimination rates in man with those in rats and dogs indicates that the toxicity of 2,4,5-T to man would lie somewhere between that to rats and dogs. The peak plasma levels attained with a dose of 5 mg/kg, which are higher in man than in either rats or dogs, are associated with a greater degree of plasma protein binding in man. Also, the volume of distribution in man of 80 ml/kg is attested to the retention of 2,4,5-T in the vascular compartment.

Fig. 4.14 illustrates simulated levels of 2,4,5-T that would be attained in the plasma of man with repeated ingestion. If 0.25 mg/kg were ingested daily, a level equalling that attained by ingesting a single dose of 5 mg/kg, as in this study, would never be reached.

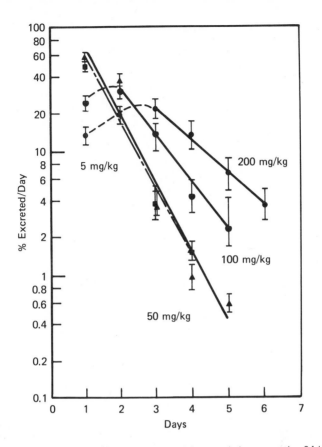

Fig. 4.9 Percent administered ^{14}C activity excreted by rats during successive 24-h intervals following a single oral dose of ^{14}C-2,3,5-T at 5, 50, 100 or 200 mg/kg. Each point represents a mean and S.E.

Additional studies on 2,4,5-T have demonstrated that it is actively secreted by the kidney (Hook et al., 1974). This process of elimination is saturable at high doses and the capacity for excretion in dogs is more limited than in rats. As indicated previously, when doses of 2,4,5-T are given that exceed the capacity for renal excretion, the compound finds its way into more tissues and cells, is eliminated more slowly, and undergoes a greater degree of metabolic transformation. Thus, to use the toxicity incurred by high doses of 2,4,5-T to make statistical estimates of the toxicity that may be incurred at low doses violates a basic *a priori* assumption.

The nonlinear chemobiokinetics of toxic doses of 2,4,5-T is an example for many other compounds (Gehring et al., 1976). Indeed, it is likely that for most compounds, toxicity may coincide with the saturation of

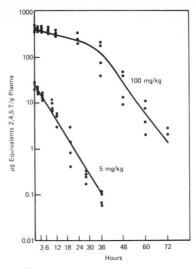

Fig. 4.10 Concentration of ^{14}C activity expressed as μg equivalents 2,4,5-T/g plasma of rats following a single intravenous dose of ^{14}C-2,4,5-T at 5 or 100 mg/kg.

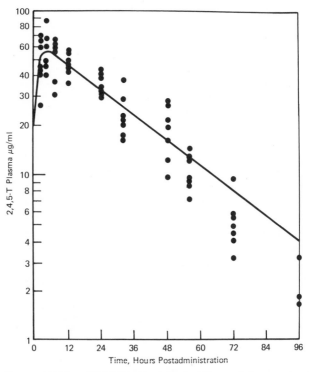

Fig. 4.11 The concentration of 2,4,5-T in blood plasma of human beings as a function of time following a single oral dose of 5 mg/kg. The points are values of 7 different subjects.

154

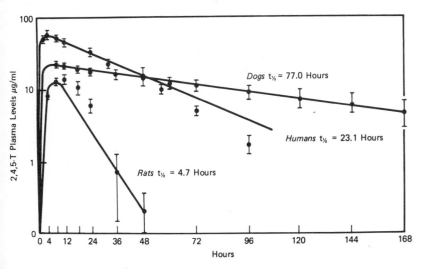

Fig. 4.12 The concentration of 2,4,5-T in blood plasma of dogs, human beings and rats following a single oral dose of 5 mg/kg. Each point represents a mean and SE.

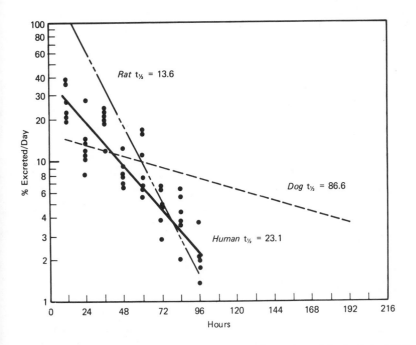

Fig. 4.13 Percent of administered 2,4,5-T excreted by rats, dogs and man following a single oral dose of 5 mg/kg.

155

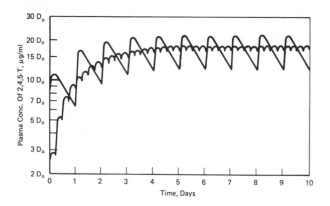

Fig. 4.14 Predicted plasma concentrations of 2,4,5-T in human beings ingesting a dose of D_0 in units of mg/kg every 24 h (curve with large peaks) or a dose of $\frac{1}{4} D_0$ every 6 h (curve with small peaks).

the detoxification process, operative at low doses. Recently, Gillette (1974a,b) has given special consideration to the chemobiokinetics of reactive metabolites of chemicals that react with macromolecules (DNA, RNA, and protein) causing toxic effects. The concepts presented in these papers are very important to the toxicologist because they indicate possible threshold mechanisms for toxicity, in particular chronic toxicity.

4.10 Linear Chemobiokinetics Used to Assess Potential for Bioaccumulation of 2,3,6,7-tetrachlorodibenzo-*p*-dioxin (TCDD)

TCDD is a highly toxic compound formed as an unwanted contaminant in the manufacture of 2,4,5-trichlorophenol (Schwetz et al., 1973). Use of trichlorophenol to manufacture 2,4,5-trichlorophenoxyacetic acid may result in contamination of 2,4,5-T with TCDD. The physicochemical properties of TCDD suggest that exposure to small amounts may result in the persistent accumulation of the highly toxic material and, eventually, in toxic effects. To elucidate the propensity of TCDD to accumulate in the body, a series of pharmacokinetic studies was conducted (Rose et al., 1975). In these studies, one group of rats was given a single oral dose of ^{14}C-TCDD at 1 μg/kg and the excretion of ^{14}C activity in urine, expired air, and faeces was determined. Other groups of rats were given orally 0.01, 0.1 or 1.0 μg of ^{14}C-TCDD/kg/day, from Monday to Friday, for up to 7 weeks. In addition to determining the amounts of ^{14}C activity excreted in the urine and faeces of these rats, the amounts remaining in the body were calculated as a function of time and the levels of ^{14}C-activity residing in various tissues after 1, 3, and 7 weeks of administration were determined.

Since the overall recovery of ^{14}C in rats given a single oral dose of ^{14}C-TCDD was 97 $\pm$ 8%, the amounts of ^{14}C activity remaining in the bodies of the rats as a function of time was calculated by subtracting the cumulative amount excreted from the original dose. The resulting body burdens of ^{14}C are depicted in Fig. 4.15. The halftime for elimination of ^{14}C from the body ranged from 21 to 39 days. All of the ^{14}C activity was eliminated via the faeces.

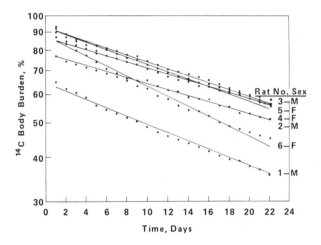

Fig. 4.15 Percent of the ^{14}C activity remaining in the body of rats following a single oral dose of ^{14}C-TCDD at 1 µg/kg.

The concentration of ^{14}C activity in the bodies of rats given 0.1 or 1.0 µg/kg/day, from Monday to Friday, for 7 weeks as a function of time are shown in Fig. 4.16. The data show clearly that, with repeated exposure, the concentration of ^{14}C activity in the body increases but the rate of increase decreases with time and the amount in the body begins to plateau, even though exposure continues.

The average overall recovery of administered ^{14}C was 97.7 $\pm$ 9% of the cumulative dose of ^{14}C. Mathematical analyses of the data presented in Fig. 4.16 revealed a rate constant for excretion of TCDD of 0.0293 $\pm$ 0.0050 days^{-1} which corresponds to a half-time of 23.7 days. The fraction of each dose absorbed was 0.861 $\pm$ 0.078. Using these values, it may be calculated that the ultimate steady state body burden would be 21.3 D_0 for rats given a daily dose of D_0, 5 consecutive days weekly for an infinite number of weeks.

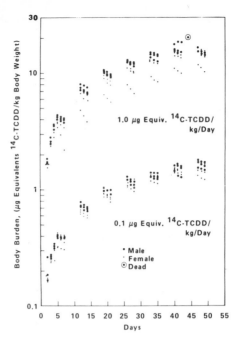

Fig. 4.16 The concentration of microgram equivalents TCDD in the body of rats given oral doses of 0.1 and 1.0 μg/kg/day of ^{14}C-TCDD, from Monday to Friday, for 7 weeks.

If D_0 were administered every day for an infinite time, the ultimate steady state body burden would be 29.0 D_0. Within the 7 weeks of this study, the rats had attained 79.1% of the ultimate steady state body burden. The time required to reach 90% of the ultimate steady state body burden would be 78.5 days.

The concentrations of ^{14}C-activity in the liver and fat of rats given ^{14}C-TCDD at concentrations of 0.01, 0.1, or 1.0 μg/kg/day, from Monday to Friday, for 1, 3, or 7 weeks are illustrated graphically in Figs. 4.17 and 4.18, respectively. Just like the body burden levels, the levels in these tissues increase at a decreasing rate and begin to plateau. It should also be noted that at each time of measurement, there is a direct relationship between the dose being administered and the level in the tissue. This latter observation is illustrated more clearly in Figs. 4.19 and 4.20, where the concentrations of ^{14}C-activity in the liver and the fat have been divided by the dose. This shows that over the range of doses given, 0.01 to 1.0 μg/kg/day, the relative degree of accumulation of ^{14}C-TCDD by these tissues is not influenced by dose.

Mathematical evaluation of the data presented in Fig. 4.17–4.20 revealed

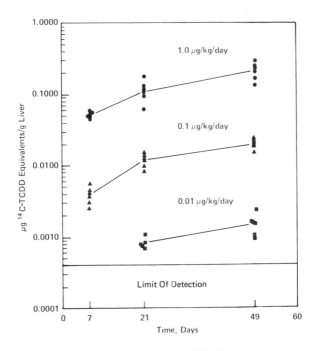

Fig. 4.17 The concentration of microgram equivalents TCDD in the liver of rats given oral doses of ^{14}C-TCDD at 0.01, 0.1, 1.0 μg/kg, from Monday to Friday, for 1, 3, or 7 weeks.

that the rates for the clearance of TCDD from liver and fat were 0.026 ± 0.000 and 0.029 ± 0.001 days^{-1} respectively. These rates are essentially the same as the rate of elimination from the body *in toto*, which is not unexpected because these tissues contained the bulk of the ^{14}C-TCDD in the body. The ultimate steady state concentrations in liver and fat that would be attained with an infinite duration of exposure are 0.250 ± 0.000 and 0.058 ± 0.003 D_0 μg TCDD/g where D_0 equals the dose being administered in μg/kg. The times required to reach specified fractions of the ultimate steady state concentrations would be identical no matter what dose, D_0, is being administered.

The ^{14}C-activity in liver tissue from rats given 0.1 or 1.0 μg/kg/day, from Monday to Friday, weekly for 7 weeks, was demonstrated by gas chromatography and by a combination of gas chromatography and mass spectrometry to be due to ^{14}C-TCDD. Also important was the finding that the ^{14}C-TCDD present in the liver was readily extractable, indicating that TCDD does not bind irreversibly with tissue. With regard to the assessment of the hazard of repeated exposure to very small amounts of TCDD, the results show that TCDD would not continue to accumulate in the body with

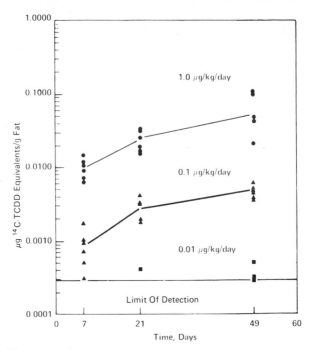

Fig. 4.18 The concentration of microgram equivalents TCDD in the fat of rats given single oral doses of ^{14}C-TCDD at 0.01, 0.1 or 1.0 μg/kg, from Monday to Friday, for 1, 3, or 7 weeks.

prolonged repeated exposure. In rats, 93% of the ultimate steady state level of TCDD in the body would be attained within 90 days. Recently, a toxicological evaluation of TCDD was conducted in rats given doses of 0.001, 0.01, 0.1 and 1.0 μg TCDD/kg/day, from Monday to Friday, for 13 weeks (Kociba et al., 1975). Perceptible adverse effects did not develop in rats given 0.001 or 0.01 μg TCDD/kg/day. Adverse effects including hepatic pathology and functional changes, atrophy of the thymus, and haematological alterations were observed in rats receiving 0.1 or 1.0 μg TCDD/kg/day. Indeed, some rats receiving 1.0 μg TCDD/kg/day died. The results of the studies on the fate and accumulation of TCDD in rats given repeated daily doses showed clearly that even with more prolonged exposure those rats which received 0.01 μg TCDD/kg/day would not continue to accumulate TCDD in the body and its tissues to the extent leading to the toxic manifestations as seen in those rats receiving 0.1 or 1.0 μg/kg/day. Since the levels of TCDD in the tissues had essentially plateaued within 90 days, more prolonged exposure would not be expected to lead to the attainment of toxic amounts of TCDD in the body or its tissues.

160

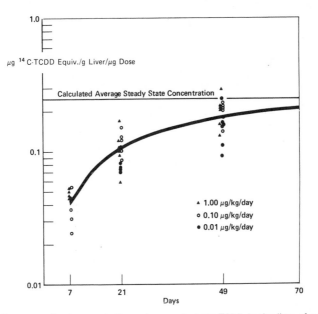

Fig. 4.19 Dose-normalized concentrations of μg equivalents TCDD in the liver of rats given ^{14}C-TCDD at 0.01, 0.1 or 1.0 g/kg/day from Monday to Friday, for 1, 3, or 7 weeks.

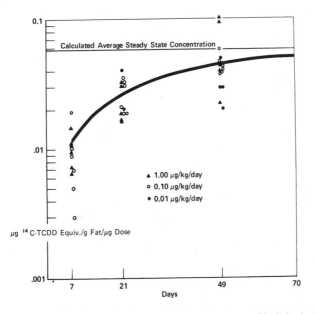

Fig. 4.20 Dose-normalized concentrations of microgram equivalents TCDD in the fat of rats given ^{14}C-TCDD at 0.01, 0.1 or 1.0 μg/kg/day from Monday to Friday, for 1, 3, or 7 weeks.

161

Table 4.1   Different types of drug-metabolizing reactions

I.   OXIDATIONS

(a)   *Microsomal oxidations*
(Ciaccio, 1971; Dahm, 1971; Daly, 1971; Gillette, 1971b; Gram, 1971; Smuckler, 1971; Weisburger & Weisburger, 1971.)

Aliphatic oxidation $\quad\quad\quad RCH_3 \longrightarrow RCH_2OH$

Aromatic hydroxylation

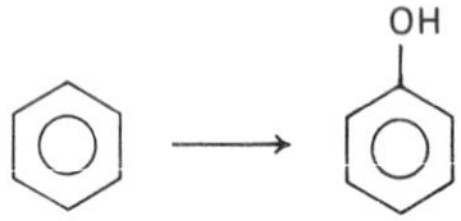

Epoxidation $\quad\quad\quad R-CH_2-CH_2-R \longrightarrow R-CH-CH-R$ (with epoxide O)

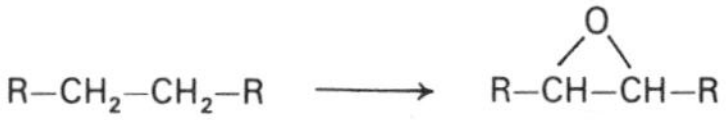

Oxidative deamination

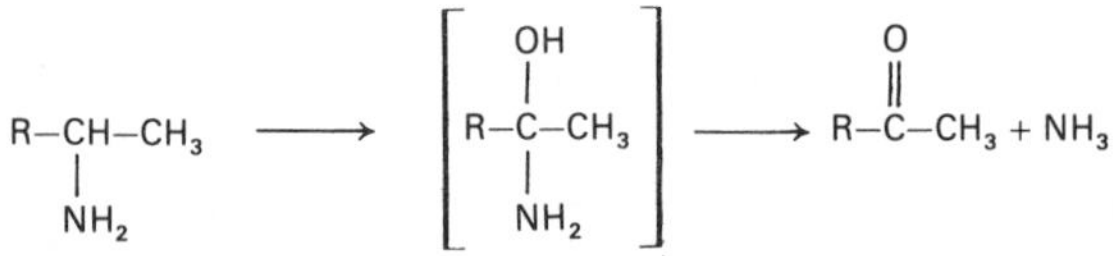

$$R-\underset{\underset{NH_2}{|}}{CH}-CH_3 \longrightarrow \left[R-\underset{\underset{NH_2}{|}}{\overset{\overset{OH}{|}}{C}}-CH_3 \right] \longrightarrow R-\overset{\overset{O}{\|}}{C}-CH_3 + NH_3$$

N-dealkylation $\quad\quad\quad R-N\Big\langle{}^{CH_3}_{CH_3} \longrightarrow R-N\Big\langle{}^{H}_{CH_3} + CH_2O$

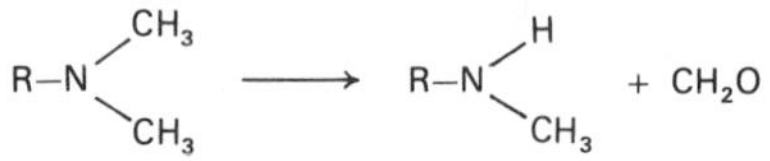

O-dealkylation $\quad\quad\quad R-O-CH_3 \longrightarrow R-OH + CH_2O$

S-dealkylation $\quad\quad\quad R-S-CH_3 \longrightarrow R-SH + CH_2O$

Metalloalkane dealkylation $\quad\quad\quad Pb(C_2H_5)_4 \longrightarrow PbH(C_2H_5)_3$

N-oxidation $\quad\quad\quad \overset{R}{\underset{R}{R-N}} \longrightarrow \overset{R}{\underset{R}{R-N}}=O + H^+$

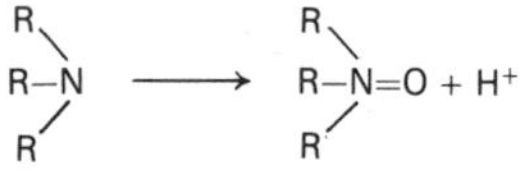

N-hydroxylation

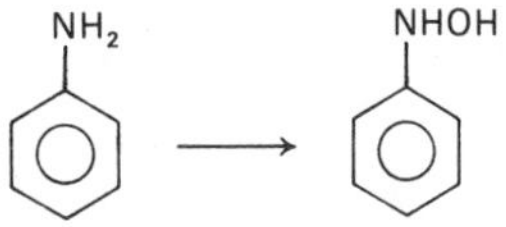

Sulfoxidation $\quad\quad\quad R-S-R \longrightarrow R-\overset{\uparrow}{\underset{}{S}}-R$ (with O above S)

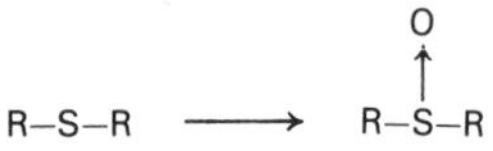

Table 4.1 Different types of drug-metabolizing reactions—*continued*

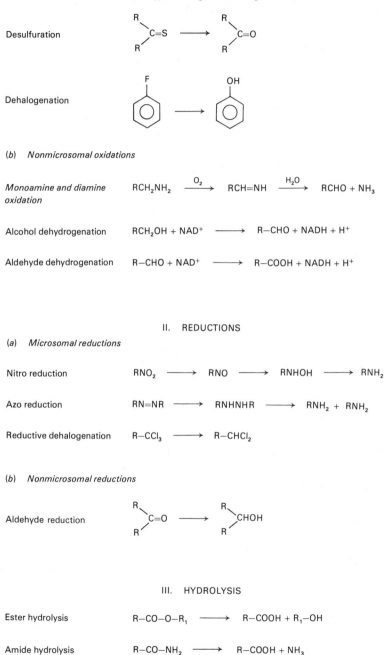

Desulfuration

Dehalogenation

(*b*) *Nonmicrosomal oxidations*

Monoamine and diamine oxidation $RCH_2NH_2 \xrightarrow{O_2} RCH{=}NH \xrightarrow{H_2O} RCHO + NH_3$

Alcohol dehydrogenation $RCH_2OH + NAD^+ \longrightarrow R{-}CHO + NADH + H^+$

Aldehyde dehydrogenation $R{-}CHO + NAD^+ \longrightarrow R{-}COOH + NADH + H^+$

II. REDUCTIONS

(*a*) *Microsomal reductions*

Nitro reduction $RNO_2 \longrightarrow RNO \longrightarrow RNHOH \longrightarrow RNH_2$

Azo reduction $RN{=}NR \longrightarrow RNHNHR \longrightarrow RNH_2 + RNH_2$

Reductive dehalogenation $R{-}CCl_3 \longrightarrow R{-}CHCl_2$

(*b*) *Nonmicrosomal reductions*

Aldehyde reduction

III. HYDROLYSIS

Ester hydrolysis $R{-}CO{-}O{-}R_1 \longrightarrow R{-}COOH + R_1{-}OH$

Amide hydrolysis $R{-}CO{-}NH_2 \longrightarrow R{-}COOH + NH_3$

Table 4.1   Different types of drug-metabolizing reactions—*continued*

IV.   CONJUGATION

(*a*)   *UDPGA-mediated conjugations*

O-glucuronide formation
    ether type:

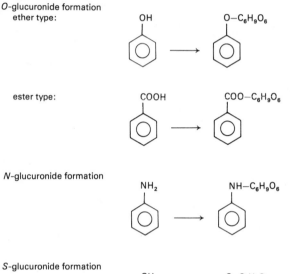

    ester type:

N-glucuronide formation

S-glucuronide formation

(*b*)   *PAPS-mediated conjugation*

Sulfate ester formation

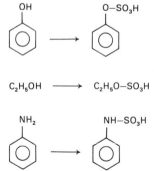

Table 4.1   Different types of drug-metabolizing reactions—*continued*

(*c*)   *Methylations*

N-methylation

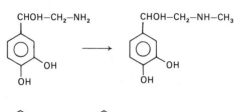

O-methylation

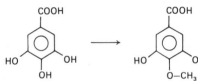

S-methylation $C_2H_5SH \longrightarrow C_2H_5S-CH_3$

(*d*)   *Acetylations*

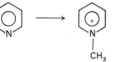

(*e*)   *Peptide conjugations*

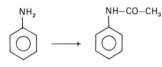

(*f*)   *Glutathione conjugations*

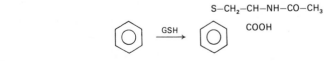

Table 4.2   Methods for the determination of several mixed-function oxidase activities

(a)	Aryl hydrocarbon hydroxylation (using 3,4-benzpyrene as substrate) (Nebert & Gelboin, 1968a,b; Wattenberg et al., 1962)
(b)	Aliphatic side-chain hydroxylation (of pentobarbital) (Cooper & Brodie, 1955)
(c)	4-hydroxylation (of aniline) (Brodie & Axelrod, 1948; Chabra et al., 1972; Gilbert & Golberg, 1965; Henderson & Kersten, 1970; Hilton & Santorelli, 1970; Imai et al., 1966; Kato & Gillette, 1965; Schenkman et al., 1967; Sternsen & Hes, 1975)
(d)	N-hydroxylation (of aniline) (Herr & Kiese, 1959)
(e)	N-oxidation (determination of amine oxides) (Fok & Ziegler, 1970; Ziegler et al., 1973)
(f)	Nitro reduction (Fouts & Brodie, 1957; Hietbrink & DuBois, 1965)
(g)	N-demethylation (of aminopyrine) (Brodie & Axelrod, 1950; Chrastil & Wilson, 1975; Cochin & Axelrod, 1959; Dewaide & Henderson, 1968; Feuer et al., 1971; Kinoshita et al., 1966; Klinger, 1974; La Du et al., 1955; MacMahon, 1962; Nash, 1953; Pederson & Aust, 1970; Poland & Nebert, 1973; Schoene et al., 1972)
(h)	N-demethylation (of benzphetamine) (Hewick & Fouts, 1970a,b; Liu et al., 1975; Lu et al., 1969; Nash, 1953)
(i)	N-demethylation (of ethylmorphine) (Anders & Mannering, 1966)
(j)	O-demethylation (of O-nitroanisole) (Christensen & Wissing, 1972; Kinoshita et al., 1966; Netter, 1960; Netter & Seidel, 1964; Schoene et al., 1972; Zannoni, 1971)
(k)	O-dealkylation (of ethylumbelliferone) (Ullrich & Weber, 1972)

REFERENCES

AITIO, A. (1973) Glucuronide synthesis in the rat and guinea pig lung. *Xenobiotica*, **3**: 13–22.

AL-KASSAB, S., BOYLAND, E., & WILLIAMS, K. (1963) An enzyme from rat liver catalysing conjugations with glutathione; replacement of nitro groups. *Biochem. J.*, **87**: 4–9.

ALLEN, J. R., NORBOCK, D. H., & HSU, I. C. (1974) Tissue modifications in monkeys as related to absorption, distribution and excretion of polychlorinated biphenyls. *Arch. environ. Contam. Toxicol.*, **2**: 86–95.

ANDERS, M. W. & MANNERING, G. J. (1966) Inhibition of drug metabolism. I. Kinetics of the inhibition of the *N*-demethylation of ethylmorphine by 2-diethylaminoethyl 2, 2-diphenylvalerate HCl (SKF 525A) and related compounds. *Mol. Pharmacol.*, **2**: 319–327.

ARIAS, I. M. (1962) Chronic unconjugated hyperbilirubinaemia without overt signs of haemolysis in adolescents and adults. *J. clin. Invest.*, **41**: 2233–2245.

ASSICOT, M. & BOHUON, C. (1969) A simple and rapid fluorimetric determination of catechol-*O*-methyl transferase activity. *Life Sci.*, **8**: 93–100.

AXELROD, J. (1971) Methyltransferase enzymes in the metabolism of physiologically active compounds and drugs. In: Brodie, B. B. & Gillette, J. R., ed. *Concepts in biochemical pharmacology*, Berlin, Springer-Verlag, Vol. 2, pp. 609–619.

AXELROD, J. & DALY, J. W. (1968) Phenol-*O*-methyl transferase. *Biochim. Biophys. Acta*, **159**: 472–478.

AXELROD, J. & TOMCHICK, R. (1958) Enzymatic *O*-methylation of epinephrine and other catechols. *J. biol. Chem.*, **233**: 702–705.

BAKER, R. C., COONS, L. B., & HODGSON, E. (1973) Low speed preparation of microsomes: a comparative study. *Chem. biol. Interactions*, **6**: 307–316.

BECKETT, A. H. & HOSSIE, R. D. (1971) Buccal absorption of drugs. In: Brodie, B. B. & Gillette, J. R., ed. *Concepts in biochemical pharmacology*, Berlin, Springer-Verlag, Vol. 1, pp. 25–46.

BOND, E. J. & DE MATTEIS, F. (1969) Biochemical changes in rat liver after administration of carbon disulfide with reference to microsomal changes. *Biochem. Pharmacol.*, **18**: 2531–2549.

BONNICHSEN, R. K. & BRINK, N. G. (1955) Liver alcohol dehydrogenase. In: Colowick, S. P. & Kaplan, N. O., ed. *Methods in enzymology*, New York, Academic Press, Vol. 1, pp. 495–500.

BOOTH, J., BOYLAND, E., & SIMS, P. (1961) An enzyme from rat liver catalysing conjugations with glutathione. *Biochem. J.*, **79**: 516–524.

BORCHARDT, R. T. (1974) A rapid spectrophotometric assay for catechol-*O*-methyl transferase. *Anal. Biochem.*, **58**: 382–389.

BORGÅ, O., AZARNOFF, D. L., & SJÖQVIST, F. (1968) Species differences in the plasma-protein binding of desipramine. *J. Pharm. Pharmacol.*, **20**: 571.

BOYD, G. S. & SMELLIE, R. M. S. (1972) *Biological hydroxylation mechanism*. New York, Academic Press.

BOYLAND, E. (1971) Mercapturic acid conjugation. In: Brodie, B. B. & Gillette, J. R., ed. *Concepts in biochemical pharmacology*, Berlin, Springer-Verlag, Vol. 2, pp. 584–608.

BOYLAND, E. & CHASSEAUD, L. F. (1967) Enzyme-catalysed conjugations of glutathione with unsaturated compounds. *Biochem. J.*, **104**: 95–102.

BOYLAND, E. & WILLIAMS, K. (1965) A new enzyme catalysing the conjugations of epoxides. *Biochem. J.*, **94**: 190–197.

BRAUER, R. W. (1959) Mechanisms of bile secretion. *J. Am. Med. Assoc.*, **169**: 1462–1466.

BROCH, O. J., JR & GULDBERG, H. C. (1971) On the determination of catechol-*O*-methyl transferase activity in tissue homogenates. *Acta Pharmacol. Toxicol.*, **30**: 266–277.

BRODIE, B. B. (1964) Physicochemical factors in drug absorption. In: Binns, T. B., ed. *Absorption and distribution of drugs*, Baltimore, Williams & Wilkins, pp. 16–48.

167

BRODIE, B. B. & AXELROD, J. (1948) The estimation of acetanilide and its metabolic products, aniline, *N*-acetyl-*p*-aminophenol and *p*-aminophenol (free and total conjugates) in biological fluids and tissues. *J. Pharmac. exp. Ther.*, **94:** 22–28.

BRODIE, B. B. & AXELROD, J. (1950) The fate of aminopyrine (Pyramidon) in man and methods for the estimation of aminopyrine and its metabolites in biological material. *J. Pharmac. exp. Ther.*, **99:** 171–184.

BRODIE, B. B. & HOGBEN, C. A. M. (1957) Some physicochemical factors in drug action. *J. Pharm. Pharmacol.*, **9:** 345–347.

BURCHELL, B., DUTTON, G. J., & NEMETH, A. M. (1972) Development of phenobarbital-sensitive control mechanisms for uridine diphosphate glucuronyl-transferase activity in chick liver. *J. cell. Biol.*, **55:** 448–456.

CHASE, G. D. & RABINOWITZ, J. L. (1968) *Principles of radioisotope methodology*, 3rd ed. Minneapolis, Burgess Publishing Company.

CHABHRA, R. S., GRAM, T. E., & FOUTS, J. R. (1972) A comparative study of two procedures used in the determination of hepatic microsomal aniline hydroxylation. *Toxicol. appl. Pharmacol.*, **22:** 50–58.

CHIGNELL, C. F. (1971) Physical methods for studying drug-protein binding. In: Brodie, B. B. & Gillette, J. R., ed. *Concepts in biochemical pharmacology*, Berlin, Springer-Verlag, Vol. 1, pp. 187–212.

CHRASTIL, J. & WILSON, J. T. (1975) A sensitive colorimetric method for formaldehyde. *Anal. Biochem.*, **63:** 202–207.

CHRISTENSEN, F. & WISSING, F. (1972) Inhibition of microsomal drug-metabolizing enzymes from rat liver by various 4-hydroxy-coumarin derivatives. *Biochem. Pharmacol.*, **21:** 975–984.

CIACCIO, E. I. (1971) Intimate study of drug action. II. Fate of drugs in the body. In: Dipalma, J. R., ed. *Drills pharmacology in medicine*, New York, McGraw–Hill, pp. 36–66.

COCHIN, J. & AXELROD, J. (1959) Biochemical and pharmacological changes in the rat following chronic administration of morphine, nalorphine and normorphine. *J. Pharmac. exp. Ther.*, **125:** 105–110.

COLLINS, T. F. X. & WILLIAMS, C. H. (1971) Teratogenic studies with 2,4,5-T and 2,4-D in the hamster. *Bull. environ. Contam. Toxicol.*, **6:** 559–567.

CONNEY, A. H. (1967) Pharmacological implications of microsomal enzyme induction. *Pharmacol. Rev.*, **19:** 317–366.

CONNEY, A. H. & BURNS, J. J. (1962) Factors influencing drug metabolism. *Adv. Pharmacol.*, **1:** 31–54.

CONNEY, A. H., COUTINHO, C., KOECHLIN, B., SWARM, R., CHERIPHO, J. A., IMPELLIZERI, C., & BARUTH, H. (1974) From animals to man: metabolic considerations. *Clin. Pharmacol. Ther.*, **16:** 176–182.

COOPER, J. R. & BRODIE, B. B. (1965) Enzymatic oxidation of pentobarbital and thiopental. *J. Pharmacol. exp. Ther.*, **120:** 75–87.

COTZIAS, G. C. & DOLE, V. P. (1951) Metabolism of amines. I. Microdetermination of aminoamine oxidase in tissues. *J. biol. Chem.*, **190:** 665–672.

COURTNEY, D. K., GAYLOR, D. W., HOGAN, M. D., FLAK, H. L., BATES, R. R., & MITCHELL, I. (1970) Teratogenic evaluation of 2,4,5-T. *Science*, **168:** 864–866.

COURTNEY, D. K. & MOORE, J. A. (1971) Teratology studies with 2,4,5-trichlorophenoxy-acetic acid and 2,3,7,8-tetrachlorodibenzo-*p*-dioxin. *Toxicol. appl. Pharmacol.*, **20:** 396–403.

CREASEY, N. H. (1956) Factors which interfere with the manometric assay of monoamine oxidase. *Biochem. J.*, **64:** 178–183.

DAHM, P. A. (1971) Oxidative desulfuration and dealkylation of selected organophosphate insecticides. In: Brodie, B. B. & Gillette, J. R., ed. *Concepts in biochemical pharmacology*, Berlin, Springer-Verlag, Vol. 2, pp. 362–366.

DALY, J. (1971) Enzymatic oxidation of carbon. In: Brodie, B. B. & Gillette, J. R., ed. *Concepts in biochemical pharmacology*, Berlin, Springer-Verlag, Vol. 2, pp. 285–311.

DAVIES, D. S., GIGON, P. L., & GILLETTE, J. R. (1969) Species and sex differences in electron transport systems in liver microsomes and their relationship to ethylmorphine demethylation. *Life Sci.*, **8**: 85–91.

DAVSON, H. & DANIELLI, J. F. (1952) *The permeability of natural membranes*, 2nd ed. Cambridge, Cambridge Univ. Press.

DEITRICH, R. A. & ERWIN, V. G. (1969) Spectrophotometric assay for monoamine oxidase. *Anal. Biochem.*, **30**: 395–402.

DEWAIDE, J. H. & HENDERSON, P. T. (1968) Hepatic *N*-demethylation of aminopyrine in rat and trout. *Biochem. Pharmacol.*, **17**: 1901–1907.

DRILL, V. A. & HERATJKA, T. (1953) Toxicity of 2,4-dichlorophenoxyacetic acid and 2,4,5-trichlorophenoxyacetic acid. *Arch. ind. Hyg. occup. Med.*, **7**: 61–67.

DUTTON, G. J. (1966) The biosynthesis of glucuronides. In: Dutton, G. J. ed. *Glucuronic acid, free and combined*. New York, Academic Press.

DUTTON, G. J. (1971) Glucuronide-forming enzymes. In: Brodie, B. B. & Gillette, J. R., ed. *Concepts in biochemical pharmacology*, Berlin, Springer-Verlag, Vol. 2, pp. 378–400.

DUTTON, G. J. & STOREY, I. D. E. (1962) Glucuronide-forming enzymes. In: Colowick, S. P. & Kaplan, N. O., ed. *Methods in enzymology*, New York, Academic Press, Vol. 5, pp. 159–164.

ESTABROOK, R. W. (1971) Cytochrome P-450. Its function in the oxidative metabolism of drugs. In: Brodie, B. B. & Gillette, J. R., ed. *Concepts in biochemical pharmacology*, Berlin, Springer-Verlag, Vol. 2, pp. 264–284.

ESTABROOK, R. W., FRANKLIN, M. R., COHEN, B., SHIGAMATSU, A., & HILDEBRANDT, A. G. (1971) Influence of hepatic microsomal mixed function oxidation reactions on cellular metabolic control. *Metabolism*, **20**: 186–199.

ESTABROOK, R. W., GILLETTE, J. R., & LEIBMAN, K. C. (1972) *Microsomes and drug oxidations*. Baltimore, Williams & Wilkins.

FEUER, G., SOSA-LUCERO, J. C., LUMB, F., & MODDEL, G. (1971) Failure of various drugs to induce drug metabolizing enzymes in extrahepatic tissues of the rat. *Toxicol. appl. Pharmacol.*, **19**: 579–589.

FLYNN, E. J., LYNCH, M., & ZANNONI, V. G. (1969) Species differences in hepatic microsomal electron transport. *Fed. Proc.*, **28**: 483.

FLYNN, E. J., LYNCH, M., & ZANNONI, V. G. (1972) Species differences and drug metabolism. *Biochem. Pharmacol.*, **21**: 2577–2590.

FOK, A. K. & ZIEGLER, D. M. (1970) Estimation of amine oxides in the presence of hepatic microsomes. *Biochem. Biophys. Res. Commun.*, **41**: 534–540.

FOREMAN, H. (1971) Translocation of drugs into bone. In: Brodie, B. B. & Gillette, J. R., ed. *Concepts in biochemical pharmacology*, Berlin, Springer-Verlag, Vol. 1, pp. 249–257.

FOUTS, J. R. (1970) The stimulation and inhibition of hepatic microsomal drug-metabolising enzymes with special reference to the effects of environmental contaminants. *Toxicol. appl. Pharmacol.*, **17**: 804–809.

FOUTS, J. R. & BRODIE, B. B. (1957) The enzymatic reduction of chloramphenicol, *p*-nitrobenzoic acid and other aromatic nitro compounds in mammals. *J. Pharmacol. exp. Ther.* **119**: 197–207.

FOUTS, J. R. & POHL, H. J. (1971) Further studies on the effects of metal ions on rat liver microsomal reduced nicotinamide adenine dinucleotide phosphate-cytochrome P-450 reductase. *J. Pharmacol. exp. Ther.*, **179**: 91–100.

GARATTINI, S., MARCUCCI, F., & MUSSINI, E. (1975) Biotransformation of drugs to pharmacologically active metabolites. In: Gillette, J. R. & Mitchell, J. R., ed. *Concepts in biochemical pharmacology*, Berlin, Springer-Verlag, Vol. 3, pp. 113–119.

GEHRING, P. J. & BUERGE, J. (1969) The distribution of 2,4-dinitrophenol relative to its cataractogenic activity in ducklings and rabbits. *Toxicol. appl. Pharmacol.*, **15**: 574–592.

GEHRING, P. J., KRAMER, C. D., SCHWETZ, B. A., ROSE, J. Q., & ROWE, V. K. (1973) The fate of 2,4,5-trichlorophenoxyacetic acid (2,4,5-T) following oral administration to man. *Toxicol. appl. Pharmacol.*, **26**: 352–361.

GEHRING, P. J., BLAU, G. E., & WATANABE, P. G. (1976) Pharmacokinetic studies in evaluation of the toxicological and environmental hazard of chemicals. In: *Advances in modern toxicology—Newer concepts in safety evaluation.* Washington, Hemisphere Publ. Corp.

GIBSON, J. E. & BECKER, B. A. (1967) Demonstration of enhanced lethality of drugs in hypoexcretory animals. *J. pharm. Sci.,* **56:** 1503–1505.

GIGON, P. L., GRAM, T. E., & GILLETTE, J. R. (1969) Studies on the rate of reduction of hepatic microsomal cytochrome P-450 by reduced nicotinamide adenine dinucleotide phosphate. Effect of drug substrates. *Mol. Pharmacol.,* **5:** 109–122.

GILBERT, D. & GOLBERG, L. (1965) Liver response tests. III. Liver enlargement and stimulation of microsomal processing enzyme activity. *Food Cosmet. Toxicol.,* **3:** 417–432.

GILLETTE, J. R. (1963) Metabolism of drugs and other foreign compounds by enzymatic mechanisms. *Arzneimittel Forsch.,* **6:** 11–73.

GILLETTE, J. R. (1971a) Factors affecting drug metabolism. *Ann. NY Acad. Sci.,* **179:** 43–66.

GILLETTE, J. R. (1971b) Reductive enzymes. In: Brodie, B. B. & Gillette, J. R. ed. *Concepts in biochemical pharmacology,* Berlin, Springer-Verlag, Vol. 2, pp. 349–361.

GILLETTE, J. R. (1971c) Effects of various inducers on electron transport systems associated with drug metabolism by liver microsomes. *Metabolism,* **20:** 215–227.

GILLETTE, J. R. (1973a) Overview of drug-protein binding. *Ann. NY Acad. Sci.,* **226:** 6–17.

GILLETTE, J. R. (1973b) The importance of tissue distribution in pharmacokinetics. *J. Pharmacol. Biopharm.,* **1:** 497–519.

GILLETTE, J. R. (1974a) A perspective on the role of chemically reactive metabolites of foreign chemicals in toxicity. I. Correlation of changes in covalent binding of reactivity metabolites with changes in the incidence and severity of toxicity. *Biochem. Pharmacol.,* **23:** 2785–2794.

GILLETTE, J. R. (1974b) A perspective on the role of chemically reactive metabolites of foreign compounds in toxicity: II. Alterations in the kinetics of covalent binding. *Biochem. Pharmacol.,* **23:** 2927–2938.

GILLETTE, J. R. (1975) Other aspects of pharmacokinetics. In: Gillette, J. R. & Mitchell, J. R., ed. *Concepts in biochemical pharmacology,* Berlin, Springer-Verlag, Vol. 3, pp. 35–85.

GILLETTE, J. R., CHAN, T. W., & TERRIERE, L. C. (1966) Interactions between DDT analogues and microsomal epoxidase systems. *J. agric. Food Chem.,* **14:** 540–545.

GILLETTE, J. R. DAVIS, D. C., & SASAME, (1972) Cytochrome P-450 and its role in drug metabolism. *Annu. Rev. Pharmacol.,* **12:** 57–84.

GILLETTE, J. R., MITCHELL, J. R., & BRODIE, B. B. (1974) Biochemical mechanisms of drug toxicity. *Annu. Rev. Pharmacol.,* **14:** 271–288.

GOLDSTEIN, A., ARONOW, L., & KOLMAN, S. M. (1974) Principles of drug action. In: *The basis of pharmacology,* 2nd ed., New York, Wiley, pp. 106–205.

GRAM, T. E. (1971) Enzymatic *N-, O-* and *S-*dealkylation of foreign compounds by hepatic microsomes. In: Brodie, B. B. & Gillette, J. R., ed. *Concepts in biochemical pharmacology,* Berlin, Springer-Verlag, Vol. 2, pp. 334–348.

GRAM, T. E. (1973) Comparative aspects of mixed function oxidation by lung and liver of rabbits. *Drug. Metabol. Rev.,* **2:** 1–32.

GREGORY, J. D. (1960) The effect of borate on the carbazole reaction. *Arch. Biochem. Biophys.,* **89:** 157–159.

GREGORY, J. D. & LIPMANN, F. (1957) The transfer of sulfate among phenolic compounds with 3,5-diphosphoadenosine as co-enzyme. *J. Biol. Chem.,* **229:** 1081–1090.

GRIFFITHS, M. H. (1968) The metabolism of *N*-triphenylmorphine in the dog and rat. *Biochem. J.,* **108:** 731–740.

HART, L. G. & FOUTS, J. R. (1965) Further studies on the stimulation of hepatic microsomal drug metabolizing enzymes by DDT and its analogues. *Arch. exp. Pathol.,* **249:** 486–500.

HEIRWEGH, K. P. M., VAN DER VIJER, M., & FEVERY, J. (1972) Assay and properties of digitonin-activated bilirubin uridine diphosphate glucuronyl-transferase from rat liver. *Biochem. J.*, **129:** 605–618.

HENDERSON, P. TH. & KERSTEN, K. J. (1970) Metabolism of drugs during liver regeneration. *Biochem. Pharmacol.*, **19:** 2343–2351.

HERR, F. & KIESE, M. (1959) [Determination of nitrosobenzol in the blood.] *Arch. exp. Path. Pharmakol.*, **235:** 351–353 (in German).

HEWICK, D. S. & FOUTS, J. R. (1970a) Effects of storage on hepatic microsomal cytochromes and substrate-induced difference spectra. *Biochem. Pharmacol.*, **19:** 457–472.

HEWICK, D. S. & FOUTS, J. R. (1970b) The metabolism *in vitro* and hepatic microsomal interactions of some enantiomeric drug substrates. *Biochem. J.*, **117:** 833–841.

HIDAKA, H., NAGATSU, T., & YAGI, K. (1967) A rapid and simple assay of serotonin sulfokinase activity. *Anal. Biochem.*, **17:** 388–392.

HIETANEN, E. (1974) Effect of sex and castration on hepatic and intestinal activity of drug-metabolizing enzymes. *Pharmacology*, **12:** 84–89.

HIETANEN, E. & VALINIO, H. (1973) Interspecies variations in small intestinal and hepatic drug hydroxylation and glucuronidation. *Acta Pharmacol. Toxicol.*, **33:** 57–64.

HIETBRINK, B. E. & DUBOIS, K. P. (1965) Influence of X-radiation on development of enzymes responsible for desulfuration of an organic phosphorothioate and reduction of *p*-nitrobenzoic acid in the livers of male rats. *Radiat. Res.*, **22:** 598–603.

HILTON, J. & SARTORELLI, A. C. (1970) Induction by phenobarbital of microsomal mixed oxidase enzymes in regenerating liver. *J. biol. Chem.*, **245:** 4187–4192.

HOFFMAN, D. G., WORTH, H. M., & ANDERSON, R. C. (1968) Stimulation of hepatic microsomal drug-metabolizing enzymes by $\alpha\alpha$-bis *p*-chlorophenyl-3-pyridine methanol and a method for determining no-effect levels in rats. *Toxicol. appl. Pharmacol.*, **12:** 464–472.

HOFFMAN, D. F., WORTH, H. M., & ANDERSON, R. C. (1970) Stimulation of hepatic drug-metabolizing enzymes by chlorophenothane (DDT); the relationship to liver enlargement and hepatotoxicity in the rat. *Toxicol. appl. Pharmacol.*, **16:** 171–178.

HOLTZMAN, J. L., GRAM, T. E., GIGON, P. L., & GILLETTE, J. R. (1968) The distribution of the components of mixed function oxidase between the rough and the smooth endoplasmic reticulum of liver cells. *Biochem. J.*, **110:** 407–412.

HOOK, J. B., BAIBIE, M. D., JOHNSON, J. T., & GEHRING, P. J. (1974) *In vitro* analysis of transport of 2,4,5-trichlorophenoxyacetic acid (2,4,5-T) by rat and dog kidney. *Food Cosmet. Toxicol.*, **12:** 209–218.

HUCKER, H. B. (1970) Species differences in drug metabolism. *Annu. Rev. Pharmacol.*, **10:** 99–118.

IMAI, Y., ITO, A., & SATOR, R. R. (1966) Evidence for biochemically different types of vesicles in the hepatic microsomal fraction. *J. Biochem.*, **60:** 417–428.

ISSELBACHER, K. J. (1956) Enzymatic mechanisms of hormone metabolism. II. Mechanism of hormonal glucuronide formation. In: Pincus, G., ed. *Recent progress in hormone research*, New York, Academic Press, pp. 134–151.

JENNE, J. W. & BOYER, P. D. (1962) Kinetic characteristics of the acetylation of isoniazid and *p*-aminosalicylic acid by a liver enzyme preparation. *Biochim. Biophys. Acta*, **65:** 121–127.

JOHNSON, M. K. (1966) Metabolism of iodomethane in the rat. *Biochem. J.*, **98:** 38–43.

JOLLOW, P. J., MITCHELL, J. R., ZAMPOGLIONE, N., & GILLETTE, J. R. (1974) Bromobenzene-induced liver necrosis: protective role of glutathione and evidence for 3,4-bromobenzene oxide as the hepatotoxic metabolite. *Pharmacology*, **11:** 151–169.

KATO, R. & GILLETTE, J. R. (1965) Effect of starvation on NADPH-dependent enzymes in liver microsomes of male and female rats. *J. Pharmacol. exp. Ther.*, **150:** 279–284.

KATZ, M. & POULSEN, B. J. (1971) Absorption of drugs through the skin. In: Brodie, B. B. & Gillette, J. R., ed. *Concepts in biochemical pharmacology*, Berlin, Springer-Verlag, Vol. 1, pp. 103–174.

KEBERLE, H., HOFFMAN, K., & BERNHARD, K. (1962) The metabolism of glutethimide (Doridnene). *Experientia (Basel)*, **18**: 105–111.

KEEN, P. (1971) Effect of binding to plasma proteins on the distribution, activity and elimination of drugs. In: Brodie, B. B. & Gillette, J. R., ed. *Concepts in biochemical pharmacology*, Berlin, Springer-Verlag, Vol. 1, pp. 213–233.

KINOSHITA, F. K., FRAWLEY, J. P., & DuBois, K. P. (1966) Quantitative measurement of induction of hepatic microsomal enzymes by various dietary levels of DDT and toxaphene in rat. *Toxicol. appl. Pharmacol.*, **9**: 505–513.

KLINGER, W. (1974) Optimal conditions for the first step of amidopyrine-*N*-demethylation by 900 × g liver supernatant of newborn and adult rats. *Acta Biol. Med. Germ.*, **33**: 181–186.

KUNTZMAN, R. (1969) Drugs and enzyme induction. *Annu. Rev. Pharmacol.*, **9**: 21–36.

KURZ, H. & FRIEMEL, G. (1967) [Species-specific differences in the binding of plasma proteins.] *Arch. Pharmakol. exp. Path.*, **257**: 35–36 (in German).

LA DU, B. N. & SNADY, H. (1971) Esterases of human tissues. In: Brodie, B. B. & Gillette, J. R., ed. *Concepts in biochemical pharmacology*, Berlin, Springer-Verlag, Vol. 2, pp. 477–499.

LA DU, B. N., GAUDETTE, L., TROUSOF, N., & BRODIE, B. B. (1955) Enzymatic dealkylation of aminopyrine (Pyramidon) and other alkylamines. *J. biol. Chem.*, **214**: 741–752.

LA DU, B. N., MANDEL, G. H., & WAY, E. L. (1972) *Fundamental of drug metabolism and drug disposition*. Baltimore, Williams & Wilkins.

LEVI, A. J., GATMAITAN, Z., & ARIAS, I. M. (1969) Two hepatic cytoplasmic protein fractions, Y and Z, and their possible role in hepatic uptake of bilirubin, sulfobromophthalein, and other anions, *J. clin. Invest.*, **48**: 2156–2167.

LEVINE, R. R. (1970) Factors affecting gastrointestinal absorption of drugs. *Digest Dis.* **15**: 171–188.

LEVY, G. & GIBALDI, M. (1972) Pharmacokinetics of drug action. *Annu. Rev. Pharmacol.*, **12**: 85–98.

LEVY, G. & GIBALDI, M. (1975) Pharmacokinetics. In: Gillette, J. R. & Mitchell, J. R., ed. *Concepts in biochemical pharmacology*, Berlin, Springer-Verlag, Vol. 3, pp. 1–34.

LITWACK, G., KETTERER, B., & ARIAS, I. M. (1971) Ligondin: a hepatic protein which binds steroids, bilirubin, carcinogens and a number of exogenous organic anions. *Nature (Lond.)*, **234**: 466–467.

LIU, S. J., RAMSEY, R. K., & FALLON, H. J. (1975) Effects of ethanol on hepatic microsomal drug-metabolizing enzymes in the rat. *Biochem. Pharmacol.*, **24**: 369–378.

LU, A. Y. H. & LEVIN, W. (1974) The resolution and reconstitution of the liver microsomal hydroxylation system. *Biochim. Biophys. Acta*, **344**: 205–240.

LU, A. Y. H., STROBEL, H. W., & COON, M. J. (1969) Hydroxylation of benzphetamine and other drugs by a solubilized form of cytochrome P-450 from liver microsomes: lipid requirement for drug demethylation. *Biochem. Biophys. Res. Commun.*, **36**: 545–551.

LUCIS, O. J., SCHACKH, Z. A., & EMBIL, J. A., JR (1970) Cadmium as a trace element and cadmium-binding components in human cells. *Experientia (Basel)*, **26**: 1109–1112.

MACCAMAN, R. E. (1965) Microdetermination of catechol-*O*-methyl transferase. *Life Sci.*, **4**: 2353–2359.

MCLEAN, A. E. M. (1971) Conversion by the liver of inactive molecules into toxic molecules. In: Aldridge, W. N., ed. *Mechanism of toxicity*, London, Macmillan, pp. 219–228.

MACMAHON, R. E. (1962) The competitive inhibition of the *N*-demethylation of butynamine by 2,4-dichloro-6-phenolphenoxy-ethylamine (DPEA). *J. Pharmacol. exp. Ther.*, **138**: 382–386.

MACMAHON, R. E. (1971) Enzymatic oxidation and reduction of alcohols, aldehydes and ketones. In: Brodie, B. B. & Gillette, J. R., ed. *Concepts in biochemical pharmacology*, Berlin, Springer-Verlag, Vol. 2, pp. 500–517.

MAHER, J. R., WHITNEY, J. M., CHAMBERS, J. S., & STANONIS, D. J. (1957) The quantitative determination of isoniazid and para-aminosalicylic acid in body fluids. *Am. Rev. Tuberc.*, **76**: 852–861.

172

MANNERING, G. J. (1968) Significance of stimulation and inhibition of drug metabolism. In: Burger, A., ed. *Selected pharmaceutical testing methods*, New York, Marcel Dekker, pp. 51–119.

MANNERING, G. J. (1971a) Inhibition of drug metabolism. In: Brodie, B. B. & Gillette, J. R., ed. *Concepts in biochemical pharmacology*, Berlin, Springer-Verlag, Vol. 2, pp. 452–476.

MANNERING, G. J. (1971b) Properties of cytochrome P-450 as affected by environmental factors: qualitative changes due to administration of polycyclic hydrocarbons. *Metabolism*, **20**: 228–245.

MARK, L. C. (1971) Translocation of drugs and other exogenous chemicals into adipose tissue. In: Brodie, B. B. & Gillette, J. R., ed. *Concepts in biochemical pharmacology*, Berlin, Springer-Verlag, Vol. 1, pp. 258–275.

MARSELOS, M. & HÄNNINEN, O. (1974) Enhancement of D-glucuronolactone and acetaldehyde dehydrogenase activities in the rat liver by inducers of drug metabolism. *Biochem. Pharmacol.*, **23**: 1457–1466.

MARSH, C. A. (1963) Metabolism of D-glucuronolactone in mammalian systems; conversion of D-glucuronolactone into D-glucaric acid by tissue preparations. *Biochem. J.*, **87**: 82–90.

MARSHALL, E. K., JR (1948) Determination of para-amino-salicylic acid in blood. *Proc. Soc. Exp. Biol. Med.*, **68**: 471–472.

MASON, H. S. (1957) Mechanism of oxygen metabolism. *Adv. Enzymol.*, **19**: 79–233.

MILLER, E. C. & MILLER, J. A. (1971a) The mutagenicity of chemical carcinogens: correlations, problems and interpretations. In: Hollaender, A., ed. *Chemical mutagens*, New York, Plenum, Vol. 1, pp. 83–119.

MILLER, J. A. & MILLER, E. C. (1971b) Chemical carcinogenesis: mechanisms and approaches to its control. *J. Natl Cancer Inst.*, **47**: v-xiv.

NASH, T. (1953) The colorimetric estimation of formaldehyde by means of the Hantsch reaction. *Biochem. J.*, **55**: 416–421.

NEBERT, D. W. & GELBOIN, H. V. (1968a) Substrate inducible microsomal aryl hydroxylase. I. Assay and properties of induced enzymes. *J. Biol. Chem.*, **243**: 6242–6249.

NEBERT, D. W. & GELBOIN, H. V. (1968b) Substrate inducible microsomal aryl hydroxylase. II. Cellular responses during enzymic induction. *J. Biol. Chem.*, **243**: 6250–6261.

NETTER, K. J. (1960) [A method for the direct measurement of O-demethylization in liver microsomes and its application to the inhibitory effects of SKF 525A on microsomes.] *Arch. Pharmacol.*, **238**: 292–300 (in German).

NETTER, K. J. & SEIDEL, G. (1964) An adaptively stimulated O-demethylating system in rat liver microsomes and its kinetic properties. *J. Pharmacol. exp. Ther.*, **146**: 61–65.

NOTTON, W. R. & HENDERSON, P. TH. (1975) The influence of N-hexane treatment on the glucuronic acid pathway and activity of some drug-metabolizing enzymes in the guinea pig. *Biochem. Pharmacol.*, **24**: 127:131.

OBATA, F., USHIWATA, A., & NAKAMURA, Y. (1971) Spectrophotometric assay of mono-amine oxidase using 2,4,6-trinitrobenzene-1-sulfonic acid. *J. Biochem.*, **69**: 349–354.

OGATA, M., TOMOKUNI, K., & TAKATSUKA, Y. (1969) Quantitative determination in urine of hippuric acid and *m*- or *p*-methyl hippuric acid, metabolites of toluene and *m*- or *p*-xylene. *Brit. J. ind. Med.*, **26**: 330–334.

OMURA, T. & SATO, R. (1964a) The carbon monoxide-binding pigment of liver microsomes: I. Evidence for its hemoprotein nature. *J. biol. Chem.*, **239**: 2370–2378.

OMURA, T. & SATO, R. (1964b) The carbon monoxide-binding pigment of liver microsomes: II. Solubilization, purification and properties. *J. biol. Chem.*, **239**: 2379–2385.

OTSUKA, S. & KOBAYASHI, Y. (1964) A radioisotopic assay for monamine oxidase determinations in human plasma. *Biochem. Pharmacol.*, **13**: 995–1006.

PAPPENHEIMER, J. R. (1953) Passage of molecules through capillary walls. *Physiol. Rev.*, **33**: 387–423.

173

PARKE, D. V. (1968) *The biochemistry of foreign compounds*. New York, Pergamon Press.

PEDERSON, T. C. & AUST, S. D. (1970) Aminopyrine demethylase: kinetic evidence for multiple microsomal activities. *Biochem. Pharmacol.*, **19**: 2221–2230.

PIPER, W. N., ROSE, J. Q., LENG, M. L. & GEHRING, P. J. (1973) The fate of 2,4,5-trichlorophenoxyacetic acid (2,4,5-T) following oral administration to rats and dogs. *Toxicol. appl. Pharmacol.*, **26**: 339–351.

PITTS, R. F. (1963) *Physiology of the kidney and body fluids. Yearbook*, Chicago, Medical Publishers Inc.

PLAA, G. L. (1975) The enterohepatic circulation. In: Gillette, J. R. & Mitchell, J. R., ed. *Concepts in biochemical pharmacology*, Berlin, Springer-Verlag, Vol. 3, pp. 130–149.

PLACE, V. A. & BENSON, H. (1971) Dietary influences on therapy with drugs. *J. Mond. Pharm.*, **14**: 261–278.

POLAND, A. P. & NEBERT, D. W. (1973) A sensitive radiometric assay of aminopyrine N-demethylation. *J. Pharmacol. exp. Ther.*, **184**: 269–277.

POTTS, A. M. (1964) The reaction of uveal pigments *in vitro* with polycyclic compounds. *Invest. Ophthalmol.*, **3**: 405–416.

PRESCOTT, L. F. (1975) Pathological and physiological factors affecting drug absorption, distribution, elimination and response in man. In: Gillette, J. R. & Mitchell, J. R., ed. *Concepts in biochemical pharmacology*, Berlin, Springer-Verlag, Vol. 3, pp. 234–257.

PRICE, H. L., KOVNAT, P. J., SOFER, J. N., CONNER, E. H., & PRICE, M. L. (1960) The uptake of thiopental by body tissues and its relation to the duration of narcosis. *Clin. Pharmacol. Ther.*, **1**: 16–22.

QUASTEL, J. H. (1965) Molecular transport at cell membranes. *Proc. Roy. Soc. Br.*, **163**: 169–186.

QUINN, G. P., AXELROD, J., & BRODIE, B. B. (1958) Species, strain and sex differences in metabolism of hexobarbitone, aminopyrine, antipyrine and aniline. *Biochem. Pharmacol.*, **1**: 152–159.

RALL, D. P. (1971) Drug entry into brain and cerebrospinal fluid. In: Brodie, B. B. & Gillette, J, R., ed. *Concepts in biochemical pharmacology*, Berlin, Springer-Verlag, Vol. 1, pp. 240–248.

RASMUSSEN, F. (1971) Excretion of drugs by milk. In: Brodie, B. B. & Gillette, J. R., ed. *Concepts in biochemical pharmacology*, Berlin, Springer-Verlag, Vol. 1, pp. 390–402.

REMMER, H., SCHENKMAN, J., ESTABROOK, R. W., SASAME, H., GILLETTE, J. R., NARASHIMHULU, S., COOPER, D. Y., & ROSENTHAL, O. (1966) Drug interaction with hepatic microsomal cytochrome. *Mol. Pharmacol.*, **2**: 187–190.

RENKIN, E. M. (1964) Transport of large molecules across capillary walls. *Physiologist*, **7**: 13.

REYES, H., LEVI, A. J., GATMAITAN, Z., & ARIAS, I. M. (1971) Studies on Y and Z, two hepatic cytoplasmic organic anion-binding proteins: Effect of drugs, chemicals, hormones and cholestosis. *J. Clin. Invest.*, **50**: 2242–2251.

RODOMSKI, J. L., DEICHMANN, W. B., & CLIZER, E. E. (1968) Pesticide concentrations in the liver, brain and adipose tissue of terminal hospital patients. *Food Cosmet. Toxicol.*, **6**: 209–220.

ROLL, R. (1971) Investigations concerning the teratogenic effect of 2,4,5-T in mice. *Food Cosmet. Toxicol.*, **9**: 671–676.

ROSE, J. Q., RAMSEY, J. C., WENTZLER, T. G., HUMMEL, R. A., & GEHRING, P. J. (1975) The fate of 2,3,7,8-tetrachlorodibenzo-p-dioxin (TCDD) following single and repeated oral doses to the rat. *Toxicol. appl. Pharmacol.*, **36**: 209–226.

ROSENBLUM, C. (1965) Non-metabolite residues in radioactive tracer studies. In: Roth, L. J., ed. *Isotopes in experimental pharmacology*, Chicago, University of Chicago Press, pp. 353–360.

ROTH, L. J. (1971) The use of autoradiography in experimental pharmacology. In: Brodie, B. B. & Gillette, J. R., ed. *Concepts in biochemical pharmacology*, Berlin, Springer-Verlag, Vol. 1, pp. 286–316.

Rowe, V. K. & Hymas, T. A. (1954) Summary of toxicological information of 2,4-D and 2,4,5-T type herbicides and an avaluation of the hazards to livestock associated with their use. *Am. J. Vet. Res.*, **15**: 622–629.

Roy, A. B. (1971) Sulfate conjugation enzymes. In: Brodie, B. B. & Gillette, J. R., ed. *Concepts in biochemical pharmacology*, Berlin, Springer-Verlag, Vol. 2, pp. 536–563.

Sauerhoff, M. W., Braun, W. H., Blau, G. E., & Gehring, P. J. (1975) The dose-dependent pharmacokinetic profile of 2,4,5-trichlorophenoxyacetic acid following intravenous administration to rats. *Toxicol. appl. Pharmacol.*, **36**: 491–501.

Schanker, L. S. (1962a) Passage of drugs across body membranes. *Pharmacol. Rev.*, **14**: 501–530.

Schanker, L. S. (1962b) Concentrative transfer of an organic cation from blood into bile. *Biochem. Pharmacol.*, **11**: 253–254.

Schanker, L. S. (1963) Passage of drugs across the gastrointestinal epithelium. In: Hogben, C. A. M., ed. *Proceedings of the 1st International Pharmacological Meeting*, Oxford, Pergamon Press, Vol. 4, pp. 120–130.

Schanker, L. S. (1965) Hepatic transport of organic cations. In: Taylor, W., ed. *The biliary system*. Oxford, Blackwell.

Schanker, L. S. (1971) Absorption of drugs from the gastrointestinal tract. In: Brodie, B. B. & Gillette, J. R., ed. *Concepts in biochemical pharmacology*, Berlin, Springer-Verlag, Vol. 1, pp. 9–24.

Schanker, L. S., Shore, P. A., Brodie, B. B., & Hogben, C. A. M. (1957) Absorption of drugs from the stomach. I. The rat. *J. Pharmacol. exp. Ther.*, **120**: 528–539.

Scheline, R. R. (1968) Drug metabolism by intestinal microorganisms. *J. pharm. Sci.*, **57**: 2021–2037.

Schenkman, J. B., Remmer, H., & Estabrook, R. W. (1967) Spectral studies of drug interaction with hepatic microsomal cytochrome. *Mol. Pharmacol.*, **3**: 113–123.

Schoene, B., Fleischmann, R. A., Remmer, H., & Oldershausen, H. F. (1972) Determination of drug-metabolizing enzymes in needle biopsies of human liver. *Eur. J. clin. Pharmacol.*, **4**: 65–73.

Scholtan, W. (1963) On the protein binding of long-acting sulfonamides. *Chemotherapia*, **6**: 180–195.

Schwetz, B. A., Norris, J. M., Sparschu, G. L., Rowe, V. K., Gehring, P. J., Emerson, J. K., & Gerbig, C. G. (1973) Toxicology of chlorinated dibenzo-*p*-dioxins. *Environ. Health Perspect.* (*Experimental issue*), **5**: 87–100.

Settle, W., Hegeman, S., & Featherstone, R. M. (1971) The nature of drug-protein interaction. In: Brodie, B. B. & Gillette, J. R., ed. *Concepts in biochemical pharmacology*, Berlin, Springer-Verlag, Vol. 1, pp. 175–186.

Shore, P. A., Brodie, B. B., & Hogben, C. A. M. (1957) The gastric secretion of drugs—a pH partition hypothesis. *J. Pharmacol. exp. Ther.*, **119**: 361–369.

Shulert, A. R. (1961) Physiological disposition of hydralazine (1-hydrazinophthalazine) and a method for its determination in biological fluids. *Arch. int. Pharmacodyn.*, **132**: 1–15.

Smith, R. L. (1971a) Excretion of drugs in bile. In: Brodie, B. B. & Gillette, J. R., ed. *Concepts in biochemical pharmacology*, Berlin, Springer-Verlag, Vol. 1, pp. 354–389.

Smith, R. L. (1971b) The role of the gut flora in the conversion of inactive compounds to active metabolites. In: Aldridge, W. N., ed. *Mechanism of toxicity*, London, Macmillan, pp. 229–247.

Smith, R. L. (1973) *The excretory function of bile: the elimination of drugs and toxic substances in bile*. London, England, Chapman & Hall.

Smuckler, E. A. (1971) Metabolism of halogenated compounds. In: Brodie, B. B. & Gillette, J. R., ed. *Concepts in biochemical pharmacology*, Berlin, Springer-Verlag, Vol. 2, pp. 367–377.

Sparschu, G. L., Dunn, F. L., Lisowe, R. W. & Rowe, V. K. (1971) Study of the effects of high levels of 2,4,5-trichlorophenoxyacetic acid on fetal development in the rat. *Food Cosmet. Toxicol.*, **9**: 527–530.

SPERBER, I. (1963) Drugs and membranes. In: Hogben, C. A. M., ed. *Proceedings of the 1st International Pharmacological Meeting*, Oxford, Pergamon Press, Vol. 4.

STERRSON, L. A. & HES, J. (1975) Electrochemical method for the determination of aniline hydroxylation. *Anal. Biochem.*, **67**: 74–80.

STOTZ, E., STEINBERG, M. S., COHEN, S. N., & WEBER, W. W. (1969) Acetylation of 5-hydroxytryptamine by isoniazide *N*-acetyltransferase. *Biochim. Biophys. Acta*, **184**: 210–212.

STOWE, C. M. & PLAA, G. L. (1968) Extrarenal excretion of drugs and chemicals. *Annu. Rev. Pharmacol.*, **8**: 337–356.

STRICKLAND, R. D., GREGORY, D. H., & LYNCH, J. L. (1974) A method for assaying hepatic morphine UDP-glucuronyl transferase. *Biochem. Med.*, **11**: 180–188.

STURMAN, J. A. & SMITH, M. J. H. (1967) The binding of salicylate to plasma proteins in different species. *J. Pharm. Pharmacol.*, **19**: 621–623.

SUGA, T., OHATA, I., KUMAOKA, H., & AKAGI, M. (1967) Studies on mercapturic acids: investigation of glutathione-conjugating enzyme by the method of thin-layer chromatography. *Chem. Pharmacol. Bull.*, **15**: 1059–1064.

TABOR, H., MEHLER, A. H., & STADTMAN, E. R. (1953) The enzymatic acetylation of amines. *J. biol. Chem.*, **204**: 127–138.

TAKAHASHI, H. & TAKAHARA, S. (1968) A sensitive fluorimetric assay for monoamine oxidase based on the formation of 4,6-quinolinediol from 5-hydroxykynurenamine. *J. Biochem.*, **64**: 7–11.

TEORELL,T. (1937a) Kinetics of distribution of substances administered to the body: I. The extra-vascular modes of administration. *Arch. int. Pharmacodyn.*, **57**: 205–226.

TEORELL, T. (1937b) Kinetics of distribution of substances administered to the body: II. The intra-vascular modes of administration. *Arch. int. Pharmacodyn.*, **57**: 227–240.

TUFVESSON, G. (1970) Fluorimetric determination of amine oxidase activity in human blood serum with kynuramine as substrate. *Scand. J. clin. Lab. Invest.*, **26**: 151–154.

ULLRICH, V. & WEBER, P. (1972) The *O*-dealkylation of 7-ethoxycoumarin by liver microsomes: a direct fluorimetric test. *Z. Physiol. Chem.*, **353**: 1171–1177.

WAGNER, J. P. (1968) Pharmacokinetics. *Ann. Rev. Pharmacol.*, **8**: 67–94.

WAGNER, J. P. (1971) *Biopharmaceutics and relevant pharmacokinetics*. Hamilton, Drug Intelligence Publications.

WATTENBERG, L. W. & LEONG, J. L. (1971) Tissue distribution studies of polycyclic hydrocarbon hydroxylase activity. In: Brodie, B. B. & Gillette, J. R., ed. *Concepts in biochemical pharmacology*, Berlin, Springer-Verlag, Vol. 2, pp. 422–430.

WATTENBERG, L. W., LEONG, J. L., & STRAND, P. J. (1962) Benzpyrene hydroxylase activity in the gastrointestinal tract. *Cancer Res.*, **22**: 1120–1125.

WEBER, W. W. (1970) *N*-acetyltransferase (mammalian liver). In: Tabor, H. & Tabor, C. W., ed. *Methods in enzymology*, 17B. New York, Academic Press.

WEBER, W. W. (1971) Acetylating, deacetylating and amino acid-conjugating enzymes. In: Brodie, B. B. & Gillette, J. R., ed. *Concepts in biochemical pharmacology*, Berlin, Springer-Verlag, Vol. 2, pp. 564–583.

WEBER, W. W. & COHEN, S. N. (1968) The mechanism of isoniazid acetylation by human *N*-acetyltransferase. *Biochim. Biophys. Acta*, **151**: 276–278.

WEBER, W. W., COHEN, S. N., & STEINBERG, M. S. (1968) Purification and properties of *N*-acetyltransferase from mammalian liver. *Ann. NY Acad. Sci.*, **151**: 734–741.

WEINER, I. M. (1971) Excretion of drugs by the kidney. In: Brodie, B. B. & Gillette, J. R., ed. *Concepts in biochemical pharmacology*, Berlin, Springer-Verlag, Vol. 1, pp. 328–353.

WEISBURGER, H. H. & WEISBURGER, E. R. (1971) *N*-oxidation enzymes. In: Brodie, B. B. & Gillette, J. R., ed. *Concepts in biochemical pharmacology*, Berlin, Springer-Verlag, Vol. 2, pp. 312–333.

WEISBURGER, H. H., GRANTHAM, P. H., & WEISBURGER, E. R. (1964) Metabolism of *N*-2-fluorenylacetamide in the hamster. *Toxicol. appl. Pharmacol.*, **6**: 427–433.

WEISSBACH, H., SMITH, T. E., FALY, J. W., WITKOP, B., & UDENFRIEND, S. (1960) A rapid spectrophotometric assay of monoamine oxidase based on the rate of disappearance of kynuramine. *J. Biol. Chem.*, **235**: 1160–1163.

WILLIAMS, C. H., JR & KAMIN, H. (1962) Microsomal triphosphopyridine nucleotide-cytochrome c reductase of liver. *J. Biol. Chem.*, **237**: 587–595.

WILLIAMS, R. T. (1965) The influence of enterohepatic circulation on toxicity of drugs. *Ann. NY Acad. Sci.*, **123**: 110–124.

WILLIAMS, R. T. (1967a) The biogenesis of conjugation and detoxication products. In: Bernfield, P., ed. *Biogenesis of natural compounds*, 2nd ed., Oxford, Pergamon Press, pp. 589–639.

WILLIAMS, R. T. (1967b) Comparative patterns of drug metabolism. *Fed. Proc.*, **26**: 1029–1039.

WILLIAMS, R. T. (1971) Introduction: Pathways of drug metabolism. In: Brodie, B. B. & Gillette, J. R., ed. *Concepts in biochemical pharmacology*, Berlin, Springer-Verlag, Vol. 2, pp. 226–242.

WITIAK, D. T. & WHITEHOUSE, M. W. (1969) Species differences in the albumin binding of 2,4,6-trinitrobenzaldehyde, chlorphenoxyacetic acids, 2-(4'-hydroxybenzeneazo) benzoic acid and some other drugs; the unique behaviour of rat albumin. *Biochem. Pharmacol.*, **18**: 971–977.

WITSCHI, H. (1975) Exploitable biochemical approaches for evaluation of toxic lung damage. In: Hayes, W. J. Jr., ed. *Essays in toxicology*, New York, Academic Press, Vol. 6, pp. 125–191.

YUKI, H. & FISHMAN, W. H (1963) A carbazole method for the differential analysis of glucuronate, glucosiduronate and hyaluronate. *Biochim. Biophys. Acta*, **69**: 576–578.

ZAKIM, D. & VESSEY, D. A. (1973) Techniques for the characterization of UDP-glucuronyl-transferase, glucose-6-phosphatase and other tightly bound microsomal enzymes. In: Glick, D., ed. *Methods of biochemical analysis*, New York, Wiley, Vol. 21, pp. 2–37.

ZANNONI, V. G. (1971) Experiments illustrating drug distribution and excretion. In: La Du, B. N., Mandel, H. G., & Way, E. L., ed. *Fundamentals of drug metabolism and drug disposition*, Baltimore, Williams & Wilkins, pp. 583–590.

ZANNONI, V. G., FLYNN, E. J., & LYNCH, M. (1972) Ascorbic acid and drug metabolism. *Biochem. Pharmacol.*, **21**: 1377–1392.

ZELLER, E. A. (1971) Amine oxidases. In: Brodie, B. B. & Gillette, J. R., ed. *Concepts in biochemical pharmacology*, Berlin, Springer-Verlag, Vol. 2, pp. 518–535.

ZIEGLER, D. M., MCKEE, E. M., & POULSEN, L. L. (1973) Microsomal flavo-protein-catalyzed *N*-oxidation of arylamines. *Drug Metab. Disposition*, **1**: 314–320.

5. MORPHOLOGICAL STUDIES

5.1 Introduction

Morphological studies are often the corner stones of toxicity experiments. The variety of such studies leads to many different approaches from the viewpoint of pathology, and skill and flexibility in working procedures seem to be far more important than a strict schedule.

On the other hand, it is advisable to have some general guidelines on pathological procedures for routine quality testing for toxicity, even though specific questions may often be posed, special experiments may have to be carried out, and special animals, techniques, and examinations used in order to elucidate certain problems.

This chapter deals with the various phases of morphological studies with a view to providing some general recommendations concerning the procedures to be followed. It must be emphasized, however, that these recommendations are only a guide, and that it will be the pathologist's special responsibility to see that studies are carried out in the way most likely to ensure optimum results.

5.2 General Recommendations

Gross necropsy facilities should be in close proximity to those of the pathologist. The autopsy room must be equipped with adequate dissection tables, dissection materials, running water, drains, lighting, ventilation, and facilities for disinfection. In addition, gross photography facilities are necessary. Cooling facilities must be available for the storage of dead animals until necropsy, but the animals should not be frozen (Sontag et al., 1975). To carry out proper experiments and to prevent the loss of a considerable number of animals by cannibalism or autolysis, it is essential that animals be observed at least once a day, including Saturdays and Sundays. Animals in moribund condition should be killed.

For the trimming of fixed tissues, a well-ventilated area, preferably with an exhaust hood, and running water and drains, is required.

The histology laboratory should be separated from the autopsy room and should be equipped with tissue-processing equipment, microtomes, cryostat, embedding and staining facilities, and supplies (Sontag et al., 1975). Storage facilities are necessary for the fixed tissues, as well as for the tissue block and histological slide files. The facilities should be vermin-proof and temperature controlled or at least cool.

Veterinary or medical pathologists with experience in laboratory animal pathology or others with appropriate training and experience should be responsible for all pathology procedures. In addition, the pathologist should participate in the design and conduct of experiments.

Histology technicians with appropriate training and experience in the histological field will guarantee good histotechnical work, whereas technicians trained and experienced in laboratory animal dissection will be of great help in performing necropsies. Technicians must be able to recognize and adequately describe gross abnormalities.

Personnel should be available at the weekends to perform necropsies on animals found dead or killed *in extremis*.

5.3   Gross Observations

Gross pathology can be performed in most cases by experienced technicians under the guidance of the pathologist. They should follow a certain scheme of necropsy technique and must be able to recognize abnormalities. A checklist should be used to ensure that all organs and tissues are inspected and dissected. Information on clinical signs must be available. Abnormalities found must be recorded on autopsy cards. The descriptions must be clear and provide details such as location, size, colour, texture, number, etc.

A great number of lesions will be within the scale of known abnormalities for the animal species and breed used. Lesions found beyond this normal scale should always be examined by the pathologist himself. It is advisable for all new lesions, especially those attributable to the treatment, to be photographed.

Dead animals should be necropsied unless cannibalism or autolysis precludes this. Autolysis should not readily be accepted as an excuse for not performing an autopsy. An inadequate gross necropsy cannot be replaced by microscopic examination, no matter how well performed. On the other hand, a well-performed gross necropsy may provide optimum information for microscopic examination and may, in certain cases, facilitate more selective microscopic examination.

Several ways of killing animals are available and the methods depend on the facilities, the purpose of the experiment, and the species used. Sacrifice of animals by anaesthesia (by ether or barbiturates) is widely used as well as asphyxiation by carbon dioxide. In rodents, the blood of the body can be removed by cardiac puncture or puncturing the abdominal aorta, and in dogs by puncture of the common carotid artery. Alternatively in small rodents decapitation can be performed, though this may result in blood aspiration and damage to certain tissues or organs. On the other hand decapitation will probably give more constant results with respect to the total blood loss, and consequently lead to fairly consistent organ weights.

5.3.1 Autopsy techniques

It is difficult, if not impossible, to prescribe working procedures or techniques that will be adequate in all conditions. Often, observations made when the animals were alive or experience with other structurally-related compounds may focus attention on certain organs or tissues. Sometimes fixation by perfusion is necessary for proper examination of specific tissues (for example, the central nervous system).

Large numbers of animals should not be sacrificed at any one time, if too few technicians are available to perform the necropsies. Animals should be killed in sequence, especially where it is necessary to sample tissues for biochemical, enzyme-histochemical, or analytical studies. However, organs and tissues should be weighed as soon as possible after death to ensure that they have not dried out and that they can be fixed quickly. Special procedures may shorten the time needed for full autopsy especially in the case of small rodents. The exact organization of working procedures depends largely on the facilities and labour available, but good preparation and teamwork are crucial factors.

Sacrifice should be carried out so that animals of the experimental and control groups are killed at approximately the same time of day, thus preventing the introduction of variations in physiological status dependent on circadian rhythm. In certain cases, however, this may not be feasible.

Special care is necessary when test elements or compounds are analysed after sacrifice. At times it may be necessary to kill the animals in a given order to prevent contamination (e.g. sacrifice of the control first, followed by the lowest dose level, then the intermediate dose level, and finally the high-dose level).

Autopsy techniques have already been described (Roe, 1965) and only a general outline of the procedures is given.

5.3.2 Rat, mouse, guineapig, rabbit, monkey

The necropsy starts with external examination including the body orifices. Thereafter, the animals are fixed on their backs. After a median incision, the skin is partly removed and the subcutis, superficial lymph nodes, salivary glands, and mammary glands can be inspected and dissected. The abdomen can be opened and the negative pressure of the thorax may be checked and the thorax opened.

Thyroid and thymus can then be inspected and dissected.

Trachea, lungs, and heart are removed en bloc. The heart is detached, but the trachea and lungs remain intact to provide easy handling for inflation of the lungs with fixative (see under fixation methods).

Abdominal organs are removed. The examination of liver and kidney should include making a routine number of parallel slices of the organs to examine their cut surfaces. The gastrointestinal tract should be removed from the abdominal cavity and opened. In chronic toxicity experiments, the entire gastrointestinal tract must be opened, the mucosal surface examined, and representative parts taken for histological examination. The oesophagus and parts of the intestine can be rolled according to the Swiss roll technique in order to obtain a considerable length of mucosa musculature and serosa in the microscopic section. Brain, peripheral nerves, skeletal musculature, and bones (including a joint) are removed. The spinal cord may best be fixed *in situ*.

5.3.3 Carnivores, swine

After external examination, necropsy is performed when the animal is lying on its right side. Left front and hind legs are removed without opening the apertura thoracis superior. The skin is partly removed after a median ventral incision from mouth to os pubis. Subcutis, fat, mammary glands, salivary glands, and superficial lymph nodes may be inspected and dissected. In addition, the different joints of the legs are opened and inspected. After opening the abdomen, the thorax is checked for negative pressure and opened by removing the left side of the thoracic wall. Then the right side of the pleural cavity is inspected. The oesophagus is removed by cutting it cranially. The thoracic and abdominal organs are removed and individually inspected and opened. The nasopharynx is then opened and inspected, and the tongue, larynx, pharynx, tonsils, brain, spinal cord, peripheral nerves, and musculature collected. Most organs should be sliced in parallel slices to examine the cut surfaces.

5.4 Selection, Preservation, Preparation, and Storage of Tissues

5.4.1 Selection of tissues

Which organs and tissues should be collected for fixation is determined by the type of toxicity experiment and the compound being tested. Sufficient material should be collected to prevent the necessity of having to repeat a certain experiment. Since it is impossible to provide strict rules for selection, only a general outline will be given.

5.4.2 Oral toxicity tests

In acute toxicity experiments, restrictive microscopic examination may be necessary in certain cases. Some laboratories fix liver and kidneys, others do not. The additional information obtained from histological examination of these organs in acute experiments is, usually, limited.

In range-finding tests, restrictive pathology is common practice. Normally, the heart, liver, spleen, and kidneys and all grossly abnormal tissues are collected for fixation. When the compound tested is given by stomach tube, it is advisable to include lungs, oesophagus, and stomach in the histological study. In subacute (90-day) and chronic studies, it is advisable to select all tissues and organs for fixation in buffered formal saline. This normally includes the following organs and tissues:

brain	gall bladder (if present)
pituitary	oesophagus
thyroid (parathyroid)	stomach
thymus	duodenum
(trachea)	jejunum
lungs	ileum
heart	caecum
sternum (bone marrow)	colon
salivary glands	rectum
liver	urinary bladder
spleen	lymph nodes—mandibular or mesenteric
kidneys	lymph nodes—popliteal or axillary
adrenals	mammary glands
pancreas	(thigh) musculature
gonads	peripheral nerve
accessory genital organs	(eyes)
aorta	(femur—incl. joint)
(skin)	spinal cord (at three levels)
	(exorbital lachrymal glands)

The tissues mentioned between brackets are sometimes considered to be optional. In addition, all tissues containing grossly observed lesions should be fixed.

The same selection is usually made in carcinogenicity tests. In both chronic toxicity and carcinogenicity experiments, it is also very important to collect all organs and tissues of animals that have died or have been killed *in extremis*. Prompt examination of the tissues of these animals may provide valuable information leading to a more meaningful pathological examination of animals, that die or are sacrificed later on, or at the end of the experiment.

In cases where only part of an organ or tissue is taken, it is important that the same part of that organ or tissue be selected at approximately the same site in all animals.

5.4.3   Inhalation toxicity studies

In acute inhalation studies, it may be worth while, in some cases, to select lungs for fixation and subsequent microscopic examination, as well as liver and kidneys. In most cases, however, this seems unnecessary since the pulmonary lesions are usually of the same type (hyperaemia and oedema) and can be detected by gross inspection.

Examination of the entire respiratory tract is necessary in subacute inhalation studies. This includes nasal cavity, pharynx, larynx, trachea, main bronchi, and lungs. The exact orientation of these organs for trimming, embedding, and sectioning is of prime importance and needs special attention. More organs and tissues may be selected in the inhalation studies, selection usually being effected in the same way as for oral studies.

5.4.4   Dermal toxicity studies

In acute dermal toxicity studies, it is advisable to perform microscopic pathology on liver and kidneys. The presence of degenerative changes in these organs indicates that the compound is active transdermally. Examination of the skin is also advisable.

In subacute dermal toxicity studies, the organs and tissues are selected in the same way as that described for oral tests. Of course, the skin deserves special attention in that both treated areas and normal skin in comparable areas are selected.

5.4.5   Special studies

In the case of sensitization or irritation studies, the selection of tissues depends completely on the type of test. In eye irritation studies, the examination of eye and conjunctivae seems adequate whereas in a Landstainer–Draize test, and especially in a maximization test, the skin may be examined. In all these cases, it may, or may not, be necessary to select more tissues.

5.5   Preservation of Tissues

Preservation of tissues can be performed by immersion, inflation or distension, and perfusion. Immersion is most commonly used, but in some circumstances may not result in satisfactory preservation. Microscopic examination of the lungs, for example, cannot be done adequately if they have not been inflated or have not been fixed by perfusion. When the central nervous system is a target organ, it is an absolute necessity to use perfusion to ensure proper fixation, as fixation by immersion leads to many artifacts that are indistinguishable from certain degenerative changes. When animals in long-term tests are killed *in extremis*, it is advisable to use fixation by perfusion. Perfusion is usually essential for electron microscope studies of tissues.

With perfusion, the best conditions for microscopic examination are obtained while effective gross examination remains possible. All tissues should be fixed in 10% neutral buffered formalin or another appropriate fixative.

5.5.1 Immersion

Immersion is the most used and usually the most appropriate method of preservation in toxicity experiments. The tissues are placed in the preservative and fixed for 24–48 h. Fixation at higher temperatures (40–50°C), in a vacuum, or by use of microwaves (Gordon & Daniel, 1974) may shorten the fixation time considerably. Tissues thicker than 0.5 cm should not be fixed. The preservative/tissue ratio is very important and must be greater than 10:1 (volume fixation fluid/volume tissue) to obtain acceptable fixation. The fixation of intact animals with opened abdomen should not be carried out. All tissues and organs must be fixed separately, and some may need special attention. Skin and peripheral nerves must be fixed in a straight (but not stretched) and flat position. To achieve this, these tissues can first be attached to a piece of thick filter paper. The spinal cord can best be fixed *in situ* before it is taken out. Special fixing solutions may be used in certain cases such as Bouin's fixative for the fixation of ovaries, testes, thyroid, and adrenals or Zenker's solution for the fixation of the eyes.

As certain organs (pituitary, thyroid, ovaries, adrenals, and lymph nodes) of some of the smaller rodents are rather small, they should be fixed separately in smaller jars to prevent loss; various fixatives may be used.

5.5.2 Inflation

Inflation is used to preserve lungs effectively. To prevent the formation of artifacts that may be misjudged as emphysema, it is necessary for inflation to be carried out at constant pressure (Chevalier, 1971; Fawell & Lewis,

1971). In certain cases, however, even fixation of the lungs by inflation may not be adequate and perfusion will be preferred (for example, in inhalation studies).

Inflation with fixative is also necessary for correct fixation of the urinary bladder. If the bladder is distended, urine must be replaced by fixative via the urethra using a syringe with a blunt needle. Contracted empty bladders should be partly distended with fixative. The reflux of fixative in the bladder is prevented by ligation of the urethra. Inflation may also be used for fixation of the digestive tract. Here again, ligation is necessary. In these cases, the organs have to be bisected after fixation and the interior surface inspected.

5.5.3 Perfusion

The best way to preserve tissues is by perfusion, which is usually effected by infusion in the left ventricle of the heart and by opening the sinus venosus to provide for proper circulation. Perfusion of isolated organs (liver, kidneys) is another possibility. Before perfusion, the animals are anaesthetized with a barbiturate, administered in combination with nitrate and heparin to ensure vasodilation and prevent clotting. A solution consisting of 77.5 ml sodium nitrite (1.25%) in water, 10 ml heparin (5000 IU/ml) and 12 ml pentobarbital (60 mg/ml), of which 10 ml is administered per kg body weight, is satisfactory. Then the blood is removed with an isotonic saline solution using slight overpressure. When all the blood has left the body via the sinus venosus or right atrium, the body may be perfused with the fixative.

Perfusion is sometimes not possible especially in experiments where the recording of organ weights is important (i.e. in subchronic toxicity studies). This difficulty can be solved by increasing the number of experimental animals, though this may lead to a considerable increase in costs. Perfusion of large numbers of animals is possible using simple facilities at low cost (Fig. 5.1).

5.6 Trimming

It is important that the trimming be carried out by well-trained people. It must be emphasized that knowledge of pathological phenomena is necessary, as it frequently happens that the person responsible for trimming cuts out the "good looking" areas and discards the tumours present in the organs. The tissues must be sliced in such a way that the cut surfaces

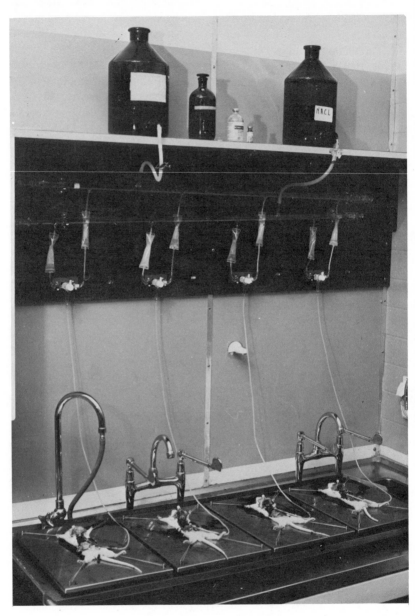

Fig. 5.1   Set up for serial perfusion.

present the largest possible area for examination. The use of a special trimming scheme during the procedure may be helpful.

The kidneys should be sectioned through the cortex and medulla, one kidney mid-longitudinally, the other mid-transversely.

The brain must be cross-sectioned at, at least, three sites: the frontal cortex with basal ganglia, parietal cortex with thalamus, and cerebellum with pons.

The lungs should be sectioned transversely, parallel to the long axis of the body. These sections must include the main bronchi and carina.

The hollow organs should be trimmed in such a way that a cross-section from mucosa to serosa is obtained.

Tumours or tumorous masses usually need to be trimmed in several portions. Preferably, tissues surrounding the tumour should be included.

When intestines are fixed as a roll, the roll can best be embedded as such, since, trimming of these rolls is practically impossible, even after fixation.

For certain organs, special trimming procedures are needed. For example, the nasal cavity should be sectioned transversely at three sites. The trimming of the larynx/pharynx is crucial in order to obtain a section that can be properly interpreted.

Trimmed tissues should have a maximum thickness of 2–3 mm for satisfactory processing.

5.7 Storage

Material not used for processing should not be discarded, but should be stored in airtight jars or plastic bags to ensure that the tissues do not dry out. Plastic bags are an excellent way of storing tissues in minimum space. The bags should be clearly and permanently labelled. The tissues should be stored, at least, until the microscopic examination has been completed and the findings adequately evaluated. If at all possible, the tissues should be stored for a long period (e.g. material from 90-day studies should be stored for 2 years and that from chronic experiments for 5–10 years), but storage facilities may prevent this. Tissue blocks and sections can be stored in a cool area for a considerable time (10 years or more).

5.8 Histological Techniques

Embedding in paraffin or polymer-containing paraffins or waxes is advisable. The embedding procedures may be shortened considerably by using automatic tissue-processing equipment and special frames in which the paraffin blocks can be made in large numbers (Fig. 5.2). Proper and exact labelling of the blocks is a necessity. The blocks may be prepared in such a way that they can be placed as they are in the microtomes.

Tissue sectioning can be performed at a thickness of 4–6 mm and sections can be stained routinely with haematoxylin and eosin or a comparable routine stain. Serial sectioning can best be done with the help of an engine-powdered microtome.

The use of semithin sections (1 μm) is of considerable importance for specific organs such as bone-marrow, kidneys, lymph nodes, spleen, and endocrine glands. These sections can now be made on special microtomes, that cut the normal paraffin blocks with glass knives. Of course, this procedure should only be followed when specific details have to be followed

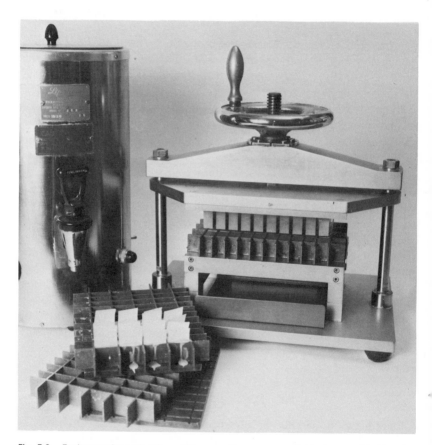

Fig. 5.2 Equipment for embedding of tissues with press to push blocks out of holder after removing the bottom plate.

during the microscopic examination. The use of semithin Epon sections yields even better results.

It will often be necessary to use special staining techniques on tissues in order to provide more information on the presence of carbohydrates, proteins, fats, elements, or certain structural organizations. Special fixation is sometimes necessary for appropriate staining. Bones and calcified tissues have to be decalcified. Eyes usually need to be fixed and embedded differently. Blood vessels may be stained with Sudan black in order to study vascular lesions.

5.9 Special Techniques

5.9.1 Enzyme histochemistry

Enzyme histochemistry is a technique used to detect the activity or presence of an enzyme in a tissue by incubating the fresh tissue in an appropriate medium, so that a fine coloured granular precipitation forms wherever the enzyme is present.

The use of the enzyme-histochemical technique is not common in toxicity testing. Nevertheless, the technique is a valuable one, since it provides information about the metabolic activity and function of the tissues. Furthermore, it introduces the possibility of correlating biochemical with histological findings that may lead to a more correct interpretation. Enzyme-histochemical investigations also make it possible to visualize certain differences in enzyme activity within the structural organization of tissues.

In some cases, a decrease in enzyme activity in certain cells is compensated for by an increase in other cells within the same organ. Such biological differences can only be detected by enzyme-histological investigation, when the results of biochemical determinations are within normal limits and no alterations are seen using conventional histological techniques. Enzyme-histological investigations can easily be incorporated in routine toxicity testing, if necessary.

Relatively small pieces of tissue are quickly frozen in an inert liquid (i.e. isopentane), or cooled in liquid nitrogen or a mixture of solid carbon dioxide and methanol. Storage of the tissues is effected at $-70\,^{\circ}C$. Cryostat sections are prepared and incubated in specially prepared media. Good reference works for the methods have been published (Barka & Anderson, 1965; Pearse, 1968, 1972). To obtain optimum information, the prepared section should be examined by semiquantitative methods.

An enzyme histochemical investigation can also be performed at the electron microscope stage (Geyer, 1973). In this case, the activity or presence of an enzyme is determined by the deposition of electron-dense material at the sites where the enzyme is located. It is evident that these delicate techniques are not easy to apply in routine toxicity testing. They may, however, be of great importance in specific studies on the biological effects of a compound on cellular components, or to detect early damage.

5.9.2 Autoradiography

Autoradiography is based on the principle that radioactive substances present in tissues are able to produce an image on a photographic film or plate. The radiations emitted by the radioactive substances must be of relatively weak energy, so that they will have a short range in tissues and emulsions. When the range is too long, developed silver grains can be found in the emulsion far away from the radioactive source.

In this respect only alpha particles, beta particles, and Auger electrons are useful since electromagnetic radiations such as gamma and X-rays give poor results due to their penetrating power.

Tritium (^{3}H) has been most frequently used in autoradiographic studies, although ^{14}C and ^{32}P are also being used as tracers.

Autoradiography, at both light microscopic and ultrastructural levels, can be used in kinetic studies on tissues by incorporating radioactive-labelled bases in DNA or RNA resulting in the production of silver grains on a photographic film covering the section. The different methods have been extensively described for nondiffusible substances (Baserga & Malamud, 1969; Rogers, 1967) as well as for diffusible substances (Roth & Stumpf, 1969).

Apart from studying the kinetics of tissues, autoradiographic techniques can also be used to study the distribution of radiolabelled compounds and their metabolites. This, again, can be done at light microscopic and ultrastructural levels.

The technique of whole-body autoradiography as developed by Ullberg et al. (1972) is a valuable tool, in this respect, since the distribution of a compound can qualitatively (or even semiquantitatively) be studied in the whole body. In addition, pieces can be cut out to use for micro-autoradiographic research.

Substances may also be labelled with fluorescent chemicals permitting their detection by illumination of the sections with ultra-violet radiation. The technique of fluorescence microscopy can also be used for the detection of certain dyes that possess autofluorescing properties. Some substances, such as the catecholamines, can be made visible by reaction with formaldehyde which converts amines into fluorescent substances (Eränko & Räisänen,

1966). Fluorescence in tissues can be measured quantitatively, thus facilitating controlled conditions (Ploem et al., 1974).

Autoradiographic studies cannot be incorporated easily into routine toxicity experiments. However, the technique may be a very important tool in special studies.

5.9.3 Immunofluorescence and immunoenzyme techniques

Immunofluorescence techniques are primarily used in determining the presence or absence of certain antibodies or antigens in tissues. Antigens are detected by binding them to specific antibodies. If a specific anti-serum is conjugated with a fluorescent dye, the specific antigen-antibody complex formed can be seen by studying the tissue section using ultraviolet radiation microscopy. This direct immunofluorescent technique can be replaced by a more sensitive indirect method in which the substance actually rendered fluorescent is not the antigen under consideration but an intermediate material the distribution of which corresponds precisely to that of the antigen being studied. Information on the principle of these techniques is available (Goldman, 1968; Nairn & Marrack, 1964).

The use of enzyme conjugates has recently been developed (Sternberger, 1974). This system is used when antigen-antibody complexes have to be localized at ultrastructural levels.

Immunofluorescence or immunoenzyme techniques will not be used in most routine toxicity experiments, but they may be of importance in special studies such as those described in Chapter 7.

5.9.5 Electron microscopy

Transmission electron microscopy is the most commonly used technique for studying the ultrastructure of tissues. Different fixation, embedding, and cutting techniques have to be used to obtain ultra-thin sections of tissues (Flauert, 1973, 1974, 1975; Hayat, 1970, 1972, 1973). At the ultra-structural level, very minute changes can be detected and they have to be distinguished from the many artifacts that can be introduced during the different processing procedures. Under optimum conditions, tissues can be examined at high magnifications.

As tissue examination by electron microscopy is very time consuming and costly, it is important only to select tissues from those experiments that justify it. Ultrastructural studies have contributed enormously to our knowledge of molecular biology. In the case of toxicology, ultrastructural studies are always carried out as a secondary investigation, and are usually applied to ultrastructurally, specific, pathological changes already studied in detail at the light microscopic level, in order to secure a better judgment of the importance of the lesion. Ultrastructural studies are also used to confirm that target organs that appear normal at a certain dose level using light microscopy, do not in fact show pathological changes.

Scanning electron microscopy (SEM) techniques, that have come into use in recent years, provide 3-dimensional images of complete biological units and also chemical information (Hayes, 1973). Here again, special processing procedures may be needed, although, in certain cases, formalin-fixed and paraffin-embedded material can be used. Natural surfaces, dissected material, sectioned tissue, and living specimens may be studied. SEM is a valuable tool in biology but, for toxicological investigations, its use is still rather restricted, apart from the possibility of obtaining quantitative chemical information. The development of analytical electron microscopy, using the principles of X-ray microanalysis, also makes it possible to correlate tissue ultrastructure and chemistry (Hayes, 1973; Weavers, 1973).

5.10 Microscopic Examination

Routine histopathological examination is very important and should be carried out correctly. First of all, the sections to be studied should be of good quality. Additional sections and special stains must be prepared if necessary. Special stains are used to study and describe individual lesions; they may also be used to examine certain organs or lesions to permit better judgment of semiquantitative comparison. For example, when haemosiderosis is found to be an important effect, special stains, based on the reaction of the dye with iron, facilitate semiquantitative analysis of the degree of the lesion.

Good microscopic equipment is necessary to perform optimum microscopic examination. Sources of ultraviolet radiation and polarized light should be available.

The microscopic examination must be carried out by well-trained pathologists or other persons trained and experienced in the field of laboratory animal pathology. The use of parapathologists for routine microscopy in toxicity and carcinogenicity experiments is extremely valuable and is important for overcoming a shortage of personnel, trained in laboratory animal pathology (Toxicol. appl. Pharmacol., 1975). Experience has shown that well-trained parapathologists can become very skilful in microscopy and in screening sections for abnormalities. With further experience, they are also able to describe certain lesions. It is the pathologist's duty to see that all lesions observed are described and interpreted correctly, and to check the sections for any lesions that may have been overlooked.

It is a serious mistake, in an experiment, to undertake microscopic examination before the results of other examinations such as biochemical determinations, haematology, and organ weights, are available, for the information obtained from these procedures may give important directions for the microscopic study. For example, an increased thyroid weight may lead to more careful examination of the thyroid for hyperplasia and may prompt histometric determinations. Lower lymph node weight may point to semiquantitative examination of these organs with regard to reduced immunocapacity (Cottier et al., 1972). Differences or changes in the blood picture call for more detailed study of the bone marrow, for example, by preparing and studying 1 μm sections, to detect suspected haemopoietic disturbances.

Gross observations should always be correlated with microscopic findings. It is a false assumption to think that a microscopic examination will be more objective when performed blindly; knowledge of clinical signs and macroscopy are indispensable for a meaningful examination. Of course, the pathologist must be careful not to let knowledge of clinical effects influence his objective evaluation of the tissues; thus, sections of the tissues considered to be involved may have to be re-examined blindly. If such a re-examination is carried out, semiquantitative scoring of the extent of the lesion will also help to detect a possible dose-effect relationship. Should there be any doubt in interpreting the significance of a lesion, it is advisable to consult other pathologists, all of whom should re-examine the slides blindly.

5.10.1 Number of animals and number of organs and tissues studied microscopically

In acute and rangefinding tests, the organs and tissues are usually fixed and examined microscopically after processing. In subacute and long-term studies, and, sometimes, in rangefinding tests, it is customary initially to examine only the tissues of the highest dose group, the control group and the target organs, if known. In addition, all grossly observed lesions are processed in the intermediate and low-level groups. If the results of the microscopic examination of the highest dose group indicate a need to examine certain organs at lower levels, this can be done at a second stage.

In chronic toxicity experiments, all males and females of the highest dose group should be examined. It is also advisable to examine all control animals completely, since this will be the only way to ascertain the incidence of tumours and other "lesions" normally occurring in the strain of animals used. Such information is indispensable for correctly evaluating the significance of changes observed in exposed animals.

In carcinogenicity experiments, where larger numbers of animals per group are usually used, some laboratories restrict microscopic examination mainly to the grossly observed abnormalities and tumours, and perform complete histological examinations on only 15–20 male and 15–20 female survivors of the highest dose group and of the control group, on the assumption that a well-performed gross examination will detect most of the tumours present. Histological examination of all tissues of 15–20 animals of each sex will give some information on the possible presence of certain pre-malignant hyperplastic or neoplastic changes not grossly observed. If such lesions are found, the histological examination should cover all animals, while small organs which may bear tumours that cannot be grossly observed (thyroid, pituitary, adrenals) must be examined histologically.

5.10.2 Description of the lesions

For the microscopic examination, it is essential to use a check-list to detect losses, especially of small organs lost in the processing procedure. All organs and tissues examined should be listed, even though no abnormalities are seen, while all lesions found should be described clearly and accurately. It is essential to describe lesions in a semiquantitative way using such words as slight, moderate, strong, and very strong to indicate the extent of the lesion; it is also essential to indicate the criteria used to investigate and classify abnormalities. It will often be necessary to re-examine certain lesions in order to obtain a well-balanced semiquantitative judgment. Several reference works may be of help in the classification of tumours and other lesions (Beveridge & Sobin, 1974; Cotchin & Roe, 1967; Ribelin & McCoy, 1965; and Turusov, 1973).

Certain lesions found by microscopic examination may, in fact, consist of several entities. In such cases, it may be important to classify these entities independently. For example, perilobular liver degeneration may be combined with bile duct proliferation, but one of the two phenomena may be more extensive than the other with respect to dose level and time. For a better interpretation, it is preferable to describe and classify such lesions independently.

5.11 Presentation, Evaluation, and Interpretation of Pathological Data

A well-performed and well-described microscopic examination is not complete if the results cannot be studied and compared easily and adequately. The lesions found in the different groups should be tabulated according to organ, group, and sex in order to facilitate comparison of the incidence of such lesions in the different groups. If, in addition, a semi-quantitative estimate of the extent of the lesions is made, it will be easy to see whether they are compound-induced and increase with time and dose.

It is important that these tables include details such as the number of animals necropsied and the number examined microscopically, per group and sex. In addition, it is advisable to state, the exact number of organs or tissues examined microscopically, since it is well known that, in every toxicity experiment, organs and tissues get lost during the processing procedure. In this way, the loss can be adequately estimated and the lesions found can be expressed against the real number of organs or tissues examined.

For correct interpretation of the tumour tables, it is advisable to include hyperplastic and preneoplastic lesions as individual groups. The table should also include the number of days that elapsed from the start of the experiment until the observation of each tumour. This first observation may be clinical, for example, when mammary, ear duct, or skin tumours are involved and the time that has elapsed can then be called the "induction time". However, usually, tumours are found after death or killing *in extremis*, or at sacrifice at the end of the experiment. Thus, in these cases, it seems most appropriate to use the term "time of observation". The inclusion of the "time of observation" of tumours in the table is of help to the investigator since it provides information on shorter or prolonged latency periods (e.g. time that has elapsed between initiation and the appearance of tumours). In addition, it reminds the reader to take into account the survival differences when expressing the results.

In long-term experiments, the number of lesions found may be quite large. Furthermore, some lesions may have been noticed during a certain period in life, when the animals died or were sacrificed *in extremis*, while others will have been noticed at the end of an experiment. When such lesions are tabulated in the same table, this information may get lost. It seems, therefore, most appropriate in such long-term experiments to pool the results of the pathological examination for certain periods, for example the first 12 months of life and then for 3- to 6-monthly intervals, and to give the results of the examination undertaken at the end of the experiment separately.

It is obvious that in preparing such tables, the use of an automated data acquisition and computer-based system will be of great help. These systems have been described for application to toxicological studies, especially for animal weights, food and drug consumption, organ weights, and bio-chemical data (Munro et al., 1972). In pathology, such systems offer considerable potential. The necessity for the correct coding of pathological changes, and the use of a code system set up so that detailed information about lesions can still be obtained, is obvious. Several systems have been described (Becker, 1973; Enlander, 1975; Smith et al., 1972), and may be adapted for this purpose.

Pathological examinations must always be evaluated and interpreted in connexion with other phenomena found. It must be decided whether lesions noticed are in fact pathological, and whether they are found in connexion with changes in other variables such as organ weights, biochemical tests, etc. If compound-induced lesions are found, they may not only be present at the highest dose level, but also at an intermediate dose level. In the latter case, it is important to determine whether there is a dose-dependent increase in the severity and extent of the lesion, a finding which would strengthen the assumption that the lesion is compound-induced. Moreover, a clear dose-response relationship permits better evaluation of the potential risk of a compound. Whenever lesions are found only at the highest dose level, the sections at all dose levels should be re-examined blindly to remove any doubt. Often the two sexes will show a different sensitivity to the action of a compound.

Problems may arise when certain lesions are found more frequently and to a greater extent in the treated groups compared with the control group and compared with the common incidence of the lesion in the strain used. The usual attitude towards this phenomenon is to consider it as an effect or response.

In the evaluation of tumour incidence, criteria such as increased tumour incidence, decrease in latency period, and the appearance of tumours in organs where they do not occur spontaneously, have to be considered. For this reason, detailed information on the spontaneous occurrence of tumours in the species and strain used is essential, particuarly when tests indicate that the compound possesses a weak carcinogenic action. Simple comparison of tumour incidence in control animals and experimental animals at one point in time may lead to erroneous conclusions, especially when only one of the above three criteria is met. Many factors other than treatment may influence the incidence of spontaneous tumours.

Statistical evaluation of the results is often necessary, but, as yet, there are no agreed procedures for comparing statistically the incidence of malignant tumours in controls and experimental groups.

REFERENCES

BARKA, T. & ANDERSON, P. J. (1965) *Histochemistry: theory, practice and bibliography.* New York, Harper & Row; London, Evanston.

BASERGA, R. & MALAMUD, D. (1969) *Autoradiography: techniques and application.* New York, Harper & Row; London, Evanston.

BECKER, H. (1973) Experiences with a test-stage free-text processing system in pathology, using display terminals. *Path. Europ.*, **8**: 307–313.

BEVERIDGE, W. I. B. & SOBIN, L. H., ed. (1974) International histological classification of tumours of domestic animals. *Bull. World Health Org.*, **50**: 1–142.

CHEVALIER, H. J. (1971) [A method for the fixation of the lungs of small animals.] *Z. Versuchstierk.*, **13**: 101–104 (in German).

COHRS, P., JAFFE, R., & MEESEN, H. (1958) [*Pathology of laboratory animals*] Berlin, Springer-Verlag, Vol. 2 (in German).

COTCHIN, E. & ROE, F. J. C. (1967) *Pathology of laboratory rats and mice.* Oxford, Edinburgh, Blackwell.

COTTIER, H., TURK, J., & SOBIN, L. (1972) A proposal for a standardized system of reporting human lymph node morphology in relation to immunological function. *Bull. World Health Organ.*, **47**: 375–408.

ENLANDER, D. (1975) Computer data-processing of medical diagnosis in pathology. *Am. J. clin. Pathol.*, **63**: 538–544.

ERÄNKO, O. & RAISANEN, L. (1966) *In vitro* release and uptake of noradrenaline in the rat iris. In: Ebler, U. S. V., Rosell, S. & Uunäs, B., ed. *Mechanism of release of biogenic amines.* New York, Pergamon Press.

FAWELL, J. K. & LEWIS, D. J. (1971) A simple apparatus for the inflation fixation of lungs at constant pressure. *Lab. Anim.*, **5**: 267–270.

FLAUERT, A. M. (1973, 1974, 1975) *Practical methods in electron microscopy.* Amsterdam, Oxford, North Holland Publ.; New York, Elsevier.

GEYER, G. (1973) [*Ultrahistochemistry, histochemical working guidelines for electron-microscopy.*] Stuttgart, Gustav Fischer Verlag (in German).

GOLDMAN, M. (1968) *Fluorescent antibody methods.* New York, London, Academic Press.

GORDON, H. W. & DANIEL, E. J. (1974) Microwave fixation of human tissues. *Am. J. med. Technol.*, **40** (10): 441–442.

HAYAT, M. A. (1970, 1972, 1973) Principles and techniques of electron microscopy. In: *Biological Applications* Vol. I, II, III, IV. New York, Van Nostrand Reinhold Company.

HAYES, T. I. (1973) Scanning electron microscopy in biology. In Koehler, J. H., ed. *Advanced techniques in biological electron microscopy*, Berlin, Heidelberg, New York, Springer-Verlag, pp. 153–214.

MUNRO, I. C., CHARBONNEAU, S. M., & WILLES, R. F. (1972) An automated data acquisition and computer-based computation system for application of toxicological studies in laboratory animals. *Lab. Anim. Sci.*, **22**: 753–756.

NAIRN, R. E. & MARRACK, J. R. (1964) *Fluorescent protein tracing.* Edinburgh, London, Livingstone.

PEARSE, A. G. E. (1968, 1972) *Histochemistry, theoretical and applied.* 3rd ed., Edinburgh, Churchill Livingstone, Vol. I & II.

PLOEM, J. S., DE STERKE, J. A., BONNET, J., & WASMUND, H. (1974) A micro-spectrofluorometer with epi-illumination operated under computer control. *J. Histochem. Cytochem.*, **22**: 668–677.

RIBELIN, W. E. & McCOY, J. R. (1965) *The pathology of laboratory animals.* Springfield, Charles Thomas.

ROE, F. J. C. (1965) Spontaneous tumours in rats and mice. *Food Cosmet. Toxicol.*, **3**: 707–720.

ROGERS, A. W. (1967) *Techniques of autoradiography.* Amsterdam, London, New York, Elsevier.

ROTH, L. J. & STUMPF, W. E. (1969) *Autoradiography of diffusible substances*. New York, London, Academic Press.

SMITH, J. E., McGAVIN, M. D., & GRONWALL, R. (1972) English-language computer-based system for storage and retrieval of pathological diagnosis. *Vet. Pathol.* **9:** 152–158.

SONTAG, J. M., PAGE, N. P., & SAFFIOTTA, U. (1975) *Guidelines for carcinogen bioassay in small rodents*. Bethesda MD, National Cancer Institute.

STERNBERGER, L. A. (1974) *Immunocytochemistry*. Englewood Cliffs, NJ, Prentice-Hall.

Toxicol. appl. Pharmacol. (1975) **31:** 1–3, A training programme for parapathologists.

TURUSOV, V. S. ed. (1973) *Pathology of tumours in laboratory animals*, Vol. 1, Lyon, IARC (Sci. Publ. No. 5).

ULLBERG, S., HAMMARSTROEM, L., & APPELGREN, L-E. (1972) Autoradiography in pharmacology. In: Cohen, Y., ed. *I.E.P.T. Section 78*, Oxford, New York, Pergamon Press, Vol. 1, pp. 221–239.

WEAVERS, B. A. (1973) The potentiality of EMMA-4, the analytical electron microscopy in histochemistry: a review. *Histochem. J.,* **5:** 173–193.

6. INHALATION EXPOSURE[a]

6.1 Introduction

Advances in technology, throughout the world, have increased the number and amount of chemicals in the atmosphere. The health effects of inhalation of these chemicals can be predicted to some extent by experimental investigation. In order to simulate environmental conditions, a special technology has evolved relating to the design and operation of inhalation chambers and the generation and characterization of aerosols and vapours. This chapter will introduce this technology and review the significance of certain biological end-points commonly measured in inhalation studies.

This chapter is not intended to be all-inclusive, nor to provide complete instructions on inhalation technology. No toxicological protocol is sufficient to cover all situations with all materials. Hence, the expertise of the individual investigator and the objectives of the investigation will govern the selection of the final protocol and the biological end-points relevant to the particular compound concerned.

The costs associated with evaluation of toxicity by the inhalation route are considerably higher than for toxicity studies using other routes of exposure because of the cost of the specialized equipment used in inhalation studies and the time required for its calibration. In general, it can be estimated that the total cost of any type of inhalation study, short- or long-term, will be two to three times that of a comparable oral study. Because of this, it is important to determine when inhalation studies should be performed and when, and if, studies by other routes would suffice. Finally, in addition to costs, other resources should be considered. In most countries, the number of laboratories capable of performing inhalation studies is limited. Thus, it is essential to develop priorities for the selection of compounds for evaluation of inhalation toxicity.

6.2 Need for Inhalation Studies

The effect of a compound depends on its concentration at the receptors of the affected organ or system. The concentration at different sites and times is a function of the route of entry. Thus the route of entry is an important factor with regard to toxicity. No good substitute model for inhalation

[a] The assistance of Dr J. O'Neil, Dr M. Amdur, and Dr W. Busey in the preparation of this chapter is gratefully acknowledged.

exposure as a means of direct exposure of the lungs has been developed, although intratracheal exposure has been frequently used, particularly in pulmonary carcinogenesis studies. The distribution kinetics are different with pulsed exposures compared with constant inhalation exposures. With pulsed exposures, such as oral, intravenous, intraperitoneal, etc., the concentration of the test material will reach a peak and then usually fall off, depending on the distribution coefficients for each compound and organ in question. With continuous exposure, concentrations in many body compartments will attain an equilibrium, depending again on the concentration of the test material and the distribution coefficient. Thus, quantitative toxicity is often quite different, depending on the route of entry.

With the exception of certain drugs, man's exposure to environmental agents comes either from skin contact, ingestion, or inhalation. Inhalation is of particular importance in occupational exposure and in exposure to air pollutants. For airborne substances, the lung is the first organ that foreign chemicals encounter and it is one of the body's first lines of defence. Chemicals that enter the lung can either exert a direct effect on the cells of the lung, or be absorbed into the systemic circulation. Blood passing from the lung to the heart and then into the peripheral circulation can carry agents directly to other organs without passing through the detoxication processes of the liver. This contrasts with oral exposure where chemicals may be absorbed into blood that immediately passes through the liver and can be metabolically transformed into either more or less toxic compounds.

Direct contact with irritants causes local inflammation in the respiratory system, the degree of which may depend on the local concentration and not on the total dose. For example, Kljačkina (1973) demonstrated that inhaled bromine acts as a specific irritant of the respiratory system whereas bromine administered orally results in changes in the nervous system.

Thus, specific reasons for performing inhalation studies include: (a) determination of specific responses of the respiratory tract; (b) assessment of the toxic hazard of agents whose principal route of exposure is via inhalation; (c) investigation into the mechanism of toxicity of inhaled materials; and (d) study of the comparative toxicity of agents administered by different routes.

6.3 Fate of Inhaled Materials

6.3.1 Nature of aerosols

The nature and characteristics of aerosols have been treated in detail elsewhere (Cadle, 1965; Mercer, 1973a,b; Raabe, 1970), but it may be useful to review a few general concepts. Aerosols consist of finely divided particles ranging in size from about 0.01 to 100 μm in diameter. The particles in a cloud are usually of many sizes and the size can be expressed as a size-frequency distribution curve which usually best fits a log-normal distribution. There are several ways to express the diameter of a particle, the common ones being count median diameter, mass median diameter, and aerodynamic mass median diameter. The last term is important as it considers each distribution as if it were made up of unit density spheres and measures its diameter as if it were acting aerodynamically like a unit density sphere. Thus, aerosol behaviour can be compared, regardless of the individual shape and density of the particles.

The division of a solid into fine particles that become airborne results in a large increase in the surface area of the material. The consequence is a generally increased chemical reactivity of the material, thus accelerating all physical and chemical processes, such as oxidation, dissolution, evaporation, absorption, and electrical activity. The physiological activity of these particles also increases. The sizes of interest from a biological standpoint range from about 0.1 to 10 μm. Larger particles do not usually enter the respiratory tract or, if they do, they are deposited in the nose.

6.3.2 Deposition

Material that enters the respiratory tract with the inspired air can either be deposited or exhaled. Many factors affect the deposition of particles or the absorption of vapours in the respiratory system. Retention of vapours is governed by the diffusion rates of the vapour, the solubility of the vapour in the various body compartments, and the degree to which these compartments have attained the equilibrium. This in turn, depends on the duration of the exposure, the concentration, and the rate of removal of the vapours. This subject has recently been reviewed by Stupfel & Mordelet-Dambrine (1974).

Many more factors govern the deposition of particulates in the respiratory tract. Roe (1968) has divided these into physical and chemical characteristics of the particle, anatomical, physiological, and pathological factors. The size, density, and shape of the particles are the physical variables that determine their aerodynamic behaviour. The Task Group on Lung Dynamics (Morrow et al., 1966) has discussed deposition as a function of particle size.

Three distinct physical processes act on particles suspended in the atmosphere to cause them to be deposited in the respiratory tract. Inertial impaction results from the tendency of particles to move in straight lines. The repeated branching and subdivision of the respiratory tract causes particles to be impacted on surfaces, particularly near the bifurcations. Inertial forces are greater with larger particles. Sedimentation due to gravity also causes particles to strike the surface of the respiratory tract. Finally, Brownian movement, particularly of smaller particles, causes them to be deposited in the lung. The effectiveness of these mechanisms depends on the anatomy of the respiratory tract, the size of the particle, and the breathing pattern. During artificially induced hyperventilation in rabbits, more material was deposited in comparison with controls (Veličkovskij & Kacnelson, 1964). Normal deposition and deposition in diseased states are discussed in detail by Albert et al. (1973), Brain & Valberg (1974), Goldberg & Laurenco (1973), Macklem et al. (1973) and Stuart (1974).

Aerosols are deposited all along the respiratory tract. Large particles (5–10 μm) are mainly deposited in the upper respiratory tract, including the nasal cavity. The depth of penetration increases as particle size decreases and particles in the 1–2 μm range are, for the most part, deposited in the alveoli. As a first approximation, 25% of inhaled particles are exhaled, 50% are deposited in the upper respiratory tract, and 25% are deposited in the lower respiratory tract (Morrow et al., 1966).

6.3.3 Clearance

Soluble particles readily dissolve at the site of deposition. Generally, they enter the bloodstream and then behave as if they had been intravenously injected. Insoluble particles can be removed from the respiratory tract by several mechanisms depending on the site of deposition. Particles that are deposited on the mucous blanket are carried towards the pharynx by the cilia and are usually swallowed or expectorated. Hence, it is impossible to completely separate respiratory exposure from gastrointestinal exposure. The rate of clearance by the mucociliary escalator has been measured in man by a number of investigators (Albert et al., 1969, 1973; Camner et al., 1972, 1973; Morrow, 1970; Sanchis et al., 1972) and animals (Albert et al., 1973; Thomas, 1969; Veličkovskij & Kacnelson, 1964; Watson et al., 1969).

Particles that are deposited in the deep non-ciliated portion of the lung clear more slowly. One mechanism responsible for alveolar clearance is phagocytosis. Although alveolar macrophages engulf particles within a few hours, there is evidence that macrophages do not carry them actively to the mucociliary escalator in the first few days following inhalation (Camner et al., 1977). Recent studies indicate that there are other mechanisms of alveolar clearance. Tucker et al. (1973) have shown alveolar clearance by normal interstitial drainage pathways. Casarett (1972) and Morrow (1973) described a possible mechanism whereby particles could move from the alveolus up to the terminal bronchiole, and then to the ciliated epithelium for removal on the mucus. Very fine particles can also enter the blood directly through the lymphatic system. Finally, particles can dissolve and be absorbed into the bloodstream. Some particles remain in the alveolar region of the lung for considerable periods of time, during which dissolution forces can operate.

6.4 Dose in Inhalation Studies

The term dose has many meanings depending on the background and expertise of the investigator. In toxicology, dose is usually defined as the mass of material introduced into the animal, and it is often divided by the body weight. Hence, toxicologists often speak of dose in mg/kg. Even this is misleading, to some extent, because the material may not interact in any way, and because of other reasons that become apparent in species comparisons. The actual dose or amount of a substance entering the internal milieu of the body depends on the concentration and the particle size of the inhaled material, the duration of the exposure, and the breathing variables of the test species. Thus, the actual absorbed dose is difficult to determine and inhalation toxicologists often refer to exposure conditions instead of dose. The exposure must be defined both in terms of concentration (C) and time (t), and is sometimes expressed as the product of these two (Ct) (MacFarland, 1968) (see also Chapter 1). While the Ct product is not a true dose, it can be used in a similar fashion. Haber (1924) recognized this and Haber's rule states that, for a fixed Ct product, the response will be the same. This rule holds reasonably well over limited ranges of C and t, but deviations occur when extreme values of the variables are examined.

More frequently, inhalation toxicologists keep the time constant and vary the concentration of the test material. Hence, they measure an LC_{50}, i.e. the median concentration to which animals are exposed for a specified time that will kill 50% of the animals within a fixed period of time after exposure. It is implicit in LC_{50} data that the durations of both the exposure and post-exposure period are standardized. Comparative LC_{50} data are often obtained for 4-h exposures and a 14-day post-exposure observation period (Carpenter et al., 1949; Pozzani et al., 1959).

6.5 Choice of Species

The ideal subject for studies relevant to man is man himself. However, human volunteers can only be used where the toxicological hazard is already reasonably well defined and accepted. Human studies have been conducted recently with chlorinated hydrocarbon solvents and common air pollutants (Andersen et al., 1974; Hazucha et al., 1973; Stewart, 1972; Stewart et al., 1970a,b, 1973). These experiments were well controlled and monitored and the exposure levels were low.

Rats, dogs, and monkeys have been the species most used for inhalation toxicity studies, although investigators have also used mice, hamsters, guineapigs, rabbits, cats, miniature swine, and donkeys. The choice of species should be made, primarily, with a view to extrapolating the experimental results to man. However, choice on this basis alone is difficult since the validity of such an extrapolation is often uncertain. When selecting the particular species for study, the following factors must be considered: the comparative morphology of the respiratory tract; the presence or absence of lung disease or susceptible states; and the similarity of biochemical and physiological responses to those in man.

6.5.1 Anatomical differences

The respiratory systems of various laboratory animals and man differ widely. As man is a primate, it is sometimes erroneously assumed that the monkey is a good model for inhalation studies, but marked differences are noted when comparing human and sub-human primate respiratory systems. In the monkey, the end airway is always a respiratory bronchiole, whereas this is rarely the case in man. Furthermore, the monkey's lung is not lobulated.

The most commonly used laboratory animals are quadrupeds, and their respiratory systems are horizontal and not vertical as in the primate. This is important because the aerodynamics of a horizontally arranged lung are different, and particle deposition will also be different. In human subjects, maximum dust deposition is in the upper portion of the lung; in experimental animals, maximum deposition in the more ventral portions of the lung is usual.

The gross anatomy of the respiratory systems of the various laboratory animals and man is quite different. In animals such as the rat and guineapig, the nose contains highly developed tortuous turbinates. In monkeys and man with relatively smaller noses, the turbinates are less complex. These differences in nasal anatomy are especially important in studies involving exposure to particulates. More particles impinge in more complex turbinate systems and will not, therefore, reach the deeper portions of the respiratory system.

The subgross anatomy of the lungs of various laboratory animals and man has been detailed and compared by McLaughlin et al. (1961a,b, 1966). The authors have grouped the common laboratory animals and man in three basic categories based on subgross pulmonary anatomy (Table 6.1). They

Table 6.1 Comparative subgross anatomy of the lung[a]

Species	Lung type	No. of lobes left	No. of lobes right	Lobulation	Respiratory bronchioles	Terminal bronchioles	Pulmonary/artery Bronchial/artery shunts	Termination of bronchial arteries	Pleura
Cow	I	3	5(4)	well developed	extremely poor development	present	present	distal airway	thick
Sheep	I	3	4	well developed	extremely poor development	present	present	distal airway	thick
Pig	I	3	4	well developed	extremely poor development	present	not present	distal airway	thick
Monkey	II	3	4	not present	very well developed	absent	not present	distal airway	thin
Dog	II	3	4	not present	very well developed	absent	not present	distal airway	thin
Cat	II	3	4	not present	very well developed	absent	not present	distal airway	thin
Guineapig	IIa	3	4	not present	fairly well developed	absent	present	distal airway	thin
Rat	IIa	1	4	not present	fairly well developed	absent	few present	distal airway	thin
Rabbit	IIa	3	4	not present	fairly well developed	absent	present	tertiary bronchus	thin
Horse	III	(3)	(4)	imperfectly developed	poorly developed	present	present	distal airway and alveoli	thick
Man	III	2	3	imperfectly developed	poorly developed	present	present	distal airway and alveoli	thick

[a] From: McLaughlin et al. (1961a,b, 1966).

grouped the various animals on the basis of lung lobulation, the presence or absence of respiratory bronchioles, the presence or absence of terminal bronchioles, pulmonary artery/bronchial artery shunts, and the termination of the bronchial arteries. Their studies indicate that the pulmonary anatomy of the horse most closely resembles that of man.

6.5.2   Physiological considerations

Pertinent differences in the lung physiology of various species must be considered in inhalation toxicology. Normal values or ranges for several species, including man, are summarized in Table 6.2 (Sanockij, 1970a).

6.5.3   Disease and susceptibility states

Most toxicological investigations are performed on healthy animals. However, epidemiological studies have indicated that during air pollution episodes the populations at greatest risk are the young, the aged, and those people with pre-existing cardiopulmonary disease. One task of the inhalation toxicologist is to identify those segments of the population that are particularly susceptible to the presence of airborne contaminants. Certain animal models of diseased or stressed states have been described (Boyd et al., 1974; Drew & Taylor, 1974; Silver et al., 1973; Taylor & Drew, 1975; see also Chapter 2) which could be used or could be adapted for use in inhalation studies. The most commonly used model of this nature is the papain-induced emphysematous animal (Gross et al., 1965; Martorana et al., 1973; Niewoehner & Kleinermann, 1973; Snider et al., 1974). Both aged and neonatal animals could be used as models of high susceptibility groups. Disease and susceptibility states are important considerations in the selection of the species and, in some cases, even the strain of animal to be investigated since it is well known that the incidence of cancer differs considerably among certain species and strains.

For example, Kuschner et al. (1975) recently reported a high incidence of respiratory tract tumours in rats after exposure to oxybis[chloromethane] (bis(chloromethyl)ether) but only a few tumours in hamsters. These tumours were about equally divided between esthesioneuroepitheliomas and bronchogenic squamous cell carcinomas. Leong et al. (1975) repeated these experiments; however, all the tumours in Leong's study were nasal tumours with no bronchogenic carcinomas. The only difference noted in the protocol was that Leong et al. used specific-pathogen-free, caesarean-derived rats, whereas Kuschner et al. used Sprague–Dawley rats, that were not specific-pathogen-free.

Table 6.2 Some physiological indices of man and animals[a]

	Man	Dog	Cat	Rabbit	Guineapig	Rat	Mouse
Body surface (m²)	1.8	0.528	0.2	0.18	0.040	0.030	0.006
Relation body surface to body weight (m²/kg)	0.0257	0.044	0.066	0.072	0.12	0.15	0.3
Basal metabolism (kJ/kg)	105	222	—	188	360	615	711
Frequency of respiration (min)	14–18	10–30	20–30	50–100	80–135	110–135	140–210
Size of alveoli (µm)	150	100	100	—	—	50	30
Surface of lungs (m²)	50	100	7.2	5.21	1.47	0.56	0.12
Relation of lung surface to body weight (m²/kg)	0.7	8.3	2.8	2.5	3.2	3.3	5.4
Inhaled air (ml)	616	40–60	—	—	1.75	0.865	0.154
Lung ventilation (ml/min)	8732	—	1000	600	155	73	25
Relation of lung ventilation to body weight (ml/min/g)	0.13	—	0.30	0.29	0.33	0.05	1.24
Consumption of oxygen (ml/kg/hr)	203.1	3600	9420	522.7	2180	2199	3910
Elimination of CO_2 (ml/kg/h)	168.8	—	—	—	—	2650	4240
Coefficient of respiration	0.82	—	—	0.83	—	0.82	0.85–1.33
Pulse frequency for 1 min	70–72	90–130	120–180	150–240	206–280	300–500	520–780

[a] From: Sanockij (1970a).

6.6 Duration of Exposure

Acute inhalation toxicity studies usually consist of a single exposure (or occasionally a few exposures) of not more than 8 h. Repeated exposure studies consist of a number of daily exposures for fixed periods of time. Occasionally, investigators terminate exposure after several days or weeks, and then maintain the animals in the colony to observe delayed development of long-term effects (Kuschner et al., 1975).

The duration of chronic studies varies considerably. One logical proposal is based on the life span of the test species (Sanockij, 1970b). If, for example, one considers that toxic signs will appear in man after an exposure over 10% of his life span (7 years), animals should also be exposed for 10% of their life span. Thus, rats should be exposed for 3–4 months, and larger animals for a somewhat longer period. Some authors (Sidorenko & Pinigin, 1970) consider that even continuous exposure for 3–4 months is insufficient to simulate lifetime exposure in man, and many studies last longer, some up to 5 years (Lewis et al., 1974). Powell & Hosey (1965) consider the minimum duration of a chronic study to be one year, the animals being exposed 6 h a day for 5 days a week. This corresponds to a significant portion of a rodent's lifetime.

Chronic studies are conducted to determine the effects of long-term exposure to compounds and particularly (in the USSR) to establish minimum effect levels (Lim_{ch}). In order to evaluate the effects of long-term exposures, such as elevated incidences of infection, emphysema, or the induction of cancer, inhalation controls should be run concurrently. Two species are usually used. Occasionally the toxic effects and the mechanism of chronic toxicity are entirely different from those manifested in acute exposures. Benzene, for example, is a central nervous system depressant at high concentrations, while, at low concentrations over long periods of exposure, it affects the hematopoietic system.

The selection of concentration for chronic studies is difficult. For example, in the USA, concentrations are chosen that do not produce mortality and produce only minimal changes in other biological indices of toxicity during limited studies. In the USSR, the concentration selected is below the Lim_{ac}. In order to investigate dose-response relationships, it is advisable to use at least three different dose levels, hoping that the highest level chosen will produce quantifiable effects and that the lowest level selected will produce minimal or even no effects. In the USSR, research workers often use as the highest level the concentration which, in single short-term exposures of human subjects, does not produce any effect during the study of reflex reactions.

When investigating the various biological indices of toxicity, it is necessary to carry out measurements more frequently during the early stages of the study (Camner et al., 1972, 1973). Studies carried out at the Institute of Labour Hygiene and Occupational Medicine of the USSR show that the time to the display of the first signs (period for initial decompensation) varies considerably. Thus, the variables are recorded at 1, 4, 8, 15, and 30 days and monthly thereafter. After terminating the exposure, the frequency of measurements may be increased again to record any early changes.

6.6.1 Intermittent versus continuous exposures

Long-term exposures are usually patterned on projected industrial experience, giving the animals a daily exposure of 6–7 h, 5 days a week (intermittent exposure), or on a possible environmental exposure, with 22–24 h of exposure per day, 7 days a week (continuous exposure), with about an hour for feeding the animals and maintaining the chambers. In both cases, the animals are usually exposed to a fixed concentration of test materials. Thus, neither situation approaches actual human experience, where concentrations of atmospheric pollutants are continuously fluctuating by one or two orders of magnitude. A major difference to consider between intermittent and continuous exposure is that with the former there is a 17–18-h period in which animals may recover from the effects of each daily exposure, and an even longer recovery period at weekends. The recovery period in some cases is extremely important as in the case of continuous versus intermittent exposure to dichlormethane (Haun, 1972).

The choice of intermittent or continuous exposure depends on the objectives of the study and on the human experience that is to be simulated. However, certain technical difficulties must be considered. For example, the advantages of continuous exposure for simulating environmental conditions may be offset by the necessity of watering and feeding during exposure, and by the need for more complicated (and reliable) aerosol and vapour generation and monitoring techniques. Intermittent systems require simpler chambers, since provision for food and water is not necessary. The contaminant dispersal systems are also simpler as they need to operate for only 6–7 h per day.

6.7 Inhalation Systems

6.7.1 Facilities required

It is more advantageous to build facilities designed specifically for inhalation studies than to modify existing buildings. High ceilings are necessary for housing exposure chambers and related equipment, such as aerosol and vapour generators, filters, flowmeters, etc. A constant supply of clean filtered air with temperature and humidity controls should be available for both the chamber rooms and the chambers themselves. Adequate floor space should provide access to at least two sides of the chambers, and the chambers themselves should be separated by a small space to avoid heat transfer between chambers.

6.7.2 Static systems

Inhalation systems can be characterized as static, when the agent is introduced into a chamber as a batch and then mixed, or dynamic, when airflow and introduction (and removal) of agent are continuous. The duration of static exposure is limited by: (a) the gradual depletion of oxygen; (b) the accumulation of carbon dioxide; (c) the accumulation of water vapour; and (d) the gradual increase in temperature inside the chamber. In spite of these limitations, static systems are of great practical usefulness in assessing acute toxicity, particularly when the supply of material is limited. Procedures similar to those described by Draize et al. (1959) are in use today for screening commercial products. Another use of static systems is for the exposure of animals to biological aerosols. It is difficult to generate a viable biological aerosol particle continuously because of the limited amount of material available; thus, material is dispersed in a large chamber, mixed, and the animals exposed through nose tubes connected to the test atmosphere (Jemski & Phillips, 1965).

6.7.3 Dynamic systems

Today, most inhalation facilities use dynamic systems where the airflow and introduction of agents are continuous. The theoretical or nominal concentration of chemicals in a chamber can be calculated as follows:

$$\text{concentration} = \frac{\text{flow of chemical}}{\text{flow of air}}$$

Many factors, including wall loss, losses on the skin and fur of animals, and uptake by the test animals, cause the actual concentration to be somewhat less than the nominal concentration. Thus, the concentration should always be measured by an appropriate instrument or technique rather than reporting the nominal concentration.

When material is introduced into a chamber, the concentration builds up exponentially according to equations originally described and verified by

Silver (1946). If perfect mixing occurs, the concentration can be calculated according to the following equation:

$$C = (w/b)(1 - \exp(-bt/a)) \qquad (1)$$

where C = the concentration of material at time t; w = amount of material introduced per minute; a = volume of the chamber; b = flow of air through the chamber.

The fraction of equilibrium concentration (w/b) attained in time t is:

$$\frac{C}{w/b} = 1 - \exp(1bt/a) \qquad (2)$$

Thus, the time required to reach 99% (t_{99}) of the equilibrium concentration is:

$$0.99 = 1 - \exp(-bt_{99}/a) \qquad (3)$$

or

$$t_{99} = 4.6052a/b$$

This equation may be given the general form:

$$t_x = Ka/b \qquad (4)$$

where x equals % nominal concentration attained in time t and

$$K = bu\left(\frac{x}{100} - 1\right)$$

Values of K for various values of x are tablulated below:

x	K
99	4.6
95	3.0
90	2.3
85	1.9
80	1.6

There are several features of interest in the above equations. Since the concentration build-up is exponential, the concentration will theoretically never reach a constant value. However, in practice, the concentration is not detectably different once the equilibration time is equal to t_{99} or longer. The clearance curve of removal of chemical from the chamber after the flow of chemical is discontinued also follows an exponential curve (Fig. 6.1). Thus, to ensure that little or no material remains in the chamber, it should be operated for t_{99} after discontinuing the flow of chemical. This procedure also

211

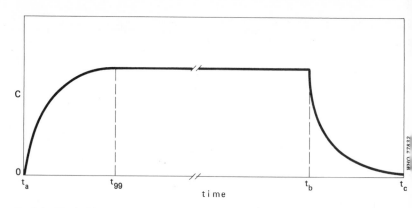

Fig. 6.1 The build-up and decay of a pollutant in a chamber. Exposures usually start at time t_a and stop at t_c. The exposure duration is recorded as t_b, the time the flow of pollutant is terminated (McFarland, 1976).

compensates for the time required for build-up of material in the chamber. Finally, it should be noted that in the general equation, t_x is only a function of the volume of the chamber and the flow of air through the chamber. Thus, if the ratio of $a/b = 1$, $t_{99} = 4.6$ min, $t_{95} = 3$ min, etc. A 150-litre chamber operated at 30 litre/min would have $a/b = 5$ and $t_{99} = 5$ (4.6 min) $= 23$ min. MacFarland (1976) has recently reviewed these principles and has also discussed ways of decreasing t_{99} by manipulating flow rate.

6.7.4 Typical whole-body systems

Inhalation exposure technology has been recently reviewed by Drew & Laskin (1973) and earlier descriptions and requirements have been given by Frazer et al. (1959), Hinners et al. (1966, 1968), and Roe (1968). The simplest inhalation system would be a box with facilities for air intake and exhaust. This concept has been used for many years in chambers similar to that described by Drew & Laskin (1973) (Fig. 6.2). In this system, a cylindrical glass battery jar is mounted in a horizontal position; a frame holds the jar and provides support for a panel which is mounted against the open end and serves as a closure. Various openings can be cut in the panel for the introduction of the pollutant and for monitoring the concentration.

Studies at the University of Rochester on the toxicity of radioactive materials contributed significantly to the development of the technology of inhalation exposure. The original test chamber was cylindrical with cones on the top and bottom. A modified chamber in the shape of a hexagon with pyramidal ends (Wilson & Laskin, 1950) is known as the "Rochester Chamber". A final modification with a square cross-section as shown

212

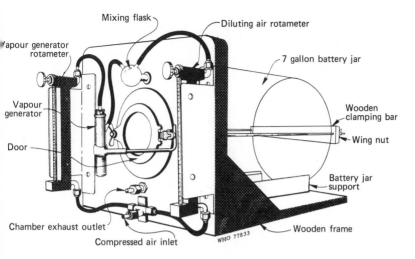

Fig. 6.2   Schematic diagram of inhalation chamber using a 7-gal (26.5 litres approx.) battery jar (Drew & Laskin, 1973).

schematically in Fig. 6.3 is known as the "NYU Chamber" (New York University Chamber) (Laskin et al., 1970). These two shapes are currently in use in several laboratories, although cubes, cylinders, spheres, modified hemispheres, and even chambers with an elliptical cross-section have all been used (Drew & Laskin, 1973). The two major considerations that influence the shape of the chamber are uniformity of distribution and wall loss of the test substance (MacFarland, 1976) with secondary importance placed on caging supports, accessibility, and costs.

A typical chamber is shown schematically in Fig. 6.3. The unit has a volume of 1.3 m³ and is about 3 m in height. The body is made of stainless steel and the windows can be made of either glass or lucite. Clean air is supplied at the top with the pollutant being injected in a perpendicular direction to the incoming airstream. Chambers with tangential pollutant introduction are also common. Airflow is usually down through the chamber and the air is removed through the side arm of a Y fitting at the bottom. Animal wastes are removed at the bottom via the building drains, usually through a trap or a valve. The trap also maintains the integrity of the system and allows operation at a pressure slightly (1–2 cm H_2O) below ambient. Chambers of this general shape have been built with volumes ranging from 128 litres up to 5 m³, although MacFarland (1976) suggests that the pollutant concentration in chambers of less than 1 m³ may not be uniform.

The size of the chamber depends on the number and size of the animals to

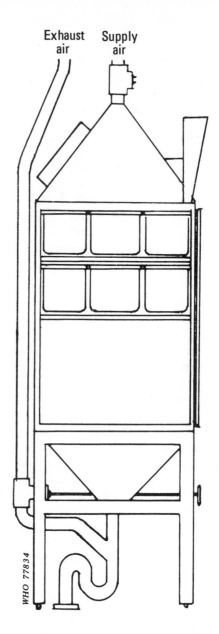

Fig. 6.3   Schematic diagram of the New York University (NYU) chamber (Drew & Laskin, 1973).

be exposed. The total animal volume should not exceed approximately 5% of the total chamber volume. Experience has shown that above 5% surface losses begin to cause excessive concentration losses and thermal considerations also begin to play a limiting role.

6.7.5 Construction materials

Inhalation chambers should be constructed of materials that do not react with the test material and are easily cleaned. The most versatile materials are stainless steel and glass. However, many other materials have been used, including aluminium, wood, wood coated with epoxy paints, lucite, and various fibre panels. The chamber should have at least two sides made almost completely of transparent material in order to view the animals during exposure. The inside surfaces should be as free as possible from perturbations and rough surfaces and edges, in order to facilitate cleaning. Openings should be included to monitor the variables needed to characterize the exposure (section 6.7.8).

6.7.6 Engineering requirements

Accurate control of airflow in the chambers is essential. The usual procedure is to supply filtered, conditioned air in excess of that required and then tap off the common supply for each chamber. In most experiments, the ratio of chamber volume to airflow ranges from 1 to about 6.

When handling hazardous materials, special safety precautions must be taken to protect operating personnel and the surrounding environment. The chambers are operated at slightly negative pressure to ensure that any leaks draw air into the system. Chamber effluents must be cleaned, usually by filters or scrubbers, or at least diluted, before being released into the environment. Stack effluents should be monitored.

Food and water must be provided in the chambers, when animals are being exposed continuously. Facilities for cleaning the chambers, while the animals are in them, are also necessary, though in many laboratories the animals are removed from the chamber for 45 min–1 h to permit it being serviced. Racks for supporting animal cages must be included and exposure cages should have all six sides made of wire mesh (stainless steel) to ensure good mixing.

6.7.7 Special systems

6.7.7.1 *Isolation units*

When handling particularly hazardous materials, additional precautions are necessary. These can be fairly simple, such as operating a battery jar in

215

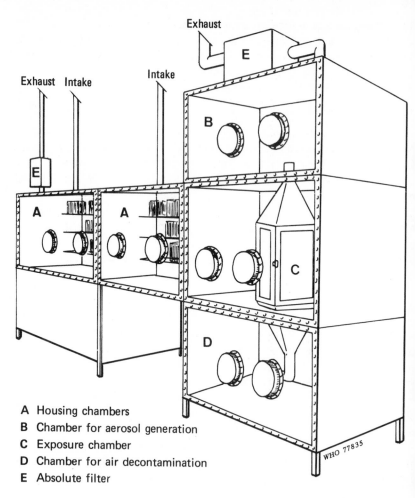

A Housing chambers
B Chamber for aerosol generation
C Exposure chamber
D Chamber for air decontamination
E Absolute filter

Fig. 6.4   Schematic drawing of New York University isolation exposure unit.

a fume hood, or complex, such as the chamber-within-a-chamber concept described by Laskin et al. (1970). In this system (Fig. 6.4) the aerosol is separated by two barriers from the operator with separate glove boxes for generation and removal of the aerosol. In addition, living quarters are provided behind a barrier with pass boxes for food and animal wastes to be moved into and out of the chamber.

6.7.7.2 *Head and nose exposures*

Early in the development of inhalation exposure systems, investigators realized the value of head or nose only exposures (Saito, 1912). Stokinger (1949) described chambers with openings for head-only exposures for several species, and Henderson (1952) described an apparatus consisting of a cylindrical chamber with openings arranged along two sides to enable nose exposure of mice to biological aerosols. Nose exposure systems are used in situations where: (*a*) skin absorption is not desirable; (*b*) the amount of test material is limited; (*c*) the material is hazardous; and (*d*) there is no need for a large chamber. They are most commonly used for acute exposures, since it is difficult to restrain the animals for long periods of time.

Nose exposure systems have been used extensively for two particular situations— exposure to radioactive aerosols and exposure to cigarette smoke. Investigators at the Lovelace Foundation for Medical Education and Research in Albuquerque have developed a series of nose exposure units (Boecker et al., 1964; Raabe et al., 1973; Thomas & Lie, 1963). The technical difficulties of exposing animals to cigarette smoke has prompted

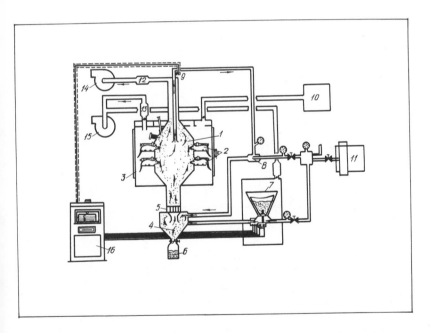

Fig. 6.5   1. Inner exposure chamber. 2. Animal containers. 3. Safety enclosure to prevent dust leakage into the laboratory. 4. Cyclone—for mixing of dust and clean air. 5. Directional grating. 6. Dust collector. 7. Dust reservoir with variable bore venturi tube. 8. Clean air invector for fine adjustment of dust concentration. 9. Sampling port. 10. Air conditioning and humidity control equipment. 11. Air reservoir and compressor. 12, 13. Filters to prevent dust leakage into the laboratory. 14, 15. Blowers. 16. Control panel (Valežnev et al., 1970).

217

the development of several systems designed specifically for this purpose (Hoffman & Wynder, 1970; Stuart et al., 1970). One device has been developed by Homburger et al. (1967) and two have been described by Dontenwill (1970). Albert et al. (1974) have developed a device to expose donkeys to cigarette smoke via nose tubes. Devices for exposing dogs to cigarette smoke have also been described (Cahan & Kirman, 1968).

A nose exposure system for exposure to dusts has been developed at the Institute of Hygiene and Occupational Medicine in Moscow (Valežnev et al., 1970) (Fig. 6.5). It consists of a completely enclosed system in which up to 40 rodents can be exposed simultaneously. A very complex system adaptable to both head-only and whole-body exposures is routinely used at the Medical Institute in Kiev (Balašov et al., 1968). A schematic diagram of this system is shown in Fig. 6.6.

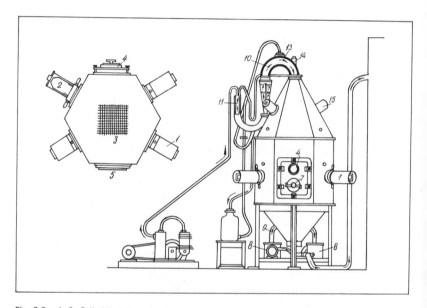

Fig. 6.6   1, 2. Cylindrical domed animal containers. 3. Grating where animals are placed during aerosol exposure. 4. Large door held to chamber with bolts. 5. Viewing window complex. 6. Accessory attachment for camera and telescope. 7. Small access door for placement and removal of animals during experiments. 8, 9. Blowers for changing air, as required. 10, 11, 12, 13, 14. Equipment for introducing samples and producing aerosols. 15. Mixing pans to prevent occurrence of deadspace (Balašov et al., 1968).

6.7.7.3   *Instantaneous exposure systems*

Occasionally, it is necessary to expose animals to a concentration of material, while avoiding the time required to attain uniform concentrations. In this case, the air in the chamber is equilibrated with the test material and the animals rapidly inserted into the chamber. Sometimes double chambers are used for this purpose. The animals are placed in the upper half and the pollutant is introduced into the lower half. When the desired concentration is reached in the lower half, a trap door opens and the animals fall into the lower half, while the mechanism immediately closes. Other investigators have described various drawer arrangements for rapid insertion of animals into test atmospheres.

6.7.8 Variables to monitor

It is necessary to monitor several variables during the operation of an inhalation chamber. The most obvious is the concentration in the chamber of the pollutant in question. This can be done continuously by automated samplers and recorded on a strip chart recorder or manually at periodic intervals using a variety of sampling techniques. When aerosols are involved, particle size should be determined. The flow of pollutant, the flow of air, and the chamber pressure should all be recorded frequently. Chamber temperature and humidity are other variables that should be monitored. It is also useful to measure the pressure drop across intake and exhaust filters in order to know when to replace them.

6.7.9 Human exposure facilities

Ethical principles will always be of first concern, when considering the exposure of human subjects to materials for toxicity evaluation. However, there are situations where controlled exposure of human beings can provide useful information with minimum risk. One of the more modern facilities has been described by Stewart et al. (1970a,b). It consists of a room approximately 6 m × 6 m × 2.7 m, completely air conditioned and operated at slightly negative pressure. Activity within this chamber is strictly sedentary and comfortable chairs and study desks are provided. Meals are served during exposures, with coffee and soft drinks available continuously. All subjects are under continuous surveillance by medical personnel and all activities are visually monitored by closed circuit television. Such facilities are particularly useful for studying psychomotor effects and other sensitive indicators of exposure to low concentrations of organic vapours.

The odour threshold concentrations used in the USSR for establishing maximum permissible concentrations for single exposures are determined in human subjects over short periods (5–10 min). Obviously such studies can only be carried out at very low concentrations considered to be safe. The minimum concentration sensed by the most sensitive individual is accepted as the odour threshold (Rjazanov, 1964).

Reflex reactions produced in man by irritating the receptive zones of the respiratory organs with subsensory concentrations of atmospheric pollutants, were established by measuring the light sensitivity of the eye, the bioelectric activity of the cerebrum, etc. (Buštueva et al., 1960; Rjazanov, 1964). Changes in encephalographic responses resulted from exposure to small concentrations of these substances. The maximum concentration that did not produce an effect on the bioelectric activity of the cerebrum was, in most cases, 3–4 times lower than the odour threshold concentration (Krotov, 1971; Sidorenko & Pinigin, 1972).

6.8 Contaminant Generation and Characterization

Extensive reviews have been published by several investigators on methods of generating and characterizing vapours and particles (Bryan, 1970; Cotabish et al., 1961; Drew & Lippmann, 1971; Lodge, 1968; Mercer, 1973a,b; Nelson, 1971; Raabe, 1970).

6.8.1 Generation of vapours

Vapours can be generated by using one of several flow-dilution devices (Cotabish et al., 1961; Drew & Lippmann, 1971; Nelson, 1971; Saltzman, 1971; Saltzman & Warburg, 1965). If the contaminant is a liquid at room temperature, a vaporization step must be included. One procedure is to use a motor-driven syringe and to apply the liquid to a wick or heated plate in a calibrated stream of air (Nelson & Griggs, 1968). Another method is to saturate the airstream with vapour and then dilute it with air to the desired concentration (Cotabish et al., 1961). A third technique, originally described by O'Keefe & Ortman (1966), consists of using permeation tubes. These are especially useful when using low concentrations of test materials for standardization procedures. In theory, there is no reason why they cannot be scaled up for use in inhalation studies.

6.8.2 Particle generators

The generation of particulate contaminants is usually more difficult than vapour generation. The contaminant may be generated from a dry powder or from a liquid and the particles generated may be of uniform size (monodisperse) or may vary greatly in size (heterogeneous).

6.8.2.1 *Heterogeneous aerosols*

The Wright dust feed (1950) is one of the better known instruments for generating aerosols from a dry powder. A gear drives the surface of a packed cylinder of finely ground powder against a scraping mechanism. A high velocity airstream disperses the powder. Proper use of the Wright dust feed is dependent upon the control of the relative humidity of the airstream and the packing density of the powder. Other devices for producing aerosols from dry powders have been described (Crider et al., 1968; Deichman, 1944; Dimmick, 1959; Stead et al., 1944). Since the particle size of the resultant aerosols depends upon the size of the original powder, elutriators and cyclones are sometimes included to limit the maximum size. Laskin et al. (1971) described generators that include such devices for producing freshly ground polyurethane aerosols.

Agglomeration, usually caused by electrical charge, is a serious problem with dry dust aerosols. The electrical behaviour of aerosols has been reviewed by Whitby & Liu (1966). A mechanical solution to agglomeration has been proposed by Drew & Laskin (1971) who described a fluidizing dust generator.

Wet dispersion generators break liquid into droplets. The liquid may be a solution or a suspension of the test material. In most cases, the liquid is drawn into filaments or films that are broken into droplets. A number of compressed air-driven generators (nebulizers), that produce droplets of many sizes, have been described (Dautrebande, 1962; Laskin, 1948; Lauterbach et al., 1956; Raabe, 1970). The resulting aerosols are polydisperse although relatively narrow size distribution can be attained with some nebulizers.

Monodisperse aerosols are occasionally needed by investigators, especially when studying regional deposition. The most popular device for dispensing uniform droplets is the spinning disc generator first described by Walton & Prewett (1949). Primary droplets thrown off the perimeter of a spinning disc are uniform in size. The liquid is fed on to the centre of the disc and accumulates at the edge until broken off by centrifugal force. Some secondary, smaller droplets are also produced but these can be separated dynamically. Several investigators have successfully used the spinning disc for inhalation studies (Albert et al., 1964; Kajland et al., 1964; Lippmann & Albert, 1967; Philipson, 1973). Another device employing a controlled condensation process originally described by LaMer & Sinclair (1943) has been found to be suitable for inhalation studies. A third principle, consisting of size specific collection, resuspension and subsequent dispersion, has also been used (Kotrappa et al., 1972).

6.8.3 Monitoring contaminant concentrations

The techniques and equipment for monitoring contaminant concentrations have been reviewed by a number of authors (Lippman, 1971;

Powell & Hosey, 1965). In many cases, the characteristics of the contaminant determine the sampling technique. Sometimes a number of techniques are available and the method of choice may depend upon the availability of equipment, cost of reagents, time for analysis, or other factors. Automated instrumentation is currently available for a number of contaminants. However, when using automatic devices, a second method, usually chemical, should be used to verify the instrument performance.

6.8.3.1 *Vapour sampling*

Two basic methods for the collection of gaseous samples are employed. The first involves the use of a gas collector, such as an evacuated flask or bottle, to obtain a definite volume of air at a known temperature and pressure. The second method involves the passage of a known volume of air through a collecting medium to remove the desired contaminants from the sampled atmosphere. The samples are then analysed by appropriate analytical techniques.

Since the assays are related to the volume of air sampled, the instrumentation for monitoring airflow or volume should be accurately calibrated. It is also important that there are no leaks in the sampling train, thus assuring that all the air measured has passed through the collecting medium.

A number of devices, currently available, measure the concentration of vapours continuously; many record the result graphically. Many detection principles are used including conductivity, colorimetry, and spectrophotometry. Recent commercial instrumentation using the principle of infrared spectrometry are especially useful. Most of these instruments have been described by Nader (1971).

6.8.3.2 *Particulate sampling*

When monitoring particulate atmospheres, mass concentration and particle size must be determined. The mass concentration can be measured by techniques similar to those used for monitoring vapours. The material can be collected, then assayed by appropriate chemical methods. Gravimetric analysis can also be performed by weighing the filter paper before and after collecting a sample. The resulting mass can be related to the volume of air that was sampled.

Particle collection techniques include filtration, impingement, thermal and electrostatic precipitation, and sedimentation. The basic principles for these techniques and specific examples of each method have been reviewed (Lippmann, 1971). These principles should be thoroughly understood prior to selection of a method for a specific contaminant.

The techniques for measuring particle size and numbers have been discussed in detail by Mercer (1973a,b). Direct methods consisting of both conventional and electron microscopy can be used. In both cases, proper sampling methods to ensure collection of a representative sample should be followed. Electrostatic and thermal precipitators or an impinger can be used. After using an impinger, the dust can be counted in a standard haematology counting cell or counted directly with a Coulter Counter.

There are two indirect methods of assessing particle size; the use of cascade impactors and the use of light scattering devices. The theory of cascade impaction has been described by Mercer (1963, 1964, 1965). The theory of light scattering devices has been reviewed by Hodkinson (1966) and commercially available instruments have been listed by Swift (1971). Many factors, including shape, opacity, and others, some unknown, affect the amount of light scattered and the measured number and size of the particles. These devices should, therefore, be used cautiously.

6.9   Other Methods of Respiratory Tract Exposure

6.9.1   *In vivo* exposures

In addition to direct inhalation, several other methods of exposing the respiratory tract have been described (Roe, 1968). Andervont (1937) originally described a thread implantation technique whereby a thread impregnated with a test compound was literally passed through a lobe of the lung. This technique was modified by Kuschner et al. (1957) who devised a pellet that could be impregnated with the test material or coated with radio-active materials. This pellet had hooks which held it in the lumen of the bronchus or bronchiole. This technique has been used to demonstrate the carcinogenicity of a number of compounds including benzo(a)pyrene, 3-methylcholanthrene, and calcium chromate (Laskin et al., 1970). A technique whereby hamsters are anaesthetized and then intratracheally intubated with various materials is in use in a number of laboratories (Laskin et al., 1970; Little & O'Toole, 1974; Saffiotti, 1970; Schreiber et al., 1972). In two laboratories, this technique has been coupled with inhalation exposures to study the potential cocarcinogenicity of various agents (Laskin & Nettesheim, 1974, personal communication).

6.9.2   *In vitro* exposures

A few *in vitro* techniques that show promise as regards elucidation of the mechanisms of toxicity of inhaled materials should be mentioned. A number of investigators (Niemeier & Bingham, 1972; O'Neill & Tierney, 1974;

Orton et al., 1973) are using various, isolated, perfused lung preparations to study toxicity. Such preparations could be particularly useful in studying the transfer of materials from the lung to the blood. These preparations are also used to study pulmonary metabolism as are lung tissue slices (O'Neil & Tierney, 1974). Finally, several laboratories are developing methods of culturing tracheal rings and sections (Griesemer et al., 1974; Lane & Miller, 1975). These preparations show great promise for toxicological evaluation (section 2.7.4).

6.10 Biological End-points and Interpretation of Changes in these End-points

Throughout the course of an inhalation study, there are a number of biological indicators to observe. The classical indices of toxicity include weight change and mortality, organ-to-body weight ratios, and both gross and microscopic changes in the morphology of the various tissues and organs. While the study is in progress, respiratory, physiological indices can be monitored and the excretion of certain chemicals in breath, urine, and faeces can also be followed. Some procedures particularly useful in inhalation toxicity studies are discussed below.

6.10.1 Morphological changes

The primary function of the lung is the exchange of oxygen and carbon dioxide between the blood and alveolar air. The walls of the alveoli are lined by a single, flattened layer of epithelial cells that are in close proximity to endothelial cells lining capillaries. The mean distance from the lumen of the capillary to the lumen of the alveolus is less than one micron. Because this distance is so small, any thickening or inflammation of the alveolar wall will severely disrupt the diffusion of gases.

The air in the alveolus arrives through a series of branching bronchi and bronchioles the specialized epithelial lining of which is instrumental in removing particulate matter from the lung. Any lesions that result in narrowing of the lumen of these bronchi and bronchioles cause a disruption in the ventilation of that portion of the lung. Chemicals affecting the specialized ciliated epithelial lining, the bronchioles, and the bronchi may interrupt the clearance mechanism, resulting in a build-up of inhaled particulates in the lung.

The type of morphological change observed in the lung as a result of the inhalation of materials depends upon the concentration of the inhaled material and the length of time for which animals are exposed. Short-term inhalation of high concentrations of certain materials may result in acute changes in the lung such as oedema, necrosis, and purulent inflammation. However, the inhalation of the same material at lower concentrations for longer periods of time may result in chronic changes such as fibrosis and even neoplasia. Table 6.3 lists a number of chemicals and the response elicited in the lung following their inhalation.

Table 6.3 Responses of the lung to various chemicals

Chemical	Bronchiolar epithelial hyperplasia	Loss of goblet cells	Oedema	Epithelial metaplasia	Fibrosis	Emphysema	Granuloma	Necrosis	Neoplasia	Bronchial constriction	Alveolar epithelial hyperplasia	Nonsuppurative alveolitis
nitrogen dioxide	×		×	×	×	×		×				
ozone	×	×	×	×	×							
allergens							×					×
sulfuric acid	×			×				×			×	
bis-chloromethyl ether									×			
silica					×		×					
coal dust					×	×						
beryllium	×			×			×		×			
cotton dust										×		
nickel compounds									×			

Techniques for quantifying morphological changes are, at best, limited. The usual practice is to assign some number to the degree of damage and then to apply statistical procedures to these numbers. These procedures are, however, subject to individual interpretation. Assessment of the degree of fibrosis is possible (Roe, 1968), although such measurements should be checked by special staining procedures.

Interpretation of any morphological changes in the lung must take into consideration the concentration and duration of exposure. Exposure to certain materials will elicit immediate acute morphological changes which, with time, tend to resolve and disappear. This phenomenon suggests that the animal is able to adapt to the effects of some chemicals, if the concentration is not too high. An example of this adaptive phenomenon is seen with ozone. Nonlethal exposures to ozone have a protective effect against subsequent lethal exposures which would result in marked pulmonary oedema (Alpert & Lewis, 1971).

6.10.2 Functional changes

There are certain advantages in using alterations in respiratory functions as indices of toxicity: (a) quantitative measurements can usually be made at concentrations far below those needed to produce morphological effects; (b) many effects may be measured at the level of reversible rather than irreversible changes; (c) such measurements may elucidate mechanisms of action of materials, and (d) in many instances similar data can be obtained from experimental animals and man.

6.10.2.1 *Measurement of respiratory frequency*

Alteration of respiratory frequency in mice may be used as a simple screening test for assessing irritant potency (Alarie, 1973). The changes produced are dose-related, which permits construction of dose-effect curves and calculation of the concentration required to produce, for example, a 50% decrease in respiratory frequency. Some irritants, mainly those affecting the upper respiratory tract, decrease frequency. Other irritants, mainly those which penetrate to the deeper areas of the lung, increase frequency. Measurement of respiratory frequency alone is a very sensitive measure of effect for those irritants that increase frequency (e.g. ozone and nitrogen dioxide), but it is a relatively insensitive measure of effect for those irritants that decrease frequency (e.g. sulfur dioxide and formaldehyde).

6.10.2.2 *Measurement of mechanics of respiration*

Alterations in pulmonary flow resistance or pulmonary compliance may be used to assess irritant potency. The method of Amdur & Mead (1958) required three basic measurements: intrapleural pressure, tidal volume, and the rate of flow of gas in and out of the respiratory tract. Intrapleural pressure is estimated by placing a fluid-filled catheter in the pleural space, while the animal is under anaesthesia. Once the catheter is positioned, no further anaesthesia is necessary. Tidal volume is obtained by placing the animal in a body plethysmograph and measuring the pressure changes as the animal breathes quietly. Rate of gas flow is obtained by electrical differentiation of the volume signal. This method provides data on both resistance and compliance, but is generally limited to single exposure studies of a few hours duration. The guineapig has been the species most commonly used for this method; however, plethysmographic studies have been successfully carried out on several other rodents including mice (Alarie, 1973), rats (Palacek, 1969) and rabbits (Davidson et al., 1966).

The method of Murphy & Ulrich (1964) does not involve surgical intervention and, thus, makes it possible to perform measurements repeatedly on the same animals. The animal is placed in a body plethysmograph to which an oscillating sine wave pressure is applied. The animal's face is fitted with a mask containing a pneumotachograph screen for measuring flow. Changes in resistance are calculated for the alterations in flow produced by the superimposed pressure oscillations. This technique has been used in toxicological studies without making compliance measurements. However, by measuring oesophageal pressure reflecting intrapleural pressure, it should be possible to estimate compliance changes. A compliance measurement is described by Mead (1960) that involves no surgical intervention.

The observed changes in respiratory mechanics are dose-related and permit the construction of dose-effect curves. These may be used to compare irritant potency or to study such things as the effect of inert particles on the reaction to irritant gases. The deep lung irritants that increase respiratory frequency tend to show a decrease in compliance as the primary alteration in the mechanical behaviour of the lung. Resistance changes with such irritants are minimal. The irritants that slow respiratory frequency tend to show an increase in resistance accompanied by a smaller decrease in compliance, as the primary alteration in pulmonary mechanics.

An increase in pulmonary flow resistance can result from a narrowing of the lumen of the bronchi mediated by constriction of the smooth muscle. The effect, in this situation, usually occurs rapidly on exposure to the irritant. In the case of a gaseous irritant, the effect is fairly rapidly reversed when irritant exposure ceases. In the case of a particulate irritant which remains in the lung, the effect is less readily reversible. Swelling of the respiratory mucosa or an increase in mucus secretion can also cause an increase in flow resistance. The effect, in this situation, usually takes some time to develop.

Much of the damage to the lung is to the small airways which change either in calibre or stability or both. It would be very useful if this damage could be detected early during an exposure before more serious disease develops. There are three tests which are promising and have been useful in human subjects. They are the maximal expiratory flow volume curve, reviewed by Hyatt & Black (1973), the alveolar closing volume (Dollfuss et al., 1967) and the frequency dependency of compliance (Woolcock et al., 1969). Animal models that provide the same data have not yet been fully developed.

6.10.3 Biochemical end-points

In the last decade, much research has centred around the elucidation of some of the biochemical aspects of the lung. It has only recently been demonstrated that the lung is capable of biotransforming many foreign chemicals and several authors have investigated the role of cytochrome P-450-dependent enzyme systems in pulmonary microsomes (Bend et al., 1972; Chhabra & Fouts, 1974; Chhabra et al., 1974; Fouts & Devereux, 1972; Harper et al., 1975; Hook et al., 1972). The importance of intermediary metabolism is now being considered (Tierney, 1974). The biochemistry of pulmonary surfactants and their role in pulmonary defence mechanisms has been reviewed by King (1974). Investigations of the lung collagen have recently been reviewed by Crystal (1974). Witschi (1975) has provided an excellent summary of biochemical approaches for the evaluation of pulmonary toxicity.

6.10.4 Other end-points in inhalation studies

Exposure by inhalation is only a means by which the substance enters the animal. This chapter has concentrated on the lung as the critical organ. However, there are end-points that are not necessarily related to the lung. Inhalation studies have recently been reported to assess the teratological effects of inhaled materials (Schwetz et al., 1975). They have also been used in behavioural studies (Weiss & Laties, 1975; Xintaras et al., 1974).

REFERENCES

ALARIE, Y. (1973) Sensory irritation of the upper airways by airborne chemicals. *Toxicol. appl. Pharmacol.*, **24:** 279–297.

ALBERT, R. E., PETROW, H. G., SALAM, A. S., & SPIEGELMAN, J. R. (1964) Fabrication of monodisperse lucite and iron oxide particles with a spinning disc generator. *Health Phys.*, **10:** 933–940.

ALBERT, R. E., LIPPMANN, M., & BRISCOE, W. (1969) The characteristics of bronchial clearance and the effects of cigarette smoking. *Arch. environ. Health*, **18:** 738–755.

ALBERT, R. E., LIPPMANN, M., PETERSON, H. T., JR, BERGER, J., SANBORN, K., & BORWAG, D. (1973) Bronchial deposition and clearance of aerosols. *Arch. intern. Med.*, **131:** 115–131.

ALBERT, R. E., BERGER, J., SANBORN, K., & LIPPMANN, M. (1974) Effects of cigarette smoke components on bronchial clearance in the donkey. *Arch. environ. Health*, **29:** 96–101.

ALPERT, S. M. & LEWIS, T. R. (1971) Ozone tolerance studies utilizing unilateral lung exposure. *J. appl. Physiol.*, **192:** 364–368.

AMDUR, M. O. & MEAD, J. (1958) Mechanics of respiration in unanaesthetized guinea pigs. *Am. J. Physiol.*, **192:** 364–368.

ANDERSEN, I., LUNDQVIST, G. R., JENSON, P. L., & PROCTOR, D. F. (1974) Human response to controlled levels of sulfur dioxide. *Arch. environ. Health*, **28:** 21–39.

ANDERVONT, H. B. (1937) Pulmonary tumours in mice: IV. Lung tumours induced by sub-cutaneous injection of 1,2,5,6-dibenzanthracene in different media and by its direct contact with lung tissue. *Public Health Rep.*, **52:** 1584.

BALAŠOV, V. E., BARTENEV, V. D., SAVICKIJ, I. V., & TRAHTENBERG, I. M. (1968) [Toxicological assessment of volatile substances leaking from synthetic materials.] *Zdorov'e, Kiev* (in Russian).

BEND, J. R., HOOK, G. E. R., EASTERLING, R. E., GRAM, T. E., & FOUTS, J. R. (1972) A comparative study of the hepatic and pulmonary microsomal mixed function oxidase systems in the rabbit. *J. Pharmacol. exp. Ther.*, **183:** 206–217.

BOECKER, B. B., AQUILAR, F. L., & MERCER, T. T. (1964) The design of a canine inhalation exposure apparatus incorporating a whole-body plethysmograph. *Health Phys.*, **10:** 1077–1089.

BOYD, M. R., BURKA, L. T., HARRIS, T. M., & WILSON, B. J. (1974) Lung-toxic furanoterpenoids produced by sweet potatoes (*Ipomoea batatas*) following microbial infection. *Biochim. Biophys. Acta*, **337:** 184–195.

BRAIN, J. D. & VALBERG, P. A. (1974) Models of lung retention based on International Congress of Radiation Protection Task Group Report. *Arch. environ. Health*, **28:** 1–11.

BRYAN, R. J. (1970) Generation and monitoring of gases for inhalation studies. In: Hanna, M. G. Jr, Nettesheim, P., & Gilbert, J. R., ed. *Inhalation carcinogenesis.* Springfield VA, Clearinghouse for Federal Scientific and Technical Information, NBS, US Dept of Commerce (CONF-691001).

BUŠTUEVA, K. A., POLEZAEV, E. F., & SOMENENKO, A. D. (1960) [A study of threshold values for reflex action of atmospheric pollutants.] *Gig. i Sanit.*, No. 1, pp. 57–61 (in Russian).

CADLE, R. D. (1965) *Particle size.* Princeton, NJ, Van Nostrand-Reinhold.

CAHAN, W. G. & KIRMAN, D. (1968) An effective system and procedure for cigarette smoking by dogs. *J. surg. Res.*, **8:** 567–575.

CAMNER, P., PHILIPSON, K., & FRIBERG, L. (1972) Tracheobronchial clearance in twins. *Arch. environ. Health*, **24:** 82–87.

CAMNER, P., MOSSBERG, B., & PHILIPSON, K. (1973) Tracheobronchial clearance and chronic obstructuve lung disease. *Scand. J. respir. Dis.*, **54:** 272–281.

229

CAMNER, P., HELLSTRÖM, P. A., LUNDBERG, M., & PHILIPSON, K. (1977) Lung clearance of 4 µm particles coated with silver, carbon and beryllium. *Arch. environ. Health*, **32**: 58–62.

CARPENTER, C. P., SMYTH, H. F., JR, & POZZANI, U. C. (1949) The assay of acute vapour toxicity and the grading and interpretation of results on 96 chemical compounds. *J. ind. Hyg. Toxicol.*, **31**: 343–346.

CASARETT, L. J. (1972) The vital sacs: alveolar clearance mechanisms in inhalation toxicology. In: Hayes, W. J., ed. *Essays in toxicology.* New York, London, Academic Press.

CHHABRA, R. S. & FOUTS, J. R. (1974) Sex differences in the metabolism of xenobiotics by extrahepatic tissue in rats. *Drug Metab. Disposition*, **2**: 375–379.

CHHABRA, R. S., POHL, R. J., & FOUTS, J. R. (1974) A comparative study of xenobiotic-metabolizing enzymes in liver and intestine of various animal species. *Drug Metab. Disposition*, **2**: 443–447.

COTABISH, H. N., McCONNAUGHEY, P. W., & MESSER, H. C. (1961) Making known concentrations for instrument calibration. *Am. Ind. Hyg. Assoc. J.*, **22**: 392–402.

CRIDER, W. L., BARKELEY, N. P., & STRONG, A. A. (1968) Dry-powder aerosol dispensing device with long-time output stability. *Rev. Sci. Instrum.*, **39**: 152–155.

CRYSTAL, R. G. (1974) Lung collagen: definition, diversity and development. *Fed. Proc.*, **33**: 2248–2255.

DAUTREBANDE, L. (1952) *Microaerosols.* New York, Academic Press, pp. 7–22.

DAVIDSON, J. T., WASSERMAN, K., LILLINGTON, G. A., & SCHMIDT, R. W. (1966) Pulmonary function testing in the rabbit. *J. appl. Physiol.*, **21**: 1094–1098.

DEICHMANN, W. B. (1944) An apparatus designed for the production of controlled dust concentrations in the air breathed by experimental animals. *J. ind. Hyg. Toxicol.*, **26**: 334–335.

DIMMICK, R. L. (1959) Jet disperser for compacted powders in the one-to-ten micron range. *Am. Med. Assoc. Arch. ind. Health*, **20**: 8–14.

DOLLFUSS, R. E., MILIC-EMILI, J., & BATES, D. V. (1967) Regional ventilation of the lung studied with boluses of 133 xenon. *Respir. Phys.*, **2**: 234–246.

DONTENWILL, W. (1970) Experimental investigations on the effect of cigarette smoke inhalation on small laboratory animals. In: Hanna, M. G. Jr, Nettesheim, P., & Gilbert, J. R., ed. *Inhalation carcinogenesis.* Springfield VA, Clearinghouse for Federal Scientific and Technical Information, NBS, US Dept of Commerce.

DRAIZE, J. H., NELSON, A. A., NEWBURGER, S. N., & KELLEY, E. A. (1959) Inhalation toxicity studies of six types of aerosol hair sprays. *Proc. Sci. Sec. Toilet Goods Assoc.*, **31**: 28–32.

DREW, J. H. & LASKIN, S. (1971) A new dust-generating system for inhalation studies. *Am. Ind. Hyg. Assoc. J.*, **32**: 327–330.

DREW, R. T. & LASKIN, S. (1973) Environmental inhalation chambers. In: Day, W. I., ed. *Methods of animal experimentation.* New York, Academic Press.

DREW, R. T. & LIPPMANN, M. (1971) Calibration of air sampling instruments: II. Production of test atmospheres for instrument calibraton. In: Lippmann, M., ed. *Air sampling instruments*, 4th ed., Cincinnati, OH, ACGIH, pp. I-1.

DREW, R. T. & TAYLOR, G. J. (1975) Cardiophysical studies with stressed animals. In: *Proceedings of the 5th Annual Conference on Environmental Toxicology, Dayton, Ohio, 1974*, US Govt Printing Office, pp. 121–129.

FOUTS, J. R. & DEVEREUX, T. R. (1972) Developmental aspects of hepatic and extrahepatic drug-metabolizing enzyme systems: microsomal enzymes and components in rabbit liver and lung during the first month of life. *J. Pharmacol. exp. Ther.*, **183**: 458–468.

FRASER, D. A., BALES, R. E., LIPPMANN, M., & STOKINGER, H. E. (1959) *Exposure chambers for research in animal inhalation.* USPHS (Public Health Monograph 57).

GOLDBERG, I. S. & LAURENCO, R. V. (1973) Deposition of aerosols in pulmonary disease. *Arch. intern. Med.*, **131**: 88–92.

GRIESEMER, R. A., KENDRICK, J., & NETTESHEIM, P. (1974) Tracheal grafts. In: *Proceedings on Experimental Respiratory Carcinogenesis, Seattle 1974*, Springer-Verlag, pp. 537–547.

GROSS, P., PFITZER, E. A., TOLKER, E., BABYAK, M. A., & KASCHAK, M. (1965) Experimental emphysema: its production with papain in normal and silicotic rats. *Arch. environ. Health*, **11**: 50–58.

HABER, F. (1924) [*Five lectures for the years 1920–1923.*] Berlin, Springer-Verlag (in German).

HARPER, C., DREW, R. T., & FOUTS, J. R. (1975) Species differences in benzene hydroxylation to phenol by pulmonary and hepatic microsomes. *Drug Metab. Disposition*, **3**: 381–388.

HAUN, C. C. (1972) Continuous animal exposure to methylene chloride. In: *Proceedings of the 2nd Annual Conference on Environmental Toxicology, Dayton, Ohio, 1971*, US Govt Printing Office, pp. 309–326.

HAZUCHA, M., SILVERMAN, F., PARENT, C., FIELD, S., & BATES, D. V. (1973) Pulmonary function in man after short-term exposure to ozone. *Arch. environ. Health*, **27**: 183–188.

HENDERSON, D. W. (1952) Apparatus for study of airborne infection. *J. Hyg. (Lond.)*, **50**: 53–68.

HINNERS, R. G., BURKART, J. K., & CONTNER, G. L. (1966) Animal exposure chambers in air pollution studies. *Arch. environ. Health*, **13**: 609–615.

HINNERS, R. G., BORKART, J. K., & PUNTE, C. L. (1968) Animal inhalation exposure chambers. *Arch. environ. Health*, **16**: 194–206.

HODKINSON, J. R. (1966) The optical measurements of aerosols. In: Davies, C. N., ed. *Aerosol science*, New York, Academic Press, pp. 287–357.

HOFFMANN, D. & WYNDER, E. L. (1970) Chamber development and aerosol dispersion. In: Hanna, M. G. Jr, Nettesheim, P., & Gilbert, J. R., ed. *Inhalation carcinogenesis*. Springfield, VA. Clearinghouse for Federal Scientific and Technical Information, NBS, US Dept of Commerce (CONF-691001).

HOMBURGER, F., BERNFELD, P., BOGDONOFF, P., KELLEY, T., & WALTON, R. (1967) Inhalation by small animals of fresh cigarette smoke generated by new smoking machine. *Toxicol. appl. Pharmacol.*, **10**: 382.

HOOK, G. E. R., BEND, J. R., HOEL, D., FOUTS, J. R., & GRAM, T. E. (1972) Preparation of lung microsomes and a comparison of the distribution of enzymes between subcellular fractions of rabbit lung and liver. *J. Pharmacol. exp. Ther.*, **182**: 474–490.

HYATT, R. E. & BLACK, L. F. (1973) The flow-volume curve: a current perspective. *Am. Rev. Respir. Dis.*, **107**: 191–199.

JEMSKI, J. V. & PHILLIPS, G. B. (1965) Aerosol challenge of animals. In: Gay, W. I., ed. *Methods of animal experimentation*, New York, Academic Press, Vol. 1, pp. 273–341.

KAJLAND, A., EDFORS, M., FRIBERG, L., & HOLMA, B. (1964) Radioactive monodisperse test aerosols and lung clearance studies. *Health Phys.*, **10**: 941–945.

KING, R. J. (1974) The surfactant system of the lung. *Fed. Proc.*, **33**: 2238–2247.

KLJAČKINA, A. M. (1973) In: *Toxicology of new industrial chemical*, Moscow, Medicina, Vol. 13, p. 23.

KOTRAPPA, P., BOYD, H. A., & WILKINSON, C. J. (1972) Technology for the production of monodisperse aerosols of oxides of transuranic elements for inhalation experiments. *Health Phys.*, **22**: 837–843.

KROTOY, YU. A. (1971) [Setting of approximate maximum permissible concentrations of atmospheric pollutants by calculation.] *Gig. i Sanit.*, **12**: 8–12 (in Russian).

KUSCHNER, M., LASKIN, S., CHRISTOFANO, E., & NELSON, N. (1957) Experimental carcinoma of the lung. In: *Proceedings of the 3rd National Cancer Conference*, Philadelphia, Lippincott, pp. 485–495.

KUSCHNER, M., LASKIN, S., DREW, R. T., CAPIELLO, V., & NELSON, N. (1975) Inhalation carcinogenicity of alpha haloethers: III. Lifetime and limited period inhalation studies with bis(chloromethyl) ether et 0.1 ppm. *Arch. environ. Health*, **30**: 73–77.

231

LaMer, V. K. & Sinclair, D. (1943) *An improved homogeneous aerosol generator.* Washington DC, US Dept of Commerce (OSRD Report No. 1668).

Lane, B. P. & Miller, S. L. (1975) Dose dependence of carcinogen-induced changes in tracheal epithelium in organ culture. In: *Proceedings of the Symposium on Experimental Respiratory Carcinogenesis, Seattle, 1974,* Springer-Verlag, pp. 507–513.

Laskin, S. (1948) *AEC Project Quarterly Report UR-38.* Rochester, NY, University of Rochester.

Laskin, S., Kuschner, M., & Drew, R. T. (1970) Studies in pulmonary carcinogenesis. In: Hanna, M. G. Jr, Nettesheim, P., & Gilbert, J. R., ed. *Inhalation carcinogenesis.* Springfield VA, Clearinghouse for Federal Scientific and Technical Information, NBS, US Dept of Commerce (CONF-691001).

Laskin, S., Drew, R. T., Capiello, V. P., & Kuschner, M. (1971) Inhalation studies with freshly generated polyurethane foam dust. In: Mercer, T. T., Morrow, P. E., & Storer, W., ed. *Assessment of airborne particles,* Springfield, IL, Thomas, pp. 382–404.

Lauterbach, K. E., Hayes, D., & Coelho, M. A. (1956) An improved aerosol generator. *Am. Med. Assoc. Arch. ind. Health,* **13:** 156–160.

Leong, B. J. K., Kociba, R. J., Jersey, G. C., & Gehring, P. J. (1975) Effects from repeated inhalation of parts per billion of bis(chloromethyl) ether in rats. *Toxicol. appl. Pharmacol.,* **33:** 175.

Lewis, T. R., Moorman, W. J., Yang, Y., & Stara, J. F. (1974) Long-term exposure to auto exhaust and other pollutant mixtures. *Arch. environ. Health,* **29:** 102–106.

Lippmann, M. & Albert, R. E. (1967) A compact electric motor-driven spinning disc aerosol generator. *Am. Ind. Hyg. Assoc. J.,* **28:** 501–506.

Lippmann, M., ed. (1971) *Air sampling instruments,* 4th ed. Cincinnati, OH, ACGIH.

Little, J. B. & O'Toole, W. F. (1974) Respiratory trace tumours in hamsters induced by benzo(a)pyrene and polonium[210] alpha radiation. *Cancer Res.,* **34:** 3026–3039.

Lodge, J. P. (1968) Production of controlled test atmospheres. In: Stern, A. C., ed. *Air pollution,* 2nd ed., New York, Academic Press, Vol. II, pp. 465.

MacFarland, H. N. (1968) Exposure chambers—design and operation. In: *Proceedings of the 7th Annual Technical Meeting of the American Association of Contamination Control, Chicago, 1968,* pp. 19–25.

MacFarland, H. N. (1976) Respiratory toxicology. In: Hayes, W. J. Jr, ed. *Essays in toxicology,* New York, San Francisco, London, Academic Press, Vol. 7, pp. 121–154.

Macklem, P. T., Hogg, W. E., & Bruton, J. (1973) Peripheral airway obstruction and particulate deposition in the lung. *Arch. intern. Med.,* **131:** 93–100.

Martorana, P. A., McKeel, N. W., Richard, J. W., & Share, N. N. (1973) Function-structure correlation studies on excised hamster lungs in papain-induced emphysema. *Can. J. Physiol. Pharmacol.,* **51:** 635–641.

McLaughlin, R. F., Tyler, W. S., & Canada, R. O. (1961a) Subgross pulmonary anatomy in various mammals and man. *J. Am. Med. Assoc.* **175:** 694–697.

McLaughlin, R. F., Tyler, W. S., & Canada, R. O. (1961b) Study of the subgross pulmonary anatomy of various mammals. *Am. J. Anat.,* **108:** 149–164.

McLaughlin, F. R., Tyler, W. S., & Canada, R. O. (1966) Subgross pulmonary anatomy of the rabbit, rat and guinea pig with additional notes on the human lung. *Am. Rev. Respir. Dis.,* **94:** 380–387.

Mead, J. (1960) Control of respiratory frequency. *J. appl. Physiol.,* **15:** 325–360.

Mercer, T. T. (1963) On the calibration of cascade impactors. *Ann. occup. Hyg.,* **6:** 1–14.

Mercer, T. T. (1964) The stage constants of cascade impactors. *Ann. occup. Hyg.,* **7:** 115–125.

Mercer, T. T. (1965) The interpretation of cascade impactor data. *Am. Ind. Hyg. Assoc. J.,* **26:** 236–241.

Mercer, T. T. (1973a) Production and characterization of aerosols. *Arch. intern. Med.,* **131:** 39–50.

MERCER, T. T. (1973b) *Aerosol technology in hazard evaluation.* New York, London, Academic Press.

MORROW, P. E. (1970) Models for the study of particulate retention and elimination in the lung. In: Hanna, M. G., Nettesheim, P. & Gilbert, J. R., ed. *Inhalation carcinogenesis.* Springfield VA, Clearinghouse for Federal Scientific and Technical Information, NBS, US Dept of Commerce (CONF-691001).

MORROW, P. E. (1973) Alveolar clearance of aerosols. *Arch. intern. Med.,* **131:** 101–108.

MORROW, P. E., HODGE, H. C., NEWMAN, W. F., MAYNARD, E. A., BLANCHET, H. J. JR, FASSET, D. W., BIRK, R. E., & MAVRODT, S. (1966) Deposition and retention models for internal dosimetry of the human respiratory tract. *Health Phys.,* **12:** 173–207.

MURPHY, S. D. & ULRICH, G. E. (1964) Multi-animal test system for measuring effects of irritant gases and vapours on respiratory function of guinea pig. *Am. Ind. Hyg. Assoc. J.,* **25:** 28–36.

NADER, J. S. (1971) Direct-reading instruments for analysing airborne gases and vapours. In: Lippmann, M., ed. *Air sampling instruments,* 4th ed., Cincinnati, ACGIH, p. J-1.

NELSON, G. O. (1971) *Controlled test atmospheres: principles and techniques.* Ann Arbor, MI, Ann Arbor Sci. Publ.

NELSON, G. O. & GRIGGS, K. E. (1968) Precision dynamic method for producing known concentrations of gas and solvent vapour in air. *Rev. Sci. Instrum.,* **39:** 927–928.

NIEMEIER, R. W. & BINGHAM, E. (1972) An isolated perfused lung preparation for metabolic studies. *Life Sci.,* **11**(II): 807–820.

NIEWOEHNER, D. R. & KLEINERMAN, J. (1973) Effects of experimental emphysema and bronchiolitis on lung mechanics and morphometry. *J. appl. Physiol.,* **35:** 25–31.

O'KEEFE, A. E. & ORTMAN, G. O. (1966) Primary standards for trace gas analysis. *Anal. Chem.,* **38:** 760–763.

O'NEIL, J. J. & TIERNEY, D. G. (1974) Rat lung metabolism: glucose utilization by isolated perfused lungs and tissue slices. *Am. J. Physiol.,* **226:** 867–873.

ORTON, T. C., ANDERSON, M. W., PICKETT, R. D., ELING, T. E., & FOUTS, J. R. (1973) Xenobiotic accumulation and metabolism by isolated perfused rabbit lungs. *J. Pharmacol. exp. Ther.,* **186:** 482–497.

PALACEK, F. (1969) Measurement of ventilatory mechanics in the rat. *J. appl. Physiol.,* **27:** 149–156.

PHILIPSON, K. (1973) On the production of monodisperse particles with a spinning disc. *Aerosol Sci.,* **4:** 51–57.

POWELL, C. H. & HOSEY, A. D. (1965) *The industrial environment, its evaluation and control* (US PHS Publ. 614).

POZZANI, U. C., WEIL, C. S., & CARPENTER, C. P. (1959) The toxicological basis of threshold limit values: 5. The experimental inhalation of vapour mixtures by rats with notes upon the relationship between single-dose oral data. *Am. Ind. Hyg. Assoc. J.,* **20:** 364–369.

RAABE, O. G. (1970) Generation and characterization of aerosols. In: Hanna, M. G. Jr, Nettesheim, P., & Gilbert, J. R., ed. *Inhalation carcinogenesis.* Clearinghouse for Federal Scientific and Technical Information, NBS, Springfield VA, US Dept of Commerce (CONF-691001).

RAABE, O. G., BENNICK, J. E., LIGHT, M. E., HOBBS, C. N., THOMAS, R. L., & TILLERY, M. T. (1973) An improved apparatus for acute inhalation exposure of rodents to radio-active aerosols. *Toxicol. appl. Pharmacol.,* **26:** 264–273.

RJAZANOV, V. A. (1964) Criteria and methods for establishing maximum permissible concentrations of atmospheric pollutants in the USSR. In: *Maximum permissible concentrations of atmospheric pollutants,* Moscow, Medicina, Vol. 8, pp. 5–21.

ROE, F. J. C. (1968) Inhalation tests. In: Boyland, E. & Goulding, R., ed. *Modern trends in toxicology,* London, Butterworth, Vol. 1.

SAFFIOTTI, U. (1970) Experimental respiratory tract carcinogenesis and its relation to inhalation exposures. In: Hanna, M. G. Jr, Nettesheim, P., & Gilbert, J. R., ed. *Inhalation carcinogenesis.* Springfield, VA, Clearinghouse for Federal Scientific and Technical Information, NBS, US Sept of Commerce (CONF-691001).

SAITO, Y. (1912) [Experimental investigations on the quantitative absorption of dust by animals at accurately known concentrations of dust in air.] *Arch. Hyg.*, **75:** 134–151 (in German).

SALTZMAN, B. E. (1971) Permeation tubes as calibrated sources of gas. In: *Proceedings of 1st Annual Conference on Environmental Toxicology, Dayton, Ohio, 1970*, US Govt Printing Office, pp. 309–326.

SALTZMAN, B. E. & WARBURG, A. F. (1965) Precision flow dilution system for standard low concentrations of nitrogen dioxide. *Anal. Chem.*, **37:** 1261–1264.

SANCHIS, J., DOLOVICH, M., CHALMERS, R., & NEWHOUSE, M. (1972) Quantification of regional aerosol clearance in the normal human lung. *J. appl. Physiol.*, **33:** 757–762.

SANOCKIJ, I. V., ed. (1970a) [*Methods for determining toxicity and hazards of chemicals.*] Moscow, Medicina, pp. 62–63 (in Russian).

SANOCKIJ, I. V. (1970b) [Complete toxicometry.] In: [*Methods for determining the toxicity and hazards of chemicals.*] Moscow, Medicina, pp. 50–54 (in Russian).

SCHREIBER, H., NETTESHEIM, P., & MARTIN, D. H. (1972) Rapid development of bronchiolo-alveolar squamous cell tumours in rats after intratracheal injection of 3-methylcholanthrene. *J. Natl Cancer Inst.*, **49:** 541–554.

SCHWETZ, B. A., LEONG, B. J. K., & GEHRING, P. J. (1975) The effect of maternally inhaled trichloroethylene, perchloroethylene, methyl chloroform and methylene chloride on embryonal and fetal development in mice and rats. *Toxicol. appl. Pharmacol.*, **32:** 84–96.

SIDORENKO, G. I. & PINIGIN, M. A. (1970) Rapid determination of maximum permissible concentrations of atmospheric pollutants. *Gig. i Sanit.*, No. 3, pp. 93–96.

SILVER, M. J., HOCH, W., KOCSIS, J. J., INGERMAN, C. M., & SMITH, J. B. (1973) Arachadonic acid causes sudden death in rabbits. *Science*, **183:** 1085–1086.

SILVER, S. D. (1946) Constant flow gassing chambers: principles influencing design and operations. *J. lab. clin. Med.*, **31:** 1153–1161.

SNIDER, G. L., HAYES, J. A., FRANZBLAU, C., KAGEN, H. M., STONE, P. S., & KORTHY, A. L. (1974) Relationship between elastolytic activity and experimental emphysema-inducing properties of papain preparations. *Am. Rev. Respir. Dis.*, **10:** 254–262.

STEAD, F. M., DERNEHL, C. U. & NAU, C. A. (1944) A dust feed apparatus useful for exposure of small animals to small and fixed concentrations of dust. *J. ind. Hyg. Toxicol.*, **26:** 90–93.

STEWART, R. D. (1972) Use of human volunteers for the toxicological evaluation of materials. In: *Symposium on an Appraisal of Halogenated Fire Extinguishing Agents.* Washington DC, National Academy of Sciences.

STEWART, R. D., DODD, H. C., GAY, H. H., & ERLEY, D. S. (1970a) Experimental human exposure to trichloroethylene. *Arch. environ. Health*, **20:** 64–71.

STEWART, R. D., PETERSON, J. E., BARETTA, E. D., BACHARD, R. T., HOSCO, M. T., & HERRMANN, A. A. (1970b) Experimental human exposure to carbon monoxide. *Arch. environ. Health*, **21:** 154–164.

STEWART, R. D., PETERSON, J. E., FISHER, T. N., HOSKO, M. J., BARETTA, E. D., DODD, H. C., & HERRMANN, A. A. (1973) Experimental human exposure to high concentrations of carbon monoxide. *Arch. environ. Health*, **26:** 1–7.

STOKINGER, H. E. (1949) Toxicity following inhalation. In Voegtlin, C. & Hodge, C., ed. *Pharmacology and toxicology of uranium compounds*, 1st ed., New York, McGraw-Hill, Vol. III.

STUART, B. O. (1974) Deposition of inhaled aerosols. *Arch. intern. Med.*, **131:** 60–75.

STUART, B. O., WILLARD, D. H., & HOWARD, E. B. (1970) Uranium mine air contaminants in dogs and hamsters. In: Hanna, M. G. Jr, Nettesheim, P., & Gilbert, J. R., ed. *Inhalation carcinogenesis.* Springfield, VA, Clearinghouse for Federal Scientific and Technical Information, NBS, US Dept of Commerce (CONF-691001).

STUPFEL, M. & MORDELET-DAMBRINE, M. (1974) Penetration of pollutants in the airways. *Bull. Physio-Path. Respir.*, **10:** 481–509.

234

SWIFT, D. L. (1971) Direct-reading instruments for analysing airborne particles. In: Lippman, M., ed. *Air sampling instruments*, 4th ed., Cincinnati, OH, ACGIH, p. T-1.

TAYLOR, G. J. & DREW, R. T. (1975) Cardiomyopathy predisposes hamsters to trichlorofluoromethane toxicity. *Toxicol. appl. Pharmacol.*, **32:** 177–183.

THOMAS, R. G. & LIE, R. (1963) *Procedures and equipment used in inhalation studies on small animals*. LF-11, Lovelace Foundation for Medical Education and Research.

THOMAS, R. L. (1969) Deposition and initial translocation of inhaled particles in small laboratory animals. *Health Phys.*, **16,** 417–428.

TIERNEY, D. G. (1974) Intermediary metabolism of the lung. *Fed. Proc.*, **33:** 2232–2237.

TUCKER, A. D., WYATT, J. H., & UNDRY, D. (1973) Clearance of inhaled particles from alveoli by normal interstitial drainage pathways. *J. appl. Physiol.*, **35,** 719–732.

VALEŽNEV, I. P., ELOVSKAJA, L. T., & MOISEJCEV, P. I. (1970) [Equipment for research on biological effects of aerosols.] *Ofic. bjull. Gos. kom. Min. SSSR po delam izobretenij i otkrytij*, No. 10, avtonskoe svidetel'stvo No. 265307 (in Russian).

VELIČKOVSKIJ, B. T. & KACNELSON, B. A. (1964) [*Etiology and pathogenesis of silicosis.*] Moscow, Medicina (in Russian).

WALTON, W. H. & PREWETT, W. C. (1949) The production of sprays and mists of uniform drop size by means of spinning disc type sprayers. *Proc. Phys. Soc. (London)*, **62:** 341–350.

WATSON, J. A., SPRITZER, A. A., AULD, J. A. & GUETTHOFF, M. A. (1969) Deposition and clearance following inhalation and intra-tracheal injection of particles. *Arch. environ. Health*, **19:** 51–58.

WEISS, B. & LATIES, V. (1975) *Behavioural toxicology*. New York, Plenum Press.

WHITBY, K. T. & LIU, B. Y. H. (1966) The electrical behaviour of aerosols. In: Davies, C. N., ed. *Aerosol Science*, New York, Academic Press.

WILSON, R. H. & LASKIN, S. (1950) *Improved design for an animal inhalation exposure unit*. Rochester, NY, University of Rochester (AEC Proj. Rep. U-116), p. 80.

WITSCHI, H. P. (1975) Exploitable biochemical approaches for the evaluation of toxic lung damage. In: Hayes, W. Jr, ed. *Essays in toxicology*, New York, Academic Press, Vol. 6.

WOOLCOCK, A. J., VINCENT, N. J., & MACKLEM, P. T. (1969) Frequency dependence of compliance as a test for obstruction in the small airways. *J. clin. Invest.*, **48:** 1097–1106.

WRIGHT, B. M. (1950) A new dust-feed mechanism. *J. Sci. Instrum.*, **27:** 12–15.

XINTARAS, C., JOHNSON, B. L., & DE GROOT, I., ed. (1974) *Behavioural toxicology*. Washington DC, US Govt Printing Office.

235

7. CARCINOGENICITY AND MUTAGENICITY

7.1 Introduction

This chapter deals with the two related but separate processes, heritable mutations and cancer. Cancer involves the conversion of normal cells to malignant cells and the development of what is usually an irreversible malignant disease process in the present generation freqently leading to a fatal outcome for the bearer of the malignancy. Heritable mutations are mutations that are transmissible to later generations and the target cells are the germ cells of either sex.

Developments in the last two decades make it possible to discuss certain aspects of mutagenesis and carcinogenesis in parallel. In other words, there is now increasing evidence that, in most cases, somatic mutations are probably involved in the conversion of normal to malignant cells. Thus, the ability of a chemical or physical agent to produce mutations is relevant both to the question of heritable mutations (mutations of the germ cell) and carcinogenicity.

There is a well-established body of knowledge that shows a close correspondence between cancer of the whole animal as studied in the laboratory and the occurrence of cancer in man; this is especially true of occupational cancer. More recently, a fairly close correlation has been shown between tests of isolated, simple, biological systems, e.g. reverse bacterial mutations and the response to carcinogens of whole animals, and human beings.

A similar situation does not exist with respect to patterns in human heritable mutations. Thus, although there is good evidence of correlation between *in vitro* tests for mutagenicity and heritable mutations in insects and experimental mammals, it can only be inferred, at present, that this also applies to man. The inference, however, is extremely strong and not subject to serious doubt. Thus, there is every reason to expect, that, in general, man will respond biologically in a manner quite similar to that of other species when exposed to mutagens that reach the germ cells. The lack of full correlation stems more from the lack of appropriate studies in man than from any uncertainty concerning the underlying biological considerations. At present, methods for the detection of mutations in man are difficult, cumbersome, and insensitive, and it is imperative to operate on the assumption that agents capable of producing germ cell mutations in laboratory studies would also be capable of producing similar mutations in man.

Thus, two quite different disease processes can have one common level of consideration, namely, their ability to produce alterations in the genetic material of cells. The following discussion is concerned with methods for carcinogenicity testing. First, the traditional lifetime exposure of the entire organism to the test compound is considered. This is followed by a discussion of various *in vitro* systems for the examination of mutagenicity including DNA damage, mutagenicity in bacteria and eukaryotic organisms, and transformation of cell cultures. (The first three of these are particularly relevant to mutagenicity of the germ cell or of the somatic cell.) Following this, the general problem of examination for heritable mutations is considered. This includes inquiries at three levels: injury to DNA, point mutations, and chromosome alterations. Whole animal and isolated test systems are available to make relevant determinations. However, the whole field of mutagenicity testing is now in a period of rapid evolution with advances being made in a number of areas. It can, therefore, be anticipated that present procedures will undergo alteration and, it is hoped, will improve within the near future.

7.2 Carcinogenicity

7.2.1 Long-term bioassays

The fact that environmental factors have a direct effect in producing cancer in man is shown by: (*a*) the unequivocal evidence of the chemical origin of occupational cancer, for example, urinary bladder tumours in workers exposed to aromatic amines, lung cancers in workers exposed to bis(chloromethyl)ether, etc.; (*b*) the well-documented cases of iatrogenic cancer; (*c*) the positive correlation between cigarette smoking and lung cancer; (*d*) the differences in cancer incidence in urban and rural populations and (*e*) the results of studies on migrants showing that for some types of cancer they acquire incidences similar to those found in the host countries. Results obtained in experimental studies on carcinogenesis confirm the direct carcinogenic effect of chemicals. However, there is not necessarily a correlation between acute toxicity and carcinogenicity; a chemical with a high acute toxicity may not have any, or only a very low carcinogenic potential. Conversely, a chemical that produces a very minor, or no evident toxic effect in acute or subacute experiments may be a very powerful carcinogen. Knowledge of the acute and subacute toxicity of the test chemical however, is important in order to permit better planning of the experiment. For instance, the premature death of the test animals, due to unforeseen side-effects, may thus be avoided.

237

7.2.1.1 *Species, strain, and sex selection, and size of groups*

The description of methods and recommended procedures in this chapter applies to long-term testing in rodents and specifically to the mouse, rat, and Syrian golden hamster (FDA, 1971; NCI, 1976; Weil, 1972; Weisburger, 1975; Weisburger & Weisburger, 1967). Rodents have been preferred to other species because of their susceptibility to tumour induction, their relatively short life span, the limited cost of their maintenance, their widespread use in pharmacological and toxicological studies, the availability of inbred strains and, as a consequence of these characteristics, the large amount of information available on their physiology and pathology. Nonrodents, in particular dogs and primates, have rarely been used in the past; though used more at the present time, their much higher cost of maintenance, the long period of observation, and the impracticability of using sufficiently large numbers put nonrodents at a disadvantage for long-term bioassays. Also, comparative studies on the metabolism of various chemicals have not indicated necessarily that primates and dogs are closer to man in this respect that rodents. Nevertheless, many of the procedures for long-term bioassays in rodents are applicable to assays in nonrodents.

Long-term bioassays of the carcinogenicity of environmental chemicals are carried out to assess a possible risk to man and to estimate the need for primary preventive measures. Because of the urgent nature of these problems, it is recommended that a compound of unknown activity should be tested on two animal species. Although a positive (that is, carcinogenic) effect in one species is considered as adequate warning, only negative findings in two species can be regarded as adequate negative evidence.

Among rodents, the species of choice are undoubtedly the mouse, the rat, and the Syrian golden hamster. The European hamster has recently been introduced, particularly for studies in lung pathology, but its use cannot be recommended for routine testing. Guineapigs and rabbits have been used occasionally but they have few of the advantages of smaller rodents combined with the disadvantages implied by a much longer life span, higher cost of maintenance, and the scarcity or absence of inbred strains.

Of the three rodent species of choice, the mouse and the rat have been more widely used than the hamster. However, the last species has proved to be an excellent tool for revealing carcinogenic effects in the respiratory tract and urinary bladder. Furthermore, hamster cells are widely used for *in vitro* transformation assays, and, since in most cases these assays require the back transplantation of the cells in syngenic hosts, the use of the hamster has recently been extended. The hamster is generally randomly bred but a pure strain is becoming available.

The use of inbred strains undoubtedly has the advantage of making available animals with known characteristics such as an average life span, and a spontaneous tumour rate with little variability. Random-bred animals or, even better, animals bred with maximum avoidance of inbreeding, are considered more resistant to infections and perhaps more liable than many inbred strains to reveal any carcinogenic effect on an unsuspected target organ. It is common experience that carcinogenic activity is more easily recognized by the increased frequency and earlier appearance of tumours at sites where tumours occur spontaneously. Inbred strains are often known to have one or two particularly susceptible organs and the induction of tumours in these organs could, in part, be regarded as an intensification of whatever underlies the spontaneous occurrence of tumours in that organ. A carefully planned experiment must take this possibility into account, and preference should be given to strains with a low incidence of tumours. Noninbred strains are inconvenient in that, in many cases, background tumour incidence in untreated controls is unpredictable. Moreover, experimental groups initiated at different times can rarely be compared with each other since inter- as well as intragroup variation may be considerable.

Hybrid mice of two known inbred strains are excellent as they are particularly robust and long-lived, but they are, of course, more difficult to obtain and are likely to be more expensive than inbred strains.

In selecting the species, it is important to be aware that there are, within each species, particular susceptibilites; for instance, it is easier to induce liver tumours in the mouse than in the rat, and conversely it is much easier to induce subcutaneous tumours in the rat than in the mouse. The skin of the mouse and the rabbit is possibly more sensitive to tumour induction by skin painting than that of the rat and the hamster, particularly when polycyclic hydrocarbons are used. The hamster is more susceptible to urinary bladder carcinogenesis than the mouse and possibly the rat.

It is essential that experimental groups should be composed of an equal number of animals of each sex, since differences in response to the carcinogenic activity of chemicals are well documented. Thus, the use of one sex only would not show the full range of activity of the test chemical.

The group should be sufficiently large to permit statistical evaluation of the results. The UICC Committee on Carcinogenicity Testing (UICC, 1969) recommended that the number of animals should be such that it "would be likely to yield reasonable (e.g. 90%) statistical significance as between the main induced tumour incidence and its spontaneous incidence". A sufficient number of animals must be alive at the time that the first tumour appears and it is suggested that this number should never be less than 25 per sex.

7.2.1.2 *Route of administration*

It has been agreed that the chemical under test should be administered by the route of human exposure. This applies to food additives and food contaminants in particular, but it is equally desirable for drugs. This rule cannot always be applied to environmental or industrial chemicals. It is well known that the three main routes of exposure in man are inhalation, ingestion, and skin absorption. Inhalation is often predominant in man but in experimental carcinogenesis the inhalation route, while highly desirable in principle, has rarely been used in the past because of lack of adequately equipped laboratories. However, it is now being widely used in programmes concerning smoking and health.

When the route of exposure is *per os*, the chemical is administered either mixed in the diet or drinking water, or by gavage, the choice depending on the specific characteristics of the test chemical; a volatile compound, for example, should never be mixed in the diet while, for a drug, the route by which it will be used in man should be selected, i.e. *per os*, or by intravenous, subcutaneous or topical application.

7.2.1.3 *Inception and duration of tests*

Most commonly, tests are initiated in young adult animals from 7 to 9 weeks of age. The start of treatment soon after weaning is recommended as a routine procedure. One objective of carcinogenicity testing is to obtain the maximum possible carcinogenic effect of the test chemical in order to compensate for the limited number of individuals at risk. This is accomplished by employing high levels of exposure (see 7.1.4) and by starting the treatment when the animals are at their most sensitive age. For some years following the pioneer work of Pietra et al. (1961), treatment immediately after birth and within the first 24 h of life was thought to be the most sensitive model. Careful reviews of the data available have indicated that neonatal treatment alone can be recommended in some instances, but not as a general routine procedure (Della Porta & Terracini, 1969). For a single neonatal administration, only a very limited quantity of the chemical to be tested is needed and this could be advantageous, when only a small amount of the chemical is available.

The main limitation of the use of a single neonatal treatment is that the newborn animal may not have developed sufficient metabolic competence to metabolize the test chemical. Another limitation is that not all chemical carcinogens are active after one, or even a few exposures.

More recently, prenatal exposure has received considerable attention, since it has been demonstrated that some tissues, notably nervous tissue, are more susceptible to certain carcinogens during fetal life than later (Druckrey et al., 1967; Napalkov, 1973; Napalkov & Alexandrov, 1968; Tomatis, 1973). At present, however, it can only be speculated that prenatal exposure will reveal the carcinogenic effect of a chemical that would not have been revealed had treatment started at a later age. A sensitive procedure might be to integrate prenatal exposure with long-term, postnatal exposure, in order to obtain maximum sensitivity of the bioassay system. To achieve this, animals mated at the age of 8–9 weeks, should be exposed to the test chemical during the second half of pregnancy. The parents so treated can constitute a group under conventional long-term testing, if the treatment is continued after delivery. Their offspring, already exposed *in utero*, and possibly after birth through their mother's milk and excreta, should be exposed directly to the test chemical from the age of weaning onwards. In this way, two different experimental groups can be obtained: one for which exposure was started at the young adult stage (the parents) and the other for which exposure was started prenatally (the offspring) (Tomatis, 1974b).

The duration of a positive test, i.e. where exposure to the test chemical is followed by an increased incidence of tumours, depends on the time of appearance and the rapidity of growth of the induced tumours. To agree in advance on a given duration of exposure is of prime importance for negative tests. Some research workers have adopted a duration for carcinogenicity tests of 2 years in rats and 18 months in mice, while others have preferred an observation period extending over the entire life span of the animals. A long finite period—that is, not less than 2 years—is recommended in preference to the entire life span of the animals, for the following reasons: (*a*) induced tumours usually occur within this observation period; (*b*) "spontaneous" tumours appear with highest frequency late in life and their appearance may make it more difficult to evaluate the carcinogenicity of a compound, particularly if of low potency; (*c*) a few animals may far exceed the normal life span of the species and extend unnecessarily the duration of the experiment; (*d*) tests are very expensive and any justifiable abbreviation means good economy (Health & Welfare, Canada, 1973; Tomatis, 1974a; UICC, 1969; WHO, 1961).

7.2.1.4 *Dose-level and frequency of exposure*

If only one level is to be used, the highest dose allowing long survival of the majority of the animals should be chosen. The selection of this dose should be made from results obtained in subacute toxicity tests. Information on the LD_{50} of certain compounds may be available and this can be useful in deciding the level of the dose for the subacute studies.

While it would be very difficult to give a definition of the maximum tolerated dose, it seems quite reasonable to insist that it allows adequate survival of the animals and does not produce a reduction in weight of more than 10% compared with the controls (Friedman, 1974). If two dose levels are chosen, the second should be one quarter or one third of the first dose.

If the goal of the test is merely to ascertain the possible carcinogenicity of a compound, then the assay protocol should achieve the maximum sensitivity of the test; in this case, the highest tolerated dose is the most appropriate. If, however, additional information has to be collected, in particular regarding the establishment of a possible minimum effect or no-observed-effect level, then initiation of a dose-response experiment should be envisaged. In this case, a minimum of three doses, and preferably four, should be included. An advantage of including several dose levels, the lowest of which does not decrease the life span of the animals, is the possibility of collecting other data on chronic toxicity not otherwise available through a carcinogenicity test at high dose levels.

Frequency of exposure may vary according to the route chosen. If the chemical is administered in the drinking water or mixed in the diet, exposure is continuous. If the chemical is given by gavage, the frequency can be two to three times per week. Topical applications may be made daily, while subcutaneous or intravenous injections must be more widely spaced, e.g. once or twice weekly. The duration of treatment should cover almost the entire observation period.

7.2.1.5 *Combined treatment and cocarcinogenesis*

An investigation on the effect of more than one agent, given simultaneously, may approximate the actual environmental situation, where there is never exposure to a single chemical. In particular, it may be useful in revealing the carcinogenic effect of a chemical of very low carcinogenic potency and thereby help to identify situations or populations that may be exposed to an otherwise unsuspected high risk.

Response to an environmental chemical may be modified by the action of other chemicals that may either alter the rate and/or pathway of metabolism of the test chemical, or have a cocarcinogenic effect. A cocarcinogenic effect may be additive, when the chemical has a carcinogenic effect on its own which adds to the effect produced by the test chemical; it may be synergistic, when its effect, combined with that of the test chemical when given alone, exceeds the summation of the separate effects; or it may act as an incomplete carcinogen, that is, only as initiator or promoter in the two-stage carcinogenic process (UICC, 1969) (see Chapter 13).

It is also essential to keep in mind that dietary components may influence the incidence of tumours in test animals. This may occur either because of the unsuspected presence of carcinogens (such as aflatoxins or nitrosamines) or because of substances that may modify the response to the test chemical by altering, for instance, the hepatic microsomal enzyme activity.

7.2.1.6 *Positive and untreated controls*

An adequate group of untreated animals, serving as controls, should always be included in the planning of a carcinogenicity test. The size of the control group should never be smaller than the size of the treated group and, preferably, should be larger. When more than one chemical is tested simultaneously, the same control group can be used, provided that its size is appropriately increased.

Besides these controls, i.e. animals not receiving treatment, and which could be called negative controls, the inclusion of positive controls in planning an experiment has recently been recommended, i.e. inclusion of a group of animals receiving a known carcinogen at a dose level that has already produced carcinogenic effects in several laboratory studies. Such controls ensure: (*a*) more confidence in the outcome of tests carried out on compounds of unknown activity (Weisburger, 1974); (*b*) assessment of the relative carcinogenic potency of the test chemical, and (*c*) an indirect check on the reliability of the test laboratory. While it does not seem essential to include a positive control in every test, it is highly advisable for every laboratory to check the sensitivity of its bioassay system, periodically, with selected known carcinogenic chemicals. It is also advisable that a group of animals should receive only the vehicle (i.e. acetone, dimethylsulfoxide, etc.) in which the chemical under test is eventually administered.

7.2.1.7   *Test material*

Long-term studies should not be started until sufficient information on the identity and purity of the test chemical has been assembled. The importance of knowing the toxicity of impurities is well demonstrated by the case of TCDD present as an impurity in the herbicide 2,4,5-T. Drugs or food additives should be tested in the form and degree of purity intended for human consumption (Health & Welfare, Canada, 1973; National Academy of Sciences, 1960; WHO, 1961, 1969). In this case, as well as for mixtures of chemicals to which man may be exposed, it may be highly advisable to carry out additional studies in order to identify positively the carcinogenic component of the mixture.

7.2.1.8   *Survey of animals, necropsy, and histological examination*

In order to present results correctly, detailed records of all experimental procedures and surveillance of the animals during the entire observation period should be maintained. While all pertinent details of the experiment may not be published, it is a good rule for the investigator to keep them for discussion with other interested scientists (UICC, 1969). If the results are to be published, it is essential that adequate information be given on the test chemical and test animal, as well as on all observations made on the experimental and control groups (WHO, 1961). A detailed list of items to be considered is given in the UICC (1969) report.

In the case of neoplasms (Turusov, 1973, 1976), it is extremely important to give an exact description of the criteria used to classify lesions as hyperplastic, preneoplastic or neoplastic, benign or malignant. Many times, pathologists do not agree on certain diagnoses and it is far easier to interpret the results when the criteria used for classification are known. Terms such as hepatoma, which do not indicate the specific tissue of origin, should not be used (Reuber, 1974), while terms such as cholangioma or adenomatosis require additional qualification. The term should clearly indicate whether the lesion is considered malignant. Thus, specific descriptions should be given, e.g. in the case of "hepatoma" it may be either a liver cell adenoma or a hepatocellular carcinoma, while "cholangioma" may be cholangiocellular adenoma or cholangiocellular carcinoma. In addition, carcinomas may. be subdivided into well, moderately, and poorly differentiated carcinomas.

A lesion with atypical cells or with focal malignant change should be classified separately rather than under malignant tumours.

7.2.2 Short-term tests (rapid screening tests)

To date, there are no reliable alternatives to long-term bioassays for testing the carcinogenicity of chemicals; this means a delay of two years or more before a carcinogenicity bioassay yields results. However, recent advances in mutagenicity testing hold out hopes of a short-term test, at least for selecting, from among the many chemicals to be tested, those most in need of early attention. So far, about 80% of carcinogens have been shown to be mutagenic and with the continuously increasing sensitivity of the models now employed an even higher correlation is possible. At present, mutagenicity testing represents a valuable system for screening chemicals to be submitted to long-term carcinogenicity testing; it cannot replace long-term testing, until a satisfactory positive correlation is established and the possibility of false negatives eliminated.

A mutation is any heritable change in genetic material including a chemical transformation of an individual gene (point mutation) or a change involving rearrangement of parts of a chromosome (chromosome mutation). The question of whether or not a mutagenic event is a prerequisite for carcinogenesis has long been debated. Many mutagens have been shown to be carcinogenic but other known carcinogens are known not to be mutagenic. Other mechanisms not involving DNA have also been implied in the process of carcinogenesis (Pitot, 1974).

Recent short-term mutagenicity testing procedures (McCann & Ames, 1976: McCann et al., 1975; Sugimura et al., 1976) have shown greater correlation between mutagenicity and carcinogenicity; consequently, some thought is now being given to using these assays as preliminary screens for potential carcinogens. However, at the moment, the fact that a particular compound has mutagenic activity can only be considered, in terms of carcinogenicity, as indicative of potential reactivity with DNA.

7.2.2.1 *Metabolic activation, reaction with DNA, and DNA repair*

The synthetic and naturally occurring chemical carcinogens include a variety of chemicals having no common structural feature. However, it is becoming clear that the ultimate reactive forms of many chemical carcinogens are electrophilic (electron-deficient) reactants (Miller, 1970). Although some chemical carcinogens, such as direct alkylating agents and metal ions, are electrophiles *per se*, the majority require metabolic activation to reactive forms (ultimate carcinogens) (Fig. 7.1).

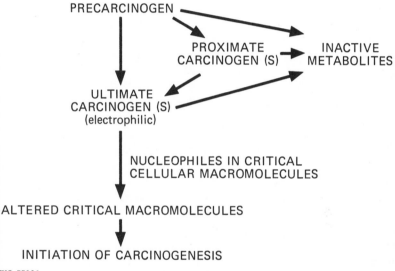

Fig. 7.1 General pathways in the activation and deactivation of chemical carcinogens (Miller & Miller, 1976).

The formation of these electrophilic reactants from exogenous chemicals, in an animal species or in an organ, is the result of the balance between *in vivo* activation and deactivation reactions carried out predominantly by enzymes localized in the endoplasmic reticulum of the cell. The ultimately available concentration of reactive metabolites seems to account for some of the organ and species specificities shown by several chemical carcinogens.

During the last decade, much progress has been made in understanding the metabolism of various classes of chemical carcinogens (polynuclear hydrocarbons, Sims & Grover, 1974; N-nitroso compounds, Magee et al., 1976; aromatic amines, Kriek, 1974; Weisburger & Weisburger, 1973; miscellaneous compounds, Miller, 1973). The activity of microsomal mixed function oxidases is influenced by various drugs or environmental chemicals, that may stimulate or inhibit the formation of the ultimate carcinogens (Conney & Burns, 1972).

These ultimate carcinogens bind covalently with cellular macro-molecules such as DNA, RNA, or proteins, which, directly or indirectly, leads to heritable changes in the affected cells. Although the critical targets of chemical carcinogens are not known, there is a great deal of evidence supporting the theory that DNA is one major target in carcinogenesis (Farber, 1973).

Some specific binding sites for the metabolites of carcinogens have been identified in the bases of DNA. The carcinogenic N-nitroso compounds are examples (Magee et al., 1976). The main site of alkylation of DNA by alkylnitroso compounds is the $N,7$ position of guanine, as with other alkylating agents. Other sites are also attacked and the significance of these DNA interactions is being investigated. The formation of 7-alkylguanine, however, seems to be of no obvious importance in the process of tumour induction, since no quantitative or qualitative correlation between the occurrence of this alkylated base in the DNA of treated animals and the carcinogenicity of nitrosamines or alkylating agents has been observed (Magee et al., 1976). Alkylation of guanine bases in DNA at the 7-position does not seem to produce mutations in bacteriophages (Loveless & Hampton, 1969), nor does it alter the coding properties of synthetic polynucleotides *in vivo* (Ludlum, 1970). Various laboratories have examined the biological importance of the alkylated $O,6$ position of guanine residues in DNA which, in consequence, is able to induce mutations in phage (Loveless, 1969). It has been shown that there is an aberrant base pairing with a polymer containing alkylated $O,6$-guanine residues (Gerchman & Ludlum, 1973). Goth & Rajewsky (1974) showed, *in vivo*, that the initial degree of alkylation at the $O,6$ position in the DNA was, apparently, not correlated with the tissue-specific carcinogenicity of ethylnitrosourea which induces brain, but not liver, tumours. However, $O,6$-ethylguanine persists much longer in brain DNA than $N,7$-ethylguanine. The $O,6$-alkyl elimination is also much slower from brain than from the liver DNA. From these findings it becomes apparent that variations in the sensitivity of different organs to the carcinogenic action of N-nitroso compounds might be attributed to different enzyme activities capable of repairing lesions in cellular DNA and/or to different rates of cell division in the target and non-target organs (Craddock, 1976; Margison et al., 1976; Pegg & Nicoll, 1976; Pegg, 1977).

Possibly these repair systems, which recognize damaged DNA, are also impaired in the case of some types of cancer in man. The skin of patients suffering from the hereditary disease xeroderma pigmentosum is extremely sensitive to sunlight and such persons have a very high incidence of skin cancer. It has been shown that the cells of the skin of these patients are deficient in the capacity to repair UV-damaged DNA and that this deficiency is caused by lack of enzymes required for the excision of damaged regions from DNA (Cleaver, 1969).

Some chemicals cause changes in the biological properties of DNA without covalent binding, e.g. by intercalation which could cause frameshift mutations. Since radioactive labelled chemicals are needed for most of these studies, technical problems associated with these methods render the tests impractical for routine screening. However, they will continue to contribute considerably to the understanding of the mechanism of interaction of a chemical or its activating metabolite with specific sites in DNA.

Initial lesions in DNA can either lead to a permanent change, such as a mutation, or can be removed by cellular repair processes. In bacteria and mammalian cells, three major repair processes can be considered. First, the photoreactivation repair process that repairs only UV damage to DNA and involves a direct enzymatic cleavage of pyrimidine dimers to monomers upon exposure of cells to visible light. This repair process is present in most prokaryotes and eukaryotes and it was recently identified in human cells (Sutherland et al., 1975). The second process, post-replication repair, which is also called recombination repair, is limited to the DNA synthesis period. Although its mechanism is not well known, it has been proposed that it is caused by the presence of damaged bases on parental DNA strands too close to the replication fork to be recognized by the third process, excision repair. Unlike post-replication repair, excision repair occurs throughout the cell cycle and is present in a large variety of organisms. During this process, damaged bases are excised, producing a single-strand break. This gap is repaired by replacing the original bases with bases complementary to those of the opposite intact strand. Various enzymes are involved in this process, namely endonuclease, a DNA exonuclease, a DNA polymerase and a DNA ligase (Cleaver, 1974).

From studies on prokaryotes, the concept arose that excision repair is error-free (Kondo, 1973). It is thought that mutations originate during semi-conservative replication as a consequence of the fact that DNA templates containing damage have not yet been or cannot be repaired by excision repair. Since DNA replication on damaged templates involves post-replication repair, this repair process is considered error-prone and responsible for mutagenesis. Whether miscoding and mutagenesis of DNA templates is the result of lack of excision repair enzymes or due to error-prone post-replicative repair is not clear at present.

The isolation of xeroderma pigmentosum-variant fibroblasts, that have normal excision repair but are deficient in post-replication repair (Maher et al., 1976) may lead to a better understanding of the role of these repair processes in mutagenesis and carcinogenesis.

Recent efforts have been devoted to the development in mammalian systems of a screening test for the detection of possible mutagens or carcinogens based on excision repair. The focus on this type of repair is mainly based on the greater availability of procedures thought to be appropriate to the problem. There are four different ways of examining this form of repair in mammalian systems and all are based on the assumption that chemical mutagens or carcinogens interact with DNA, inducing molecular alterations which result in DNA repair that can be measured as unscheduled incorporation of various DNA precursors (Cleaver, 1975; Legator & Flamm, 1973). The common basis of all these tests is the dif-ferentiation between repair and normal semiconservative synthesis of DNA.

One procedure, "unscheduled DNA synthesis", involves auto-radiography of cultured cells, and consists of the incorporation of precursors during resynthesis of short nucleotide sequences that have been eliminated from DNA strands following their damage by chemicals (Cleaver, 1973; Stich & San, 1970). This procedure permits a quantitative evaluation of DNA repair synthesis in various types of cell in a tissue and can be applied to an *in vivo* system (Stich & Kieser, 1974), thus allowing the detection of indirect mutagens and/or carcinogens.

Another process uses 5-bromodeoxyuridine (BrdU), which is an analogue of thymidine. During normal replication, the incorporation of BrdU produces a DNA with a high buoyant density; this does not occur when BrdU is incorporated in DNA during the repair synthesis. Thus, by using radiolabelled BrdU, or radiolabelled thymidine and non-labelled BrdU, it is possible to differentiate, on cesium chloride density gradients, semi-conservative replication of DNA from the repair synthesis according to the different buoyant densities.

A third procedure also uses BrdU but the differentiation between semi-conservative and repair DNA synthesis is done by different means. Cells exposed to the chemicals are incubated with BrdU and the DNA is subjected to long wavelength ultra-violet radiation. Breaks appear in the DNA at the sites of incorporation of BrdU and cause slower sedimentation of the DNA in alkaline sucrose gradients (Smith & Hanawalt, 1969). This technique appears to be a very sensitive one for measuring single-strand breaks but it still seems to be prone to artefacts and cannot be considered suitable for large-scale studies (Cleaver, 1975).

Another method involves the total suppression of normal DNA synthesis, for example, by hydroxyurea, thus the incorporation of precursors into DNA reflects only repair synthesis and not normal replication.

Some of the above techniques are time-consuming, costly and not yet standardized, so that it is difficult to adapt them for large-scale studies. The most promising approach appears to be the measurement of unscheduled DNA synthesis, but criticisms have also been made of the use of this system as an indicator of mutagenic or carcinogenic potential (Cleaver et al., 1975). One limitation is that unscheduled synthesis is an average measure of repairable damage in all cells of a population or in all sites of the DNA, whereas mutagenesis and carcinogenesis seem to depend on the amount of unrepaired damage in a small percentage of cells and in a few specific DNA sites. Due to these limitations and to the current limited understanding of these processes, none of these variables could, by themselves, be a reliable indicator of a potential mutagenic or carcinogenic chemical. However, these studies associated with studies of DNA damage as well as of the expression of this damage are essential in the understanding and development of reliable screening systems.

Metabolic activation of chemicals to electrophiles, DNA damage, and subsequent repair processes are important factors in the initiation of cancer. The phenotypic expression (tumour development) of these initial molecular changes is modulated by a number of factors (Farber, 1973) that influence the macroscopic appearance of cancer at a later stage (Pitot, 1977). However, the initial molecular changes, induced by chemical carcinogens, appear prerequisite for initiation of the cancer process. Further studies on the alteration of DNA induced by chemical carcinogens and on the repair of such lesions before cell division by tissues, whether target or not, are required to evaluate the role of DNA repair processes in chemical carcinogenesis.

7.2.2.2   In vitro *neoplastic transformation of mammalian cells*

The term transformation in such studies refers to the *in vitro* observations of various changes present in the cells treated *in vitro* with the chemicals, when compared with untreated control cells. Transformed cells may differ from control cells in various ways such as: (*a*) alteration of cellular and colony morphology; (*b*) increased plating efficiency; (*c*) agglutinability by plant lectins; (*d*) altered glycolytic patterns; (*e*) resistance to toxicity of some chemicals; (*f*) altered surface properties (contact inhibition of movement and growth, population density, growth in suspension, ability to grow in agar or other semisolid media); (*g*) sensitivity to activated macrophages and lymphocytes; (*h*) establishment of cell lines with the potential to be sub-cultured indefinitely *in vitro*; and (*i*) appearance of new antigens (Fedoroff, 1967). However, the unequivocal criterion of malignant transformation is the capacity of transformed cells to develop a malignant neoplasm when injected into a syngenic, immunosuppressed or thymus-free host, or into privileged sites (Giovannella et al., 1972; Sanford, 1965).

Recently, Sanford (1974) critically reviewed the significance of these various *in vitro* changes in relation to the acquisition of neoplastic potential. It was stressed that these criteria of neoplastic transformation cannot completely replace the *in vivo* assay for tumour production. With reference to the problems of the application of tissue culture to the rapid detection and characterization of neoplastic transformation *in vitro*, the reader is referred to the proceedings of the symposium "New Horizons for Tissue Culture in Cancer Research" (*J. Natl Cancer Inst.*, 1974).

In most *in vitro* transformation experiments the cells used have been fibroblasts. Earle & Nettleship (1943) reported the transformation by 1,2-dihydro-3-methyl-benz[j]aceanthrylene (3-methylcholanthrene) of a long-term culture of fibroblasts as demonstrated by the development of tumours after inoculation of the cells into mice. However, this observation was attributed to spontaneous transformation, since Sanford et al. (1950) observed that the cells were tumorigenic also without treatment with chemicals. The first clear demonstration of transformation of cells in culture by chemicals was that of Berwald & Sachs (1963) who observed the transformation of Syrian hamster embryo secondary cells with 3-methylcholanthrene and benzo(a)pyrene, but not with urethane or solvent. Since this report, various cells types originating from different animal species have been used for *in vitro* transformation. This topic has recently been reviewed by Heidelberger (1973) and Kuroki (1975), who critically examined the advantages and disadvantages of the various strains and lines of fibroblastic cells, namely of the Syrian hamster embryo, fibroblastic cells derived from mouse ventral prostate, cell lines derived from embryo cells of Swiss mouse BALB/c, C3H, AKR, and C57/B1 strains, Chinese hamster lung cells, as well as various tissues from organ cultures. Transformation of the above cell lines was obtained with polynuclear hydrocarbons and with chemicals that do not require metabolic activation.

Some chemical carcinogens that are active *in vivo* have failed to induce transformation, when applied directly to hamster embryo cells; this is presumably because such compounds require metabolic conversion to active intermediates that are lacking or are present in insufficient concentration in these cells. However, neoplastic transformation was detected in fibroblasts obtained from embryos whose mothers had been exposed to indirect carcinogens during pregnancy (Di Paolo et al., 1972, 1973). A similar approach was used by Borland & Hard (1974), who cultured kidney cells at various times following *in vivo* treatment of rats with N-methyl-N-nitrosomethanamine (dimethylnitrosamine). The cells isolated from treated rats showed various morphological and behavioural changes associated with transformation. Laerum & Rajewsky (1975) reported the development of glioblastomas following injection of glial cells originating from the brain of rat embryos, the mother having been treated with ethylnitrosourea during pregnancy.

Epithelial cultures from rat liver were recently established in various laboratories and used for transformation studies (Iype, 1974; Katsuta & Takaoka, 1972; Montesano et al., 1975; Weinstein et al., 1975; Williams et al., 1973). The transformation of these cells by various carcinogens that need metabolic activation was determined by the development of carcinomas after their back-transplantation into suitable hosts. Carcinomas were observed following inoculation of epithelial cells from mouse skin, or rat urinary bladder or salivary glands, treated with chemical carcinogens *in vitro* (Brown, 1973; Fusenig et al., 1973; Hashimoto & Kitagawa, 1974).

One disadvantage of these epithelial cells is that the morphological criteria for transformation of fibroblast cultures (piling up of cells, crisscross arrangement of cells etc.) do not apply possibly because normal epithelial cells have little or no locomotion and they continue to divide even when in close contact with other cells (Weinstein et al., 1975). However, the capacity for growth in soft agar appears to provide a reliable and reproducible correlation with the tumorigenicity of these cells (Weinstein et al., 1975; Montesano et al., 1977). Although, at present, this system provides only a qualitative and not a quantitative assay of *in vitro* transformation, it is the only instance of unequivocal production of carcinoma. The establishment of reliable criteria, measurable *in vitro*, for distinguishing normal from transformed epithelial cells in culture is essential for the development of quantitative systems for the transformation of these epithelial cells. Recently the neoplastic transformation of human diploid cells by chemical carcinogens has been described (Kakunaga, 1977).

Cell culture has been extremely useful in elucidating the cellular and molecular mechanism of chemical carcinogens and it holds great promise as a test for screening for the potential carcinogenicity of environmental chemicals. However, some time is needed before this test may be used for routine testing in a reproducible way.

7.2.2.3 *Mutagenicity tests*

The growing experimental evidence linking the carcinogenic activity of numerous chemicals with their capacity to be converted into electrophilic derivatives, that may also exert a mutagenic effect, has led to the suggestion that a relationship between chemical carcinogenesis and mutagenesis may exist (Miller & Miller, 1971a,b). Such a correlation has so far been limited to those changes of the genotype that appear as a consequence of structural or functional alterations of nucleic acids. Not all chemical mutagens have been shown to be carcinogenic. However, most chemical carcinogens, several of which cause cancer in man, have now been found to be mutagens, when tested by one of the mutagenicity test procedures that combine microbial, mammalian, or other animal cell systems as genetic targets with an *in vitro* or *in vivo* metabolic activation system. The growing empirical relationship between chemical mutagens and carcinogens does not imply that the two processes are identical, but it offers a promising method for the use of mutagenesis as a rapid prescreening assay for carcinogenesis (Bartsch & Grover, 1976; Bridges, 1976; Council of the Environmental Mutagenic Society, 1975; IARC, 1976; McCann & Ames, 1976; Purchase et al., 1976; Stoltz et al., 1974; Sugimura et al., 1976; WHO, 1974).

The choice of mutagen-detecting assay depends on various considerations, i.e. the chemical structure and pharmacological activity of the chemical, the type of human exposure, and the nature of the population at risk. The same considerations should be taken into account in assessing the strength of the evidence of mutagenicity and its relevance to man.

7.2.2.4 *Submammalian assay systems*

Bacterial phages have been used to test reactive forms of chemical carcinogens. Chemicals inducing point mutations can be detected by reacting the test compound with the free phage or with phage during its duplication inside bacteria (Corbett et al., 1970; Drake, 1971).

In the bacterial transformation of DNA (Freese & Strack, 1962), genetic information contained in the DNA isolated from one strain of bacteria can be transformed to that of a recipient strain. Purified bacterial DNA is readily accessible to reactive forms of mutagens. Thus, this system has been used to quantify the mutagenic potential of a number of chemicals. Extensive studies have been made on the inactivation of *Bacillus subtilis* DNA and transformation of the tryptophane-requiring strain T-3 (Herriott, 1971; Maher et al., 1968).

The reverse mutation[a] system of *Salmonella typhimurium* uses the genetically well-defined histidine-requiring mutants developed by Ames and his colleagues (Ames, 1971; Ames et al., 1972a,b, 1973; McCann et al., 1975).

These revert to prototrophy by single-base pair substitutions, e.g. strain

---

[a] Mutations in which the function of a given gene is lost are called forward mutations. Mutations that bring about the restoration of gene function are called reverse mutations or back mutations.

TA1535 or by base pair insertion (frameshift), e.g. strains TA1536, TA1537 and TA1538. Most of the theoretically possible types of mutation may be detected with a set of these test strains, where a mutation of one of the genes responsible for excision repair (UVrB) has produced a 100-fold increase in sensitivity. Penetration of larger molecules through the bacterial cell walls has also been facilitated by the use of deep-rough mutants deficient in the exterior polysaccharide coat. Two newly developed test strains TA100 and TA98 were obtained by transferring an ampicillin resistance factor (R factor) to the standard test strains TA1535 and TA1538, respectively (McCann et al., 1975). These strains are effective in detecting classes of mutagens that were not previously detected with the original strains. The tests are usually performed by adding a few crystals or a drop of solution of the test chemical in sulfinylbis[methane] (dimethylsulfoxide) or water to a uniform lawn of one of the histidine-requiring mutants on the surface of a Petri plate containing histidine-poor medium, or by incorporating the test compound, a postmitochondrial tissue fraction, cofactors (NADPH or $NADPH^+$ and glucose 6-phosphate) and the bacterial test strain in histidine-poor soft agar. For general mutagenicity screening, a liver homogenate ($9000g$ supernatant) from rats induced with a mixture of polychlorinated biphenyls (Aroclor 1254) is recommended as a metabolic activation system. For routine testing, the strains TA1535, TA1537 and TA1538 can be used in combination with the strains carrying the R factor (TA100 and TA98). This method of testing using various groups of chemicals and various experimental conditions is described in more detail by Ames et al. (1975).

Using the genetically well characterized *Escherichia coli* strains, reverse and forward mutation can be scored using nutritional resistance or fermentative markers (Bridges et al., 1972; Mohn, 1973). Prophage λ induction in *E. coli* strains by chemical mutagens activated by liver microsomal enzymes has been described as a sensitive test for the detection of potential mutagens and carcinogens (Moreau et al., 1976).

Mutagenesis has been extensively studied in *Neurospora crassa*. Heterokaryon has been developed, which is heterozygous for two closely-linked loci in the *ad*-3 region. Mutants at the *ad*-3A and *ad*-3B loci have a requirement for adenine and can be selected directly on the basis of accumulation of a reddish-purple pigment in the mycelium. The *ad*-3 mutations can be characterized by a series of simple genetic tests to distinguish point mutations from deletions and to obtain a presumptive identification of the genetic alterations in the point mutations at the *ad*-3B locus at a molecular level (de Serres & Malling, 1971).

Saccharomyces cerevisiae and *S. pombe* have been used to investigate the effects of carcinogenic and mutagenic compounds in these organisms. Mitotic gene conversion, in which a sequence of a few hundred nucleotides of one chromosome is replaced by one corresponding sequence from a homologous chromosome, can be studied in diploid cells of the yeast *S. cerevisiae* strain D-4 heteroallelic at the loci *trp*-5 and *ade*-2. This strain carries two different inactive alleles of two genes (*trp*-5 and *ade*-2) which are located on different chromosomes and the functional defects of which lead to a nutritional requirement. Mitotic gene conversion, which is increased by many types of mutagenic treatment, can transfer the intact region of one of these alleles to the defective region of the other, thus producing a hetero-zygotic diploid cell with full functional activity. The mechanism is presumably based on the formation of single-strand breaks in DNA and probably involves repair processes. Positive results are only obtained with agents or metabolites which either bind with DNA covalently or interfere with DNA metabolism. In contrast with most microbial mutation systems, mitotic gene conversion does not show a response specific to any type of mutagen. In addition to gene conversion, forward and reverse mutation can be measured with *S. cerevisiae* (Loprieno et al., 1976; Marquardt, 1974; Mortimer & Manney, 1971; Zimmerman, 1973).

7.2.2.5 *Mammalian somatic cells*

The application of cultured cell lines is somewhat restricted at present by requirements for karyotypic stability and high plating efficiency. A widely used system developed by Chu (1971) employs cell lines derived from the lung, ovary, and other tissues of Chinese hamster, which usually maintain a near-diploid chromosome number and exhibit active growth and high cloning efficiency. Two reviews discuss this topic in detail (De Mars, 1974; Thompson & Baker, 1973). Selective media have been developed to detect both forward and reverse mutations at three genetic loci involving enzymes in the salvage pathways of purines and pyrimidines. In Chinese hamster, as in man, the use of preformed hypoxanthine and guanine is controlled by an X-linked gene. Mutant cells at these loci are deficient in the enzyme hypoxanthine-guanine phosphoribosyl transferase and are resistant to certain purine analogues. Similarly, mutant cells deficient in adenosine phosphoribosyl transferase cannot metabolize preformed adenosine or its analogues for incorporation into nucleic acid. The third type of drug-resistant mutants currently studied in these and other mammalian cells are those deficient in thymidine kinase. Such cells exhibit resistance to the thymidine analogue, 5-bromodeoxyuridine. Cells carrying mutation at these loci can be selected from the wild type in an environment containing an appropriate purine or pyrimidine analogue. Revertants to the wild type can be recovered in selective media in which the cells are supplied with a natural purine or pyrimidine while the normal *de novo* pathway of purine or pyrimidine synthesis is inhibited by an antimetabolite. It has been demonstrated that Chinese hamster cells treated with physical or chemical mutagens undergo a significant increase in the frequency of forward and reverse mutations compared with the spontaneous frequency (Huberman & Sachs, 1974; Huberman et al., 1971, 1972). A liver microsomal activation system can be added for the metabolic activation of chemicals (Krahn & Heidelberger, 1975; Kuroki et al., 1977).

Forward mutations from thymidine kinase $+/-$ cells to thymidine kinase $-/-$ have been induced by treatment of cells with X-rays or chemical mutagens (mouse lymphoma L5178 Y cells). These cells can also be grown in the presence of *in vitro* or *in vivo* metabolic activation systems, which makes them suitable for host-mediated mutagenicity tests (Nahas & Capizzi, 1974).

Forward mutations to hypoxanthine-guanine phosphoribosyl transferase deficiency (resistance to 8-azaguanine) in diploid human fibroblasts in culture have been shown to occur either spontaneously or after X-radiation (Albertini & De Mars, 1973). Chemical induction of forward mutation from hypoxanthine-guanine phosphoribosyl transferase $-$ to $+$ in human lymphoblastoid cell line has also been reported (Sato et al., 1972).

7.2.2.6 *Host and tissue-(microsome) mediated assays*

These take into account the conversion of chemicals into mutagenic metabolites, and are particularly suitable for the detection of chemicals that are not mutagenic *per se* but require metabolic activation. They can be performed *in vivo* (host mediated) or *in vitro* (tissue mediated) using various indicator organisms, such as bacteria, fungi, yeast, or mammalian cells.

In the host-mediated assay, the indicator organisms are injected into the interperitoneal cavity of an animal (Legator & Malling, 1971), which is then treated with the test compound by another route. After a given length of time, the animal is killed and the indicator organism is recovered and scored for mutants. Comparison between the mutagenic action of the compound on a test strain directly and the host-mediated assay indicates whether the host can activate or inactivate the test compound. The limitations of the host-mediated assay are the high spontaneous mutation rates of the indicator organism in the host, the host's effect on cell survival and the selection of heterogenic cell populations. In order to measure a significant increase over the spontaneous mutation rate, doses well above LD_{50} have to be given to rats or mice. This type of assay is also limited since it does not identify the site of conversion to a mutagenic metabolite. Modifications have been reported (Mohn, 1973).

In the tissue-mediated assay, the indicator organisms are incubated *in vitro* in the presence of a tissue fraction plus appropriate cofactors and the test compound. The mutants are subsequently isolated and scored.

Ames et al. (1973a,b) have developed a mutagenicity assay that combines a Salmonella strain, a liver microsomal preparation, and cofactors in a soft agar layer on a Petri dish. Bartsch et al. (1975b), Czygan et al. (1973) and Malling (1974) have described a liquid incubation system where bacteria, a tissue preparation, and the test compound are incubated in liquid suspension. Test compounds that are gases at room temperature or are volatile can be assayed by exposing Petri dishes containing bacteria, tissue fraction, and cofactors to a mixture of gas and oxygen at 37°C (Bartsch et al., 1975a). The mutagenicity of urinary metabolites, excreted as conjugates in experimental animals treated with an indirect mutagen, may be detected by treating the urine with hydrolytic enzymes in the presence of a bacterial test strain or yeast, and an *in vitro* metabolic activation system (Commoner et al., 1974; Durston & Ames, 1974; Marquardt, 1974). In another modification, Huberman & Sachs (1974) used lethally irradiated rat fibroblasts that retain a drug-metabolizing capacity and cocultivated them with Chinese hamster V79 cells which are used as genetic indicators.

The mutagenicity tests previously described (7.2.2.4, 7.2.2.5, 7.2.2.6) all have individual advantages and limitations determined either by the genetic indicators or by the metabolic activation system. The use of submammalian organisms for the detection and classification of mutants, induced by chemicals, is greatly facilitated by the relatively small genome to which fine genetic mapping and biochemical analysis can be applied and by the short generation time. Huge populations of some of these organisms can be raised and they can easily be handled when analysing multiple mutations.

The relevance of such data from submammalian systems to mammalian cells is based on the assumption that the basic principles of heredity, and the structure and functions of DNA in terms of reactivity, the triplet code, transcriptional, and translational mechanisms, are essentially the same for all living cells irrespective of their evolutionary level. However, this extrapolation is hampered by lack of knowledge of repair processes that play a role in mutation fixation and expression and are insufficiently understood in mammals. It is obvious that normal human diploid cells are most desirable for this test, but current studies suggest that reliable conclusions can be drawn from results with non-human mammalian cells.

The other factor, related to the fact that many chemicals are not active *per se*, is the metabolic activation of the compounds. In many cases, reactive metabolites with a limited life span may fail to reach or react with the genetic indicator either because they are further metabolized to inactive compounds, or because they react with other cellular constituents. For this reason, mutagenicity assays in intact animals (host-mediated assays) may give negative results, as in the case of N-methyl-N'-nitro-N-nitroso-guanidine (MNNG) and acridine mustard (ICR-170), proven to be extremely potent mutagens. Metabolism in animals is affected by exogenous and endogenous factors such as chemicals causing enzyme induction and inhibition. Other modifying factors are age, sex, and strain of animals, diurnal and seasonal rhythms, differences between the fetal and adult state, mode of administration, cellular uptake, and distribution and excretion of the chemical.

The tissue-mediated mutagenicity test cannot, with certainty, reproduce the *in vivo* situation, but obvious advantages are the high sensitivity, good reproducibility, low cost, and the possibility of testing a large number of chemicals. In addition, *in vitro* testing with well-characterized genetic indicators allows the use of human tissue such as human liver to determine their ability to generate a mutagen (Bartsch, 1976).

7.2.3 Correlation between short and long-term bioassays for carcinogenicity

Short-term tests (rapid screening tests) are procedures that do not have the *in vivo* production of a visible tumour in animals as an end point. The variables used in short-term tests to detect chemical carcinogens are based on an interaction of carcinogens and/or their metabolites with macromolecules, the induction of chromosomal aberrations, mutagenesis, DNA repair, and DNA binding.

In the evaluation of these methods, the major question is which screening tests, singly or collectively, serve as reliable indicators or predictors of the potential carcinogenic hazard of the chemical. The answer can only be obtained by testing a representative number of compounds. A valid test should demonstrate that compounds with known carcinogenic properties are positive, within the limit of the test, and negative compounds are negative. If a test is required for preliminary screening, a small proportion of false negatives or positive results may be acceptable, but for a final test, no false negative results are acceptable.

Rapid screening tests should be relatively simple and inexpensive. They can be used in three ways: to trace carcinogens and/or mutagens in the complex environment of man; as a tool for prescreening chemicals to be submitted to a more lengthy set of bioassays; or for better extrapolation from experimental animal data to man and for improving the relevance of long-term bioassays in experimental animals.

Considering reproducibility, cost, the number of chemicals that can be examined in a short time, and the scientific basis of the test, tissue-mediated mutagenicity procedures using well-characterized genetic indicators and a metabolically defined *in vitro* activation system, appear at present to be the most promising short-term tests. With current methods there is still the chance of false negative results, depending on the systems used, either for lack of appropriate cofactors for activation or because of the extreme reactivity and/or toxicity of the compound or its metabolites. However, the number of false negative results in *in vitro* tissue-mediated assays is small compared with other mutagenicity test procedures (Montesano & Bartsch, 1976).

The increasing evidence of a possible correlation between mutagenicity and carcinogenicity certainly does not mean that one biological effect may be equated with another. Thus, the mutagenic activity of a chemical cannot, at present, automatically be assumed to imply a definite carcinogenic effect in man, nor can these results replace long-term carcinogenicity testing in animals.

Furthermore, it is still unknown whether all carcinogens will be found to be mutagenic, and all mutagens, carcinogenic. Examples are the strong mutagens, nitrous acid, hydroxylamine, and base analogues, for which no carcinogenic effect in animals has so far been reported; they do not act via electrophilic intermediates, a mechanism that has now been recognized for must ultimate carcinogenic forms. Nor have steroidal sex hormones, carcinogenic in animals, been reported to be mutagenic, as yet. On the other hand, various chromium salts have recently been shown to be mutagenic in bacteria (Venitt & Levy, 1974).

Development of cancer *in vivo* is determined by a variety of factors that cannot be duplicated in an *in vitro* short-term testing system because:

- (a) The concentration of ultimate reactive metabolites available to react in organs in animal species with cellular macromolecules, which is a consequence of a balance between metabolic activation and detoxication processes, is only partly reflected by *in vitro* testing procedures.
- (b) Species and organ specificity of a chemical carcinogen might be determined, in part, by organ-specific DNA repair.
- (c) Since chemical carcinogenesis is thought to be a multi-step process in which the early, apparently irreversible, initiation of a cell is followed by several subsequent stimuli provoking cellular replications, leading to an overt tumour, a short-term test capable of detecting complete carcinogens may be useful to detect initiating agents but cannot at the present time detect the action of promoting agents.

Currently used short-term tests, in particular tissue-mediated mutagenicity assays are effective in predicting, with a certain accuracy, the carcinogenic potential of chemicals (McCann & Ames, 1976; Purchase et al., 1976; Sugimura et al., 1976), but give no indication of the target organs or species specificity of their carcinogenic activity. Furthermore, the relative potency of a chemical to induce biological effects, defined as the endpoints, for the most frequently used rapid screening tests cannot at the present time be reliably correlated with its carcinogenic potency (Bartsch et al., 1977; Meselson & Russell, 1977). More data are needed to compare dose-response curves obtained in rapid screening tests on a given chemical with those of other biological effects obtained *in vivo* (long-term bioassays).

7.2.4 Significance of experimental testing for assessing the possible carcinogenic risk of chemicals to man

Experience acquired, so far, in long-term carcinogenicity testing has shown that nearly all compounds that are carcinogenic in man are also carcinogenic in one or several animal species, even though the tumour type may not be the same as in man. The concept that animal carcinogenicity data are predictive of a human carcinogenic risk and useful in preventing human cancer was accepted in 1941 in the case of 2-actylaminofluorene (AAF). This chemical was not used on a worldwide basis as an insecticide, because some experiments had already shown its carcinogenicity before it was marketed (Wilson et al., 1941); its restriction was facilitated by the existence of a number of substitutes at the time when the results of the first experiments on AAF were reported. This cautious attitude has not been consistently applied in other situations, on the grounds that the experimental data were insufficient or inadequate to evaluate the possible hazard to man. This is shown by the various relationships between experimental carcinogenicity data and possible human hazard that are considered in the adoption of preventive measures.

The first observation that some aromatic amines were involved in the causation of urinary bladder tumours in man dates from 1896; it was confirmed in 1907 and reconfirmed many times thereafter (IARC, 1974). In 1938, Hueper et al. reported the induction of bladder cancer in dogs exposed to 2-naphthalenamine (2-naphthylamine). Preventive measures were taken only in the late 1950s, when conspicuous epidemiological evidence had accumulated. In this case, the human epidemiological evidence was judged insufficient, and the experimental evidence, when it became available, was also deemed insufficient until further epidemiological findings came to hand.

The delay in taking preventive measures applies also to carcinogens on which, contrary to the case of aromatic amines, experimental evidence preceded observations of their effect in man, e.g. diethylstilbestrol, *bis*(chloromethyl)ether, and chloroethylene (vinyl chloride). (Tomatis et al. 1978; Montesano & Tomatis, 1977).

One of the main objections to carcinogenicity tests on animals is that the experimental system used tries to produce the maximum possible carcinogenic effect of the test chemical, does not reflect the human situation, and is therefore misleading. It is difficult, however, to accept this argument because, in most instances where a chemical was found by epidemiological investigations to be associated with cancer in man, the incidence was so high that the association was clear without animal studies. This has been the case for high risk groups such as occupational cancer groups. However, the risk is not confined to these groups but also applies to other populations where cancer incidence may be too low for detection by normal epidemiological methods, hence the need to carry out animal experiments under conditions that permit confident judgment of the carcinogenicity or inactivity of a chemical.

Cancer testing in animals has reached a relatively sophisticated stage and an exhaustive study of a chemical in animals is sufficient evidence of a potential cancer risk for man. An assessment of the validity of experimental results is essential for the successful prevention of cancer in man. This does not preclude further research for the development of short-term tests, but, at the present time, these cannot replace long-term carcinogenicity testing.

7.3 Heritable Mutations

As noted in the introduction, direct methods for assessing whether a chemical has the potential to cause heritable mutations in man do not exist at present. Nontheless, information relative to the possible production in man of germ cell mutations can be derived from a variety of sources. These fall into three major categories: (a) primary DNA damage involving DNA alteration, stimulation of DNA repair, gene mutations tests including mutagenicity assessment using bacterial or other microorganisms, with and without metabolic activation; (b) whole animal tests for point or gene mutations including insects, e.g. drosophila recessive, and the specific locus test in mice; (c) chromosomal mutations including cytogenetic tests in mammals, the dominant lethal test in mammals, and the heritable translocation test in rodents. Examples of the first category have already been presented. These tests provide information relevant to heritable mutations and section 7.2.2 should be consulted for fuller details. Obviously, tests employing isolated systems only provide information on mutagenic action on the specific systems tested. This information cannot be fully interpreted without evidence concerning the access of this ultimate mutagen to the germ cells.

An extensive examination of relevant test procedures for heritable mutations has recently been completed (DHEW, 1977).

.3.1 Whole-animal tests

Insects. *Drosophila melanogaster* is one of the best genetically charac-erized species and is widely used. Drosophila of either sex can be treated and mutation frequencies from successive germ cell stages may be obtained after observation of three generations. The X-lined recessive lethal test is one of the most sensitive tests with drosophila, since the X-chromosome represents about 1/5th of the whole genome. In contrast to most micro-organisms, insects possess an enzyme system that appears to metabolize foreign compounds in a fashion similar to that of vertebrates (Abrahamson & Lewis, 1971; Fahmy & Fahmy, 1972, 1973; Sobels & Vogel, 1976).

Mouse specific locus test. The specific locus test is a method of inducing, detecting, and measuring the rate of mutation at several recessive loci. It consists essentially of mating treated or untreated wild type mice, either male or female, to a strain homozygous for a number of known recessive genes. The recessive genes are such that they are readily expressed as visible phenotypes in homozygous state. If a mutation occurs in any of the test loci in the germ cells of treated animals, it may be detected in the offspring. If no mutation has occurred following treatment, the progeny from the cross will all be of the wild type (Cattanach, 1971; Russell, 1951).

Chromosomal mutations. Although the molecular basis is not un-derstood, a change in the whole chromosome, i.e. a structural chromosome aberration, occurring as a consequence of a misrepair of chromosomal breaks, may lead to deletions, duplications, and translocations. Changes in the whole chromosome complement, i.e. numerical chromosome aber-rations, arise through nondisjunction, as in failure of a pair of chromosomes to separate during gametogenesis, meiotic nondisjunction, or during mitotic division. The resulting daughter cells are either trisomic with an extra chromosome or monosomic and lacking a chromosome. Anaphase lag occurs during nuclear division in the progeny cells, and a chromosome may be either lost or gained. In somatic cells, nondisjunction and anaphase lag can lead to mosaicism.

Chromosomal damage may be studied in a number of test systems that are best divided into *in vivo* and *in vitro* systems, on the basis of their capability to metabolize the test compound (Frohberg, 1973). The short-term human lymphocyte culture *in vitro* is commonly used to assess the effects of chemicals upon chromosomes. Metabolic activation of the test compound can be achieved by addition of a liver microsomal system (Bimboes & Greim, 1976).

The micronucleus test. As an *in vivo* cytogenetic method, the micro-nucleus test is a procedure for the detection of aberrations involving ana-phase chromosome behaviour using bone-marrow erythroblasts. The test is

261

based on the formation of micronuclei from particles of chromatin material which, due to chromosome breakage or spindle disjunction, do not migrate to the poles during anaphase and are not incorporated into the telophase nuclei of the dividing cells. The procedure is to treat animals with clastogenic agents and, at an appropriate time after treatment, to aspirate bone-marrow samples into calf serum. This is then centrifuged and smears are made from the resuspended pellets of cells. The smears are air-dried and stained. The evaluation of the bone-marrow preparations involves examination of 2000–5000 erythrocytes per specimen; the total number of polychromatic and normochromatic erythrocytes with and without micronuclei are recorded (Schmid, 1973). Sister chromatid exchanges, induced by mutagens *in vivo* and *in vitro* can be scored in peripheral lymphocytes or Chinese hamster cells, using the differential straining of chromatids substituted with 5-bromo-deoxyuridine in place of thymidine (Natarajan et al., 1976; Smythe & Evans, 1976; Stetka & Wolf, 1976).

Dominant lethal tests and other in vivo *systems.* The dominant lethal test is based on the preimplantation loss of eggs or on the formation of dead embryonic implants following the injection of mutagens into a male or female mouse at a specific time before mating (Bateman & Epstein, 1971). Dominant lethal tests assume that a single mutation has occurred in the eggs or sperm, which is lethal to the embryo and heterozygous at the affected locus. However, a disturbingly high number of mutagens have given a negative response with this test. The detection of mutations arising from compounds that are metabolized to transient reactive intermediates not produced in germ cells or not reaching them from other organs may limit this test. Furthermore, chemical agents causing spermatogenic arrest or cytocidal effect on the sperms may give false positive results.

Heritable translocation in male mammals. The heritable translocation test has the important feature of measuring sexually transmissible germ cell mutations in rodent spermatogonia. Generoso et al. (1974) have described details of the technique and discussed its usefulness for the routine screening of substances that cause chromosomal mutations.

Young adult male mice are treated and females mated with the exposed males on a schedule that can be used for the comparison of the sensitivity of the different male germ cell stages. Male progeny from these matings are collected and mated for the determination of semisterility and sterility. Progeny with reduced fertility are subjected to cytogenetic analysis. The cytological examination of dividing spermatocytes, from animals treated with test chemicals that cause breaks on two nonhomologous chromosomes, yields aberrant chromosomal figures. These are recognized as rings or chains of four chromosomes as opposed to the normal bivalent chromosomal configuration.

262

A proper evaluation of this test cannot be made at this time because of insufficient data in terms of the variety of chemicals tested to date.

7.3.2 Monitoring of human populations

In spite of the variety of test systems available for detecting the mutagenic effects of chemicals, it is difficult, from the results obtained at present, to evaluate with confidence the transmissible genetic effects caused by the chemical exposure of man. However, the potential hazards of mutations are such that every effort should be made to reduce the risk.

Judgment on the potential mutagenic hazard to man should be based on various considerations such as strength of the experimental evidence of mutagenicity, the exposure pattern to the chemical, and the pharmacological properties of the compounds. This is difficult and complex. Although human studies are difficult, expensive, and often subject to misinterpretation, only studies which directly estimate the extent to which environmental factors change human genetic material give definitive answers.

Proper monitoring of the human population (Crow, 1971; Sutton, 1972) can be carried out by three main approaches:

(a) biochemical: detection of inherited protein variants;
(b) cytogenetic: screening of blood of newborn infants or of fetuses delivered by spontaneous abortion for chromosomal changes;
(c) phenotype: surveillance of genetically determined disease or anomalies.

The validity of these monitoring systems can only be properly evaluated if, and when, a mutagen is actually discovered.

7.3.3 Significance of tests for heritable mutations

As mentioned earlier, there is, at this time, no direct correlation between laboratory tests for heritable mutations and human experience. However, the available body of information from nonhuman mammals and lower life forms clearly points to the ability of chemicals to produce alterations in germ cells which are inherited in succeeding generations. Accordingly, the implications of such data for man are so persuasive that they must be taken into account in establishing safety measures for the introduction of chemicals into use. This is especially true, at this time, since techniques for detecting mutations in human populations are so insensitive that a significantly mutagenic chemical could easily escape attention.

These considerations will almost certainly lead to increasing concern in establishing regulatory and control procedures. In fact, the Environmental

Protection Agency in the USA has recently proposed preliminary guidelines for conducting tests for heritable mutations as part of the routine registration procedure for pesticides.

REFERENCES

ABRAHAMSON, S. & LEWIS, E. B. (1971) The detection of mutations in *Drosophila melanogaster*. In: Hollaender, A., ed. *Chemical mutagens, principles and methods for their detection*, Vol. 2, 461–488.

ALBERTINI, R. J. & DEMARS, R. (1973) Somatic cell mutation detection and quantification of X-ray induced mutation in cultured human diploid fibroblasts. *Mutat. Res.*, **18**, 199–244.

AMES, B. N. (1971) The detection of chemical mutagens with enteric bacteria. In: Hollaender, A., ed. *Chemical mutagens, principles and methods for their detection*, Vol. 1, pp. 267–282.

AMES, B. N., SIMS, P., & GROVER, P. L. (1972a) Epoxides of carcinogenic polycyclic hydrocarbons are frameshift mutagens. *Science*, **176**, 47–49.

AMES, B. N., GURNEY, E. G., MILLER, J. A., & BARTSCH, H. (1972b) Carcinogens as frameshift mutagens: Metabolites and derivatives of 2-acetylaminofluorene and other aromatic amine carcinogens. *Proc. Natl Acad. Sci.*, **69**: 3128–3132.

AMES, B. N., LEE, F. D., & DURSTON, W. E. (1973a) An improved bacterial test system for the detection and classification of mutagens and carcinogens. *Proc. Natl Acad. Sci.*, **70**: 782–786.

AMES, B. N., DURSTON, W. E., YAMASAKI, E., & LEE, F. D. (1973b) Carcinogens are mutagens: a simple test system combining liver homogenates for activation and bacteria for detection. *Proc. Natl Acad. Sci.*, **70**: 2281–2285.

AMES, B. N., McCANN, J., & YAMASAKI, E. (1975) Methods for detecting carcinogens and mutagens with the *Salmonella*/mammalian-microsome mutagenicity test. *Mutat. Res.*, **31**: 347–364.

BARTSCH, H. (1976) Predictive value of mutagenicity tests in chemical carcinogenesis. *Mutat. Res.*, **38**: 177–190.

BARTSCH, H. & GROVER, P. L. (1976) Chemical carcinogenesis and mutagenesis. In: Symington, T. & Carter, R. L., ed. *Scientific foundations of oncology*, London, William Heinemann Medical Books Ltd, pp. 334–342.

BARTSCH, H., MALAVEILLE, C., & MONTESANO, R. (1975a) Human, rat and mouse liver-mediated mutagenicity of vinyl chloride in *S. typhimurium* strains. *Int. J. Cancer*, **15**: 429–437.

BARTSCH, H., MALAVEILLE, C., & MONTESANO, R. (1975b) *In vitro* metabolism and microsome-mediated mutagenicity of dialkylnitrosamines in rat, hamster and mouse tissues. *Cancer Res.*, **35**: 644–651.

BARTSCH, H., MALAVEILLE, C., STICH, H. F., MILLER, E. C., & MILLER, J. A. (1977) Comparative electrophilicity, mutagenicity, DNA repair induction activity, and carcinogenicity of some *N*- and *O*-Acyl derivatives of *N*-Hydroxy-2-aminofluorene. *Cancer Res.*, **37**: 1461–1467.

BATEMAN, A. J. & EPSTEIN, S. S. (1971) Dominant lethal mutations in mammals. In: Hollaender, A., ed. *Chemical mutagens, principles and methods for their detection*, Vol. 2, pp. 541–568.

BERWALD, Y. & SACHS, L. (1963) *In vitro* transformation with chemical carcinogens. *Nature (Lond.)*, **200**: 1182–1184.

BIMBOES, D. & GREIM, H. (1976) Human lymphocytes as target cells in a metabolizing test system *in vitro* for detecting potential mutagens. *Mutat. Res.*, **35**: 155–160.

BORLAND, R. & HARD, G. C. (1974) Early appearance of "transformed" cells from the kidneys of rats treated with a "single" carcinogenic dose of dimethylnitrosamine (DMN) detected by culture *in vitro*. *Europ. J. Cancer*, **10**: 177–184.

BRIDGES, B. A. (1976) Short-term screening tests for carcinogens. *Nature (Lond.)*, **261**: 195–200.

BRIDGES, B. A., MOTTERSHEAD, R. P., ROTHWELL, M. A., & GREEN, M. H. L. (1972) Repair deficient bacterial strains suitable for mutagenicity screening tests with fungicide captan. *Chem.-Biol. Interact.*, **5**: 77–84.

BROWN, A. M. (1973) *In vitro* transformation of submandibular gland epithelial cells and fibroblasts of adult rats by methylcholanthrene. *Cancer Res.*, **33**: 2779–2789.

CATTANACH, B. M. (1971) Specific locus mutation in mice. In: Hollaender, A., ed. *Chemical mutagens, principles and methods for their detection*, Vol. 2, pp. 535–540.

CHU, E. H. Y. (1971) Induction and analysis of gene mutations in mammalian cells in culture. In: Hollaender, A., ed. *Chemical mutagens, principles and methods for their detection*, Vol. 2, pp. 411–444.

CLEAVER, J. E. (1969) *Xeroderma pigmentosum*: a human disease in which an initial state of DNA repair is defective. *Proc. Natl Acad. Sci.*, **63**: 428–435.

CLEAVER, J. E. (1973) DNA repair with purines and pyrimidines in radiation- and carcinogen-damaged normal and *Xeroderma pigmentosum* human cells. *Cancer Res.*, **33**: 362–369.

CLEAVER, J. E. (1974) Repair processes for photochemical damage in mammalian cells. In: Lett, J. T., Adler, H., & Zelle, M., ed. *Advances in radiation biology*, New York, Academic Press, Vol. 4, pp. 1–75.

CLEAVER, J. E. (1975) Methods for studying repair of DNA damaged by physical and chemical carcinogens. In: Bush, E., ed. *Methods in cancer research*, New York, Academic Press, Vol. 11, pp. 123–165.

CLEAVER, J. E., GOTH, R., & FRIEDBERG, E. C. (1975) Value of measurements of DNA repair levels in predicting carcinogenic potential of chemicals. In: Montesano, R., Bartsch, H., & Tomatis, L., ed. *Screening tests in chemical carcinogenesis*, IARC Sci. Publ. No. 12, pp. 639–661.

COMMONER, B., VITHAYATHIL, A. J., & HENRY, J. I. (1974) Detection of metabolic carcinogen intermediates in urine of carcinogen-fed rats by means of bacterial mutagenesis. *Nature (Lond.)*, **249**: 850–852.

CONNEY, A. H. & BURNS, J. J. (1972) Metabolic interactions among environmental chemicals and drugs. *Science*, **178**: 576–586.

CORBETT, T. H., HEIDELBERGER, C., & DOVE, W. F. (1970) Determination of the mutagenic activity to bacteriophage T-4 of carcinogenic and non-carcinogenic compounds. *Mol. Pharmacol.*, **6**(6): 667–679.

COUNCIL OF THE ENVIRONMENTAL MUTAGEN SOCIETY (1975) Environmental mutagenic hazards, mutagenicity screening is now both feasible and necessary for chemicals entering the environment. *Science*, **187**: 503–514.

CRADDOCK, V. M. (1976) Replication and repair of DNA in liver of rats treated with dimethylnitrosamine and with methyl methanesulphonate. In: Magee, P. N. et al., ed. *Fundamentals in cancer prevention*, Tokyo, Univ. Tokyo Press; Baltimore, Univ. Park Press, pp. 293–311.

CROW, J. F. (1971) Human population monitoring. In: Hollaender, A., ed. *Chemical mutagens, principles and methods for their detection*, Vol. 2, pp. 591–606.

CZYGAN, P. J., GREIM, H., GARRO, A. J., HUTTERER, F., SCHAFFAER, F., POPPER, H., ROSENTHAL, O., & COOPER, D. Y. (1973) Microsomal metabolism of DMN and the cytochrome activation to a mutagen. *Cancer Res.*, **33**: 2983–2986.

DELLA PORTA, G. & TERRACINI, B. (1969) Chemical carcinogenesis in infant animals. *Progr. Exp. Tumour Res.*, **11**: 334–363.

DE MARS, R. (1974) Resistance of cultured human fibroblasts and other cells to purine and pyrimidine analogues in relation to mutagenesis detection. *Mutat. Res.*, **24**: 335–364.

DHEW (1977) *Approaches to determining the mutagenic properties of chemicals: Risks to future generations*. Report of a working group of the Subcommittee on Environmental Mutagenesis.

DI PAOLO, J. A., NELSON, R. L., & DONOVAN, P. J. (1972) *In vitro* transformation of Syrian hamster embryo cells by diverse chemical carcinogens. *Nature (Lond.)*, **235**: 278–280.

DI PAOLO, J. A., NELSON, R. L., DONOVAN, P. J., & EVANS, C. H. (1973) Host-mediated *in vivo-in vitro* assay for chemical carcinogenesis. *Arch. Pathol.*, **95**: 380–385.

DE SERRES, F. J. & MALLING, H. V. (1971) Measurement of recessive lethal damage over the entire genome and at two specific loci in the *ad*-3 region of a two-component hetero-

266

karyon of *Neurospora Crassa*. In: Hollaender, A., ed. *Chemical mutagens, principles and methods for their detection*, Vol. 2, pp. 311–342.

DRAKE, J. W. (1971) Mutagen screening with virulent bacteriophages. In: Hollaender, A., ed. *Chemical mutagens, principles and methods for their detection*, Vol. 1, pp. 219–234.

DRUCKREY, H., PREUSSMAN, R., IVANKOVIC, S., & SCHMÄL, D. (1967) [Organotropic carcinogenic effects of 65 different *N*-nitroso compounds on BD-rats.] *Z. Krebsforsch.*, **69**: 103–201.

DURSTON, W. E. & AMES, B. N. (1974) A simple method for the detection of mutagens in urine: Studies with the carcinogen 2-acetylaminofluorene. *Proc. Natl Acad. Sci.*, **71**: 737–741.

EARLE, W. R. & NETTLESHIP, A. (1943) Production of malignancy *in vitro*. V. Results of injections of cultures into mice. *J. Natl Cancer Inst.*, **4**: 213–227.

FAHMY, O. G. & FAHMY, M. D. (1972) Mutagenic properties of AAF and its metabolites. *Int. J. Cancer*, **9**: 284–298.

FAHMY, O. G. & FAHMY, M. D. (1973) Mutagenic properties of benzo(a)pyrene. *Cancer Res.*, **33**: 302–309.

FARBER, E. (1973) Carcinogenesis—cellular evolution as a unifying thread: presidential address. *Cancer Res.*, **33**: 2537–2550.

FDA (1971) Panel on carcinogenesis report on cancer testing in the safety evaluation of food additives and pesticides. *Toxic. appl. Pharmacol.*, **20**: 419–438.

FEDOROFF, S. (1967) Proposed usage of animal tissue culture terms, *J. Natl Cancer Inst.*, **38**: 607–611.

FREESE, E. & STRACK, H. B. (1962) Induction of mutations in transforming DNA by hydroxylamine. *Proc. Natl Acad. Sci.*, **48**: 1796–1803.

FRIEDMAN, L. (1974) Dose selection and administration. In: Goldberg, L., ed. *Carcinogenesis testing of chemicals*, Cleveland, CRC Press, pp. 21–22.

FROHBERG, H. (1973) Critique of *in vivo* cytogenic test systems. *Agents Actions*, **3**: 119–123.

FUSENIG, N. R., SAMSEL, W., THON, W., & WORST, P. K. M. (1973) Malignant transformation of epidermal cells in culture by DMBA. In: Prunieras, M., Robert, L., & Rosenfeld, C., ed. *Differentiation of eukaryotic cells in culture*. Colloque of INSERM, Vol. 19, pp. 219–228.

GERCHMAN, L. L. & LUDLUM, D. B. (1973) The properties of O^6-methylguanine in template for RNA polymerase. *Biochim. biophys. Acta*, **308**: 310–316.

GIOVANELLA, B. C., YIM, S. O., STEHLIN, J. S., & WILLIAMS, L. J. Jr (1972) Brief communications: Development of invasive tumors in the "nude" mouse after injection of cultured human melanoma cells. *J. Natl Cancer Inst.*, **48**: 1531–1533.

GOTH, R. & RAJEWSKY, M. F. (1974) Molecular and cellular mechanisms associated with pulse-carcinogenesis in the rat nervous system by ethylnitrosourea: ethylation of nucleic acids and elimination rates of ethylated bases from the DNA of different tissues. *Z. Krebsforsch.*, **82**: 37–64.

HASHIMOTO, Y. & KITAGAWA, H. (1974) *In vitro* neoplastic transformation of epithelial cell of rat urinary bladder by nitrosamines. *Nature (Lond.)*, **252**: 497–499.

HEALTH AND WELFARE, CANADA (1973) *The testing of chemicals for carcinogenicity, mutagenicity, teratogenicity.*

HEIDELBERGER, C. (1973) Chemical oncogenesis in culture. *Adv. Cancer Res.*, **18**: 317–366.

HERRIOTT, R. M. (1971) Effects on DNA: Transforming principle. In: Hollaender, A., ed. *Chemical mutagens, principles and methods for their detection*, Vol. 1, pp. 175–218.

HUBERMAN, E. & SACHS, L. (1974) Cell-mediated mutagenesis of mammalian cells with chemical carcinogens. *Int. J. Cancer*, **13**: 326–333.

HUBERMAN, E., ASPIRAS, L., HEIDELBERGER, C., GROVER, P. L., & SIMS, P. (1971) Mutagenicity to mammalian cells of epoxides and other derivatives of polycyclic hydrocarbons. *Proc. Natl Acad. Sci.*, **68**: 3195–3199.

HUBERMAN, E., DONOVAN, P. J., & DIPAOLO, J. A. (1972) Mutation and transformation of cultured mammalian cells by *N*-acetoxy-*N*-2-fluorenylacetamide. *J. Natl Cancer Inst.* **48:** 837–840.

HUEPER, W. C., WILEY, F. H., & WOLFE, H. D. (1938) Experimental production of bladder tumours in dogs by administration of *β*-naphthylamine. *J. industr. Hyg. Toxicol.*, **20:** 46–84.

IARC (1976) *Monographs on the evaluation of carcinogenic risk of chemicals to man: some aromatic amines, hydrazine and related substances, N-nitroso compounds and miscellaneous alkylating agents.* Lyons, International Agency for Research on Cancer, Vol. 4.

IYPE, P. T. (1974) Studies on chemical carcinogenesis *in vitro* using adult rat liver cells. In: Montesano, R. & Tomatis, L., ed. *Chemical carcinogenesis essays*, IARC Sci. Publ. No. 10, pp. 119–133.

J. Natl Cancer Inst., **53:** 1427–1519 (1974) Proceedings of the Symposium "New Horizons for Tissue Culture in Cancer Research".

KAKUNAGA, T. The transformation of human diploid cells by chemical carcinogens. In: Hiatt, H. H. et al., ed. *Origins of human cancer* (1977) Cold Spring Harbor Laboratory. pp. 1537–1548.

KATSUTA, H. & TAKAOKA, T. (1972) Carcinogenesis in tissue culture. XIV. Malignant transformation of rat liver parenchymal cells treated with 4-nitroquinoline 1-oxide in tissue culture. *J. Natl Cancer Inst.*, **49:** 1563–1576.

KONDO, S. (1973) Evidence that mutations are induced by errors in repair and replication. *Genet. suppl.*, **73:** 109–122.

KRAHN, D. F. & HEIDELBERGER, C. (1975) Microsome-mediated mutagenesis in Chinese hamster cells by chemical oncogens. *Proc. Am. Assoc. Cancer Res.*, **16:** 74.

KRIEK, E. (1974) Carcinogenesis by aromatic amines. *Biochem. Biophys. Acta*, **355:** 177–203.

KUROKI, T. (1975) Contributions of tissue culture to the study of chemical carcinogenesis: A review. In: Recent topics in chemical carcinogenesis, *Gann, Monograph on Cancer Res.*, **17:** 69–85.

KUROKI, T., DREVON, C., & MONTESANO, R. (1977) Microsome-mediated mutagenesis in V-79 Chinese hamster cells by various nitrosamines. *Cancer Res.*, 1044–1050.

LAERUM, O. D. & RAJEWSKY, M. F. (1975) Neoplastic transformation of foetal rat brain cells in culture following exposure to ethylnitrosourea *in vivo. J. Natl Cancer Inst.*, **55:** 1177–1187.

LEGATOR, M. S. & FLAMM, W. G. (1973) Environmental mutagenesis and repair. *Ann. Rev. Biochem.*, 683–708.

LEGATOR, M. S. & MALLING, H. V. (1971) The host-mediated assay, a practical procedure for evaluating potential mutagenic agents in mammals. In: Hollaender A., ed. *Chemical mutagens, principles and methods for their detection*, Vol. 2, pp. 569–590.

LOPRIENO, N., BARALE, R., BARONCELLI, S., BARTSCH, H., BRONZETTI, G., CAMMELLINI, A., CORSI, C., FREZZA, D., NIERI, R., LEPORINI, C., ROSELLINI, D., & ROSSI, A. M. (1976) Induction of gene mutations and gene conversions by vinyl chloride metabolites in yeast. *Cancer Res.*, **37:** 253–257.

LOVELESS, A. (1969) Possible relevance of O^6-alkylation of deoxyguanosine to the mutagenicity and carcinogenicity of nitrosamines and nitrosamides. *Nature (Lond.)*, **233:** 206–207.

LOVELESS, A. & HAMPTON, C. L. (1969) Inactivation and mutation of coliphage T2 by *N*-methyl- and *N*-ethyl-*N*-nitrosourea. *Mutation Res.*, **7:** 1–12.

LUDLUM, D. B. (1970) Alkylated polycytidic acid templates for RNA polymerase. *Biochim. biophys. Acta*, **213:** 142–148.

MAGEE, P. N., MONTESANO, R., & PREUSSMAN, R. (1976) *N*-nitroso compounds and related carcinogens. In: Searle, C., ed. *Chemical carcinogens*, ACS monograph No. 173, pp. 491–625.

MAHER, V., MILLER, E. C., MILLER, J. A., & SZYBALSKI, W. (1968) Mutations and decreases in density of transforming DNA produced by derivatives of the carcinogens 2-acetylaminofluorene and N-methyl-4-aminoazobenzene. *Mol. Pharmacol.*, **4**: 411–426.

MAHER, V. M., CURREN, R. D., OUELLETTE, L. M., & McCORMICK, J. J. (1976) Effect of DNA repair on the frequency of mutations induced in human cells by ultraviolet irradiation and by chemical carcinogens. In: Magee, P. N., et al, ed. *Fundamentals in cancer prevention*, Tokyo, Univ. of Tokyo Press; Baltimore, Univ Park Press, pp. 363–382.

MALLING, H. V. (1974) Mutagenic activation of dimethylnitrosamine and diethyl-nitrosamine in the host-mediated assay and the microsomal system. *Mutat. Res.*, **26**: 465–472.

MARGISON, G. P., MARGISON, J. M., & MONTESANO, R. (1976) Methylated purines in the deoxyribonucleic acid of various Syrian golden hamster tissues after administration of a hepatocarcinogenic dose of dimethylnitrosamine. *Biochem. J.*, **157**: 627–634.

MARQUARDT, H. (1974) Mutation and recombination experiments with yeast as pre-screening tests for carcinogenic effects. *Z. Krebsforsch.*, **81**: 333–346.

McCANN, J. & AMES, B. N. (1976) Detection of carcinogens as mutagens in the *Salmonella*/microsome test: Assay of 300 chemicals: Discussion. *Proc. Natl Acad. Sci.*, **73**: 950–954.

McCANN, J., SPINGARN, N. E., KOBORI, J., & AMES, B. N. (1975) Detection of carcinogens as mutagens: bacterial tester strains with R factor plasmids. *Proc. Natl Acad. Sci.*, **72**: 979–983.

MESELSON, M. & RUSSELL, K. (1977) Comparisons of carcinogenic and mutagenic potency. In: Hiatt, H. H. et al. ed. *Origins of human cancer*. Cold Spring Harbor Laboratory. pp. 1473–1481.

MILLER, J. A. (1970) Carcinogenesis by chemicals: an overview—G. H. A. Clowes Memorial Lecture. *Cancer Res.*, **30**: 559–576.

MILLER, J. A. (1973) Naturally occurring substances that can induce tumors. *Proc. Natl Acad. Sci.*, **23**: 508–549.

MILLER, E. C. & MILLER, J. A. (1971a) The mutagenicity of chemical carcinogens: correlations, problems, and interpretations. In: Hollaender, A., ed. *Chemical mutagens, principles and methods for their detection*, Vol. 1, pp. 83–120.

MILLER, J. A. & MILLER, E. C. (1971b) Chemical carcinogenesis, mechanisms and approaches to its control. *J. Natl Cancer Inst.*, **47**: V–XIV.

MILLER, E. C. & MILLER, J. A. (1976) The metabolism of chemical carcinogens to reactive electrophiles and their possible mechanisms of action in carcinogenesis. In: Searle, C. E., ed. *Chemical carcinogens*, ACS Monograph 173. Washington, DC, American Chemical Society, pp. 737–762.

MOHN, G. (1973) Revertants of an *Escherichia coli* K-12 strain with high sensitivity to radiations and chemicals. *Mutat. Res.*, **19**: 349–355.

MOHN, G. & ELLENBERGER, J. (1973) Mammalian blood mediated mutagenicity test using a multi-purpose strain of *E. coli*, K-12. *Mutat. Res.*, **19**: 257–260.

MONTESANO, R. & BARTSCH, H. (1976) Mutagenic and carcinogenic N-nitroso compounds: Possible environmental hazards. *Mutat. Res.*, **32**: 179–228.

MONTESANO, R., SAINT VINCENT, L., & TOMATIS, L. (1973) Malignant transformation *in vitro* of rat liver cells by dimethylnitrosamine and N-methyl-N'-nitro-N-nitroso-guanidine. *Brit. J. Cancer*, **38**: 215–220.

MONTESANO, R., SAINT VINCENT, L., DREVON, C., & TOMATIS, L. (1975) Production of epithelial and mesenchymal tumours with rat liver cells transformed *in vitro*. *Int. J. Cancer*, **55**: 1177–1187.

MONTESANO, R., DREVON, C., KUROKI, T., SAINT VINCENT, L., HANDLEMAN, S., SANFORD, K. K., DEFEO, D. & WEINSTEIN, I. B. (1977) Test for malignant transformation of rat liver cells in culture: Cytology, growth in soft agar and production of plasminogen activator. *J. Natl Cancer Inst.*, **59**: 1651–1658.

MONTESANO, R., BARTSCH, H., & TOMATIS, L., ed. (1976) *Screening tests in chemical carcinogenesis*. IARC Sci. Publ. No. 12.

MONTESANO, R. & TOMATIS, L. (1977) Legislation concerning chemical carcinogens in several industrialized countries. *Cancer Res.*, **37:** 310–316.

MOREAU, P., BAILONE, A., & DEVORET, R. (1976) Prophage λ induction in *Escherichia coli* K12 *envA uvrB*: A highly sensitive test for potential carcinogens. *Proc. Natl Acad. Sci.*, **73:** 3700–3704.

MORTIMER, R. K. & MANNEY, T. R. (1971) Mutation induction in yeast. In: Hollaender, A., ed. *Chemical mutagens, principles and methods for their detection*, Vol. 1, pp. 289–310.

NAHAS, A. & CAPIZZI, R. L. (1974) Effect of *in vivo* treatment with *L* asparaginal on the *in vitro* uptake and phosphorylation of some anti-leukemic agents. *Cancer Res.*, **34:** 2687–2693.

NAPALKOV, N. P. (1973) Some general considerations on the problem of transplacental carcinogenesis. In: Tomatis, L. & Mohr, U., ed. *Transplacental carcinogenesis*, IARC Sci. Publ. No. 4, pp. 1–13.

NAPALKOV, N. P. & ALEXANDROV, V. A. (1968) On the effects of blastomogenic substances on the organism during embryogenesis. *Z. Krebsforsch.*, **71:** 32–50.

NATARAJAN, A. T., TATES, A. D., VAN BUUL, P. P. W., MEIJERS, M., & DE VOGEL, N. (1976) Cytogenetic effects of mutagens/carcinogens after activation in a microsomal system *in vitro*. I. Induction of chromosome aberrations and sister chromatid exchanges by diethylnitrosamine (DEN) and dimethylnitrosamine (DMN) in CHO cells in the presence of rat-liver microsomes. *Mutat. Res.*, **37:** 83–90.

MATIONAL ACADEMY OF SCIENCES (1960) Problems in the evaluation of carcinogenic hazard from use of food additives. Washington, Natl Res. Council (Publ. No. 479).

NCI (1976) NCI Technical Report Series, No. 1 (Guidelines for carcinogen bioassay in small rodents), pp. 1–65 (DHEW Publication No. (NIH) 76-701).

PEGG, A. E. (1977) Formation and metabolism of alkylated nucleosides: Possible role in carcinogenesis by nitroso compounds and alkylating agents. *Adv. Cancer Res.*, **25:** 195–269.

PEGG, T. & NICOLL, J. W. (1976) Nitrosamine carcinogenesis: The importance of the persistence in DNA of alkylated bases in the organotropism of tumour induction. In: Montesano, R., Bartsch, H., & Tomatis, L., ed. *Screening tests in chemical carcinogenesis*, IARC Sci. Publ. No. 12, pp. 571–592.

PIETRA, G., RAPPAPORT, H., & SHUBIK, P. (1961) The effects of carcinogenic chemicals in newborn mice. *Cancer*, **14:** 308–317.

PITOT, H. C. (1974) Neoplasia: A somatic mutation or a heritable change in cytoplasmic membranes? *J. Natl Cancer Inst.*, **53:** 905–911.

PITOT, H. C. (1977) The natural history of neoplasia. *Am. J. Path.*, **89:** 402–411.

PURCHASE, I. F. H., LONGSTAFF, E., ASHBY, J., STYLES, J. A., ANDERSON, D., LEFEVRE, P. A., & WESTWOOD, F. R. (1976) Evaluation of six short-term tests for detecting organic chemical carcinogens and recommendations for their use. *Nature (Lond.)*, **264:** 624–627.

REUBER, M. (1974) Criteria for tumor diagnosis and classification of malignancy. In: Golberg, L., ed. *Carcinogenesis testing of chemicals*, Cleveland, CRC Press, pp. 71–73.

ROSENKRANZ, H. S. (1973) Aspects of microbiology in cancer research. *Rev. Microbiol.*, **1622:** 383–400.

RUSSELL, W. L. (1951) X-ray induced mutations in mice. *Cold Spring Harbour Symp. Quant. Biol.*, **16:** 327–336.

SANFORD, K. K. (1965) Malignant transformation of cells *in vitro*. *Inter. Rev. Cytol.*, **18:** 249–311.

SANFORD, K. K. (1974) Biological manifestations of oncogenesis *in vitro*: a critique. *J. Natl Cancer Inst.*, **53:** 1481–1485.

SANFORD, K. K., EARLE, W. R., SHELTON, E., SCHILLING, E. L., DUCHESNE, E. M., LIKELY, G. D., & BECKER, E. M. (1950) Production of malignancy *in vitro*. XII. Further transformations of mouse fibroblasts to sarcomatous cells. *J. Natl Cancer Inst.*, **11**: 351–367.

SATO, K., SLESINSKI, R. S., & LITTLEFIELD, J. W. (1972) Chemical mutagenesis at the phosphoribosyl transferase locus in cultured human lymphoblasts. *Proc. Natl Acad. Sci.*, **69**: 1244–1248.

SCHMID, W. (1973) Chemical mutagen testing on *in vivo* somatic mammalian cells. *Agents Actions*, **3**: 77–85.

SIMS, P. & GROVER, P. L. (1974) Epoxides in polycyclic aromatic hydrocarbon metabolism and carcinogenesis. *Advances in Cancer Res.*, **20**: 165–274.

SMITH, W. E. & HANAWALT, P. C. (1969) *Molecular photobiology: Inactivation and recovery*. New York, Academic Press.

SMYTHE, D. R. & EVANS. H. J. (1976) Mapping of sister-chromatid exchanges in human chromosomes using G-Banding and autoradiography. *Mutat. Res.*, **35**: 139–154.

SOBELS, F. H. & VOGEL, E. (1976) The capacity of drosophila for detecting relevant genetic damage. *Mutat. Res.*, **41**: 95–106.

STETKA, D. G. & WOLFF, S. (1976) Sister chromatid exchange as an assay for genetic damage induced by mutagen-carcinogens. I. *In vitro* test for compounds requiring metabolic activation. *Mutat. Res.*, **41**: 333–342.

STICH, H. F. & KIESER, D. (1974) Use of DNA repair synthesis in detecting organo-tropic actions of chemical carcinogens. *Proc. Soc. Exp. Biol Med.*, **145**: 1339–1342.

STICH, H. F. & SAN, R. H. C. (1970) DNA repair and chromatid anomalies in mammalian cells exposed to 4 nitroquinoline 1-oxide. *Mutat. Res.*, **10**: 389–404.

STOLTZ, D. R., POIRIER, L. A., IRVING, C. C., STICH, H. F., WEISBURGER, J. H., & GRICE, H. C. (1974) Evaluation of short-term tests for carcinogenicity. *Toxicol. appl. Pharmacol.*, **29**: 157–180.

SUGIMURA, T., SATO, S., NAGAO, M., YAHAGI, T., MATSUSHIMA, T., SEINO, Y., TAKEUCHI, M., & KAWACHI, T. (1976) Overlapping of carcinogens and mutagens. In: Magee, P. N., Takayama, S., Sugimura, T., & Matsushima, T., ed. *Fundamentals in cancer prevention*, Tokyo, University of Tokyo Press; Baltimore, Univ. Park Press, pp. 191–215.

SUTHERLAND, B. M., RICE, M., & WAGNER, E. K.ˈ (1975) *Xeroderma pigmentosum* cells contain low levels of photoreactivating enzyme. *Proc. Natl Acad. Sci.*, **72**: 103–107.

SUTTON, H. E. (1972) Monitoring somatic mutations in human populations. In: Sutton, H. E. & Harris, M. I., ed. *Mutagenic effects of environmental contaminants*, pp. 122–128.

THOMPSON, L. H. & BAKER, R. M. (1973) Isolation of mutants of cultured mammalian cells. In: Prescott, D. M., ed. *Methods of cell biology*, New York, Academic Press, pp. 209–280.

TOMATIS, L. (1973) Transplacental carcinogenesis. In: Raven, R. W., ed. *Modern trends in oncology—1*, London, Butterworths, pp. 99–126.

TOMATIS, L. (1974a) The validity of long-term bioassays in carcinogenicity testing. Chemical and viral oncogenesis. Excerpta Medica Int. Congr. Ser. No. 350, Vol. 2, pp. 82–93.

TOMATIS, L. (1974b) Inception and duration of tests. In: Golberg, L., ed. *Carcinogenesis testing of chemicals*, Cleveland, CRC Press, pp. 23–27.

TOMATIS, L., AGTHE, C., BARTSCH, H., HUFF, J., MONTESANO, R., SARACCI, R., WALKER, E., & WILBOURN, J. (1978) Evaluation of the carcinogenicity of chemicals: A review of the monograph program of the International Agency for Research on Cancer. *Cancer Res.*, **38**: 877–885.

TURUSOV, V. S., ed. (1973, 1976) *Pathology of tumours in laboratory animals*, Vol. I, Part 1 and 2, IARC Sci. Publ. No. 5 and No. 6. Lyon.

UICC (1969) UICC Technical Report Series Vol. 2 (Carcinogenicity testing). Geneva, International Union Against Cancer, 56 pp.

VENITT, S. & LEVY, L. S. (1974) Mutagenicity of chromates in bacteria and its relevance to chromate carcinogenesis. *Nature (Lond.)*, **250**: 493–495.

271

WEIL, C. S. (1972) Statistics vs safety factors and scientific judgements in the evaluation of safety for man. *Toxicol. appl. Pharmacol.,* **21:** 454–463.

WEINSTEIN, I. B., ORENSTEIN, J. M., GEBERT, T., KAIGHN, M. E., & STADLER, V. C. (1975) Growth and structural properties of epithelial cell cultures established from normal rat liver and chemically induced hepatomas. *Cancer Res.,* **35:** 253–263.

WEISBURGER, J. H. (1974) Inclusion of positive control. In: Golberg, L., ed. *Carcinogenesis testing of chemicals,* Cleveland, CRC Press, pp. 29–34.

WEISBURGER, E. K. (1975) A critical evaluation of the methods used for determining carcinogenicity. *J. clin. Pharmacol.,* **15:** 5–15.

WEISBURGER, J. H. & WEISBURGER, E. K. (1967) Tests for chemical carcinogens. In: Busch, H., ed. *Methods in cancer research,* Academic Press, Vol. 1, pp. 307–398.

WEISBURGER, J. H. & WEISBURGER, E. K. (1973) Biochemical formation and pharmacological, toxicological and pathological properties of hydroxylamines and hydroxamic acids. *Pharmacol. Rev.* **25:** 1–66.

WHO (1961) WHO Technical Report Series No. 220 (Evaluation of carcinogenic hazards of food additives), 33 pp.

WHO (1964) WHO Technical Report Series No. 276 (Prevention of cancer).

WHO (1969) WHO Technical Report Series No. 426 (Principles for the testing and evaluation of drugs for carcinogenicity).

WHO (1974) WHO Technical Report Series, No. 546 (Assessment of the carcinogenicity and mutagenicity of chemicals), 19 pp.

WILLIAMS, G. M., ELLIOT, J. M., & WEISBURGER, J. H. (1973) Carcinoma after malignant conversion *in vitro* of epithelial-like cells from rat liver following exposure to chemical carcinogens. *Cancer Res.,* **33:** 606–612.

WILSON, R. H., DEEDS, F., & COX, A. J. (1941) The toxicity and carcinogenicity of 2-acetaminofluorene. *Cancer Res.,* **1:** 595–608.

ZIMMERMANN, F. K. (1973) Detection of genetically active chemicals using various yeast systems. In: Hollaender, A., ed. *Chemical mutagens, principles and methods for their detection,* Vol. 3, pp. 209–240.